FOURTH EDITION

PARAMEDIC CARE

PRINCIPLES & PRACTICE

VOLUME **1**

INTRODUCTION TO PARAMEDICINE

FOURTH EDITION

PARAMEDIC CARE
PRINCIPLES & PRACTICE

VOLUME 1 | **INTRODUCTION TO PARAMEDICINE**

BRYAN E. BLEDSOE, DO, FACEP, FAAEM, EMT-P

Professor of Emergency Medicine
Director, Prehospital and Disaster Medicine Fellowship
University of Nevada School of Medicine
Attending Emergency Physician
University Medical Center of Southern Nevada
Medical Director, MedicWest Ambulance
Las Vegas, Nevada

ROBERT S. PORTER, MA, EMT-P

Senior Advanced Life Support Educator
Madison County Emergency Medical Services
Canastota, New York

RICHARD A. CHERRY, MS, EMT-P

Director of Training
Northern Onondaga Volunteer Ambulance
Liverpool, New York

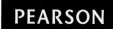

Boston Columbus Indianapolis New York San Francisco Upper Saddle River
Amsterdam Cape Town Dubai London Madrid Milan Munich Paris Montréal Toronto
Delhi Mexico City São Paulo Sydney Hong Kong Seoul Singapore Taipei Tokyo

Library of Congress Cataloging-in-Publication Data

Bledsoe, Bryan E., (Date)
  Paramedic care : principles & practice / Bryan E. Bledsoe,
    Robert S. Porter, Richard A. Cherry. — 4th ed. p. ; cm.
  Includes bibliographical references and index.
  ISBN-13: 978-0-13-211208-6 (v. 1 : alk. paper)
  ISBN-10: 0-13-211208-6 (v. 1 : alk. paper)
  I. Porter, Robert S., (Date) II. Cherry, Richard A. III. Title.
  [DNLM: 1. Emergencies. 2. Emergency Medical Services.
    3. Emergency Medical Technicians. 4. Emergency Treatment. WB 105]
  616.02'5—dc23
                                              2011034904

Publisher: Julie Levin Alexander
Publisher's Assistant: Regina Bruno
Editor-in-Chief: Marlene McHugh Pratt
Senior Managing Editor for Development: Lois Berlowitz
Editorial Project Manager: Sandra Breuer
Assistant Editor: Jonathan Cheung
Director of Marketing: David Gesell
Marketing Manager: Brian Hoehl
Marketing Specialist: Michael Sirinides
Managing Editor for Production: Patrick Walsh
Production Liaison: Faye Gemmellaro
Production Editor: Heather Willison, S4Carlisle Publishing Services

Manufacturing Manager: Ilene Sanford
Creative Director: Blair Brown
Cover and Interior Design: Kathryn Foot
Interior Photographers: Michal Heron, Ray Kemp, Richard Logan,
  Scott Metcalfe
Cover Image: © corepics/Shutterstock
Managing Photography Editor: Michal Heron
Editorial Media Manager: Amy Peltier
Media Project Manager: Lorena Cerisano
Composition: S4Carlisle Publishing Services
Printer/Binder: Courier/Kendallville
Cover Printer: Lehigh-Phoenix Color/Hagerstown

Notice

The author and the publisher of this book have taken care to make certain that the information given is correct and compatible with the standards generally accepted at the time of publication. Nevertheless, as new information becomes available, changes in treatment and in the use of equipment and procedures become necessary. The reader is advised to carefully consult the instruction and information material included in each piece of equipment or device before administration. Students are warned that the use of any techniques must be authorized by their medical advisor, where appropriate, in accordance with local laws and regulations. The publisher disclaims any liability, loss, injury, or damage incurred as a consequence, directly or indirectly, of the use and application of any of the contents of this book.

Brady
is an imprint of

PEARSON   www.bradybooks.com

10 9 8 7 6 5 4 3
ISBN 10:   0-13-211208-6
ISBN 13: 978-0-13-211208-6
V011

DEDICATION

This text is respectfully dedicated to all EMS personnel who have made the ultimate sacrifice. Their memory and good deeds will forever be in our thoughts and prayers.

BEB, RSP, RAC

DETAILED CONTENTS

Preface to Volume 1   xi
Acknowledgments   xiii
About the Authors   xv

CHAPTER 1 ● Introduction to Paramedicine   1

Introduction   3
Description of the Profession 3 | The Modern Paramedic 4 | Paramedic Characteristics 4 | The Paramedic: A True Health Professional 5
Expanded Scope of Practice   6
Critical Care Transport 6 | Helicopter EMS 6 | Tactical EMS 7 | Primary Care 7 | Industrial Medicine 8 | Sports Medicine 8 | Corrections Medicine 8 | Hospital Emergency Departments 9

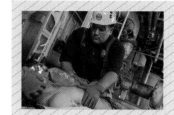

CHAPTER 2 ● EMS Systems   12

Introduction   14
History of EMS   14
Early Development 15 | The Twentieth Century 17 | The Twenty-First Century 20
Today's EMS SYSTEMS   22
Chain of Survival 22 | Levels of Licensure/Certification 22 | Education 23 | Local- and State-Level Agencies 23 | Medical Oversight 23 | Public Information and Education 24 | Communications 25 | Education and Certification 27 | Licensure/Certification 27 | National Registry of EMTs 28 | Professional Organizations 28 | Professional Journals and Magazines 28 | The Internet 28 | Patient Transportation 28 | Receiving Facilities 30 | Mutual Aid and Mass-Casualty Preparation 31 | Quality Assurance and Improvement 31 | Research 34 | Evidence-Based Medicine 35 | System Financing 36

CHAPTER 3 ● Roles and Responsibilities of the Paramedic   40

Introduction   41
Primary Responsibilities   41
Preparation 41 | Response 42 | Scene Size-Up 42 | Patient Assessment 43 | Recognition of Illness or Injury 43 | Patient Management 43 | Appropriate Disposition 44 | Patient Transfer 45 | Documentation 46 | Returning to Service 46
Additional Responsibilities   46
Administration 47 | Community Involvement 47 | Support for Primary Care 47 | Citizen Involvement in EMS 47 | Personal and Professional Development 47
Professionalism   48
Professional Ethics 48 | Professional Attitudes 48 | Professional Attributes 49 | Continuing Education 52

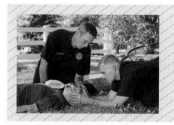

CHAPTER 4 ● Workforce Safety and Wellness   55

Introduction   56
Prevention of Work-Related Injuries   57
Basic Physical Fitness   57
Core Elements 57 | Nutrition 58 | Habits and Addictions 60 | Back Safety 60

Personal Protection from Disease   62
    Infectious Diseases 62 | Standard Safety Precautions 62 | Infection Control
    Measures 62
Death and Dying   67
    Loss, Grief, and Mourning 67 | What to Say 68 | When It Is Someone You Know 69
Stress and Stress Management   69
    Phases of Stress Response 70 | Shift Work 71 | Signs of Stress 71 | Common
    Techniques for Managing Stress 71 | Specific EMS Stresses 72 | Mental Health
    Services 73 | Disaster Mental Health Services 73
General Safety Considerations   73
    Interpersonal Relations 73 | Roadway Safety 74

CHAPTER 5 ● EMS Research 78

Introduction   80
Research and the Scientific Method   80
Types of Research   82
    Quantitative versus Qualitative Research 82 | Prospective versus Retrospective Studies 83
Experimental Design   83
    Specific Study Types 83 | Study Validity 86
Ethical Considerations in Human Research   87
    Institutional Review Boards 87
An Overview of Statistics   87
    Descriptive Statistics 88 | Inferential Statistics 88 | Quantitative and Qualitative
    Statistics 90 | Other Types of Data 90
Format of a Research Paper   90
How a Research Paper Is Published   91
Accessing the Scientific Literature   91
What to Look for When Reviewing a Study   91
Applying Study Results to Your Practice   94
Participating in Research   94
Evidence-Based Decision Making   96

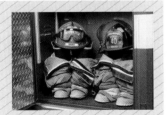

CHAPTER 6 ● Public Health 99

Introduction   100
Basic Principles of Public Health   100
Accomplishments in Public Health   101
Public Health Laws   101
Epidemiology   101
    EMS Public Health Strategies 102
Public Health and EMS   103
    Organizational Commitment 103 | EMS Provider Commitment 105
Prevention in the Community   107
    Areas of Need 107 | Implementation of Prevention Strategies 108

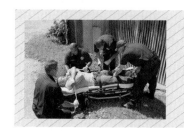

CHAPTER 7 ● Medical/Legal Aspects of Prehospital Care 112

Introduction 114

Legal Duties and Ethical Responsibilities 114

    The Legal System 115 | Anatomy of a Civil Lawsuit 115 | Laws Affecting EMS and the Paramedic 116

Legal Accountability of the Paramedic 117

    Negligence and Medical Liability 117 | Special Liability Concerns 120

Paramedic-Patient Relationships 121

    Confidentiality 121 | Consent 122 | Legal Complications Related to Consent 126 | Reasonable Force 126 | Patient Transportation 127

Resuscitation Issues 127

    Advance Directives 127 | Death in the Field 130

Crime and Accident Scenes 130

Duty to Report 130

Documentation 131

Employment Laws 131

CHAPTER 8 ● Ethics in Paramedicine 135

Introduction 136

Overview of Ethics 136

    Relationship of Ethics to Law and Religion 137 | Making Ethical Decisions 137 | Codes of Ethics 138 | Impact of Ethics on Individual Practice 138 | The Fundamental Questions 138 | Fundamental Principles 138 | Resolving Ethical Conflicts 139

Ethical Issues in Contemporary Paramedic Practice 141

    Resuscitation Attempts 141 | Confidentiality 143 | Consent 144 | Allocation of Resources 144 | Obligation to Provide Care 144 | Teaching 145 | Professional Relations 145 | Research 146

CHAPTER 9 ● EMS System Communications 148

Introduction 151

Effective Communications 151

Basic Communication Model 152

Verbal Communication 152

    Reporting Procedures 153 | Standard Format 153 | General Radio Procedures 153

Written Communication 154

Terminology 154

The Importance of Communications in EMS Response 155

    The Sequence of Communications in an EMS Response 155

Information and Communications Technology 159

    Technology Today 160 | New Technology 165

Public Safety Communications System Planning and Funding 167

Public Safety Communications Regulation 168

Introduction 172

Uses for Documentation 173

    Medical 173 | Administrative 173 | Research 173 | Legal 174

General Considerations 174

    Medical Terminology 174 | Abbreviations and
Acronyms 176 | Times 176 | Communications 176 | Pertinent Negatives 176 |
Oral Statements 182 | Additional Resources 182

Elements of Good Documentation 182

    Completeness and Accuracy 182 | Legibility 184 | Timeliness 184 | Absence
of Alterations 184 | Professionalism 185

Narrative Writing 185

    Narrative Sections 185 | General Formats 187

Special Considerations 188

    Patient Refusals 188 | Services Not Needed 189 | Multiple-Casualty Incidents 189

Consequences of Inappropriate Documentation 191

Electronic Patient Care Records 191

Closing 193

Precautions on Bloodborne Pathogens and Infectious Diseases 195

Suggested Responses to "You Make the Call" 197

Answers to Review Questions 203

Glossary 205

Index 213

Modern EMS is based on sound principles and practice. Today's paramedic must be knowledgeable in all aspects of EMS. This begins with a fundamental understanding of EMS operations and basic medical science. The paramedic curriculum follows the medical model. Students are first educated in the basic sciences. They are then introduced to the clinical sciences, reinforcing the basic science knowledge attained earlier. We have followed the *National EMS Education Standards* and the accompanying *Paramedic Instructional Guidelines* to provide the appropriate introductory material in *Volume 1, Introduction to Paramedicine*.

This volume provides paramedic students with the principles of advanced prehospital care and EMS operations. The first four chapters detail EMS systems and paramedic roles and responsibilities with added emphasis on personal wellness and injury and illness prevention. The next chapters deal with EMS research and the importance of evidence-based medicine, the EMS role in public health, the medical/legal aspects of emergency care, and ethics in paramedicine. The final two chapters of this volume deal with EMS system communications and documentation of patient care.

OVERVIEW OF THE CHAPTERS

CHAPTER 1   Introduction to Paramedicine introduces the paramedic student to the world of paramedicine. It summarizes the importance of professionalism and the expanding roles of the paramedic.

CHAPTER 2   EMS Systems reviews the history of EMS and provides an overview of EMS today. It details the aspects of EMS system design and operation. It emphasizes the importance of medical direction in all aspects of prehospital care.

CHAPTER 3   Roles and Responsibilities of the Paramedic is a detailed discussion of the expectations and responsibilities of the modern paramedic. It emphasizes the various aspects of professionalism as they pertain to the paramedic.

CHAPTER 4   Workforce Safety and Wellness presents material crucial to the survival of the paramedic in EMS. It addresses such important issues as prevention of work-related injuries, personal protection from disease, and safety concerns. It discusses physical fitness and nutrition. It discusses ways of dealing with death and dying, details the role of stress in EMS, and presents important coping strategies.

CHAPTER 5   EMS Research discusses the importance of research and evidence-based practices in EMS. It emphasizes ethical considerations in human research. Additionally, it explains how to read, evaluate, and participate in research.

CHAPTER 6   Public Health discusses the increasingly important role of EMS in public health, public education, and prevention of illness and injury—stopping injuries and illnesses before they happen.

CHAPTER 7   Medical/Legal Aspects of Prehospital Care is a detailed treatise on law and emergency care. In addition to an overview of the law and the legal system, this chapter discusses how the legal system can impact the paramedic. It also provides important tips on how the paramedic can avoid liability in a malpractice action.

CHAPTER 8   Ethics in Paramedicine presents the fundamentals of medical ethics. As EMS becomes more sophisticated, the paramedic will be faced with an ever-increasing number of ethical dilemmas. This chapter provides the paramedic student with an overview of medical ethics so as to be able to make sound decisions when confronted with ethical problems.

CHAPTER 9   EMS System Communications discusses communication as the key component linking all phases of an EMS run, discusses the current state of EMS communications, and presents anticipated advances in EMS communications and communications technology.

CHAPTER 10   Documentation explains how to write a prehospital care report (PCR), including examples of narrative report-writing styles, and discusses the elements and uses of electronic patient care records.

WHAT'S NEW IN THE FOURTH EDITION?

The Fourth Edition of *Paramedic Care: Principles & Practice* is the most extensive revision to date and reflects the dynamic and evolving world of paramedicine.

GLOBAL CHANGES/FEATURES
- Text follows the *National EMS Education Standards* and the *Paramedic Instructional Guidelines.*
- Terminology is consistent throughout the new Instructional Guidelines Gs (e.g., primary assessment).
- Reflects current 2010 American Heart Association Emergency Cardiac Care Guidelines.
- Embraces evidence-based emergency care with footnoted peer-review references to the major applicable world literature on the topic.
- Extensive review and editing.
- New design offers a fresh and professional text designed for the modern paramedic student.
- Extensive changes throughout are related to increased concerns about the detrimental effects of hyperoxia and the trend to limited oxygen administration.
- Terminology changed, when applicable, to assure consistency and reflect terms used in the AHA standards as well as the Instructional Guidelines.
- Reformatted into 7 volumes
  - *Volume 1: Introduction to Paramedicine*
  - *Volume 2: Paramedicine Fundamentals*
  - *Volume 3: Patient Assessment*
  - *Volume 4: Medicine*
  - *Volume 5: Trauma*
  - *Volume 6: Special Patients*
  - *Volume 7: Operations*

ACKNOWLEDGMENTS

CHAPTER CONTRIBUTORS

We wish to acknowledge the remarkable talents of the following people who contributed to Volume 1. Individually, they worked with extraordinary commitment. Together, they form a team of highly dedicated professionals who have upheld the highest standards of EMS instruction.

Jeff Brosius, BS, NREMT-P (Ret.)
Denver, CO: Chapter 10

Paul E. Ganss, MS, NREMT-P, NCEE
*EMS Education Program Director,
University of Missouri–Kansas City
School of Medicine, Kansas City, MO:
Chapter 2*

Kevin McGinnis, MPS, EMT-P, Chief/CEO
*North East Mobile Health Services,
Scarborough, ME: Chapter 9*

Wes Ogilvie, JD, MPA, LP
*Adjunct Faculty, University of Nevada
School of Medicine, Austin, TX:
Chapter 7*

Michael O'Keefe, MS, NREMT-P
*Assistant Director of Emergency
Medicine Research, University of Vermont,
Burlington, VT: Chapter 5*

INSTRUCTOR REVIEWERS

The reviewers of this edition of *Paramedic Care: Principles & Practice, Volume 1* have provided many excellent suggestions and ideas for improving the text. The quality of the reviews has been outstanding, and the reviews have been a major aid in the preparation and revision of the manuscript. The assistance provided by these EMS experts is deeply appreciated.

Ronald R. Audette, NREMT-P
*Vice President
Educational Resource Group LLC
East Providence, RI*

Troy Breitag, BS, NREMT-P, Fire Lt.
*Department Supervisor – Med/Fire Rescue
Lake Area Technical Institute
Watertown, SD*

Joshua Chan, BA, NREMT-P
*EMS Educator
Cuyuna Regional Medical Center
Crosby, MN*

**Thomas E. Ezell, III, NREMT-P,
CCEMT-P, CHpT**
*Fire/Rescue Captain (Ret.)
James City County Fire Department
Williamsburg, VA*

Sean P. Haaverson, AA, NR/CCEMT-P
*EMS Faculty
Central New Mexico Community College
Albuquerque, NM*

L. Kelly Kirk, III, AAS, BS, EMT-P
*Director of Distance Education
Randolph Community College
Asheboro, NC*

Paul Salway, CCEMT-P, NREMT-P
*Firefighter/EMT-P
South Portland Fire Department
South Portland, ME*

R. Thomy Windham, BS
*Director
Pee Dee Regional Community Training
Center
Florence, SC*

We also wish to express appreciation to the following EMS professionals who reviewed the third edition of Paramedic Care: Principles & Practice. *Their suggestions and perspectives helped to make this program a successful teaching tool.*

Mike Dymes, NREMT-P
*EMS Program Director
Durham Technical Community College
Durham, NC*

**Wes Hamilton, RN, BSN, CCRN, CFRN,
CTRN, NREMT-P, FP-C**
*Clinical Educator
Clinical Care Services Division
Air-Evac Lifeteam
West Plains, MO*

Sean Kivlehan, EMT-P
*St. Vincent's Hospital, Manhattan
New York, NY*

Darren P. Lacroix, AAS, EMT-P
*Del Mar College
Emergency Medical Service Professions
Corpus Christi, TX*

**Mike McEvoy, PhD, REMT-P,
RN, CCRN**
*EMS Coordinator
Saratoga County, NY*

Greg Mullen, MS, NREMT-P
*National EMS Academy
Lafayette, LA*

Deborah L. Petty, BS, EMT-P I/C
*Training Officer
St. Charles County Ambulance District
St. Peter's, MO*

**B. Jeanine Riner, MHSA, BS, RRT,
NREMT-P**
*GA Office of EMS and Trauma
Atlanta, GA*

Michael D. Smith, LP
*Kilgore College
Longview, TX*

Allen Walls
*Department of Fire & EMS
Colerain Township, OH*

Brian J. Wilson, BA, NREMT-P
*Education Director
Texas Tech School of Medicine
El Paso, TX*

PHOTO ACKNOWLEDGMENTS

All photographs not credited adjacent to the photograph or in the photo credit section below were photographed on assignment for Brady/Pearson Education.

Organizations

We wish to thank the following organizations for their valuable assistance in creating the photo program for this edition:

Canandaigua Emergency Squad
Canandaigua, NY

Flower Mound Fire Department
Flower Mound, TX

Children's Hospital St. Louis/BJC Health Care
St. Louis, MO

Christian Hospital/BJC Health Care
St. Charles, MO

MedicWest Ambulance
Las Vegas, NV

Tyco Health Care/Nellcor Puritan Bennet
Pleasanton, CA

Wolfe Tory Medical
Salt Lake City, UT

Models

Thanks to the following people from the Flower Mound Fire Department, Flower Mound, Texas, who provided locations and/or portrayed patients and EMS providers in our photographs.

FAO/Paramedic Wade Woody

FF/Paramedic Tim Mackling

FF/Paramedic Matthew Daniel

FF/Paramedic Jon Rea

FF/Paramedic Waylon Palmer

FF/EMT Jesse Palmer

Captain/EMT Billy McWhorter

BRYAN E. BLEDSOE, DO, FACEP, FAAEM, EMT-P

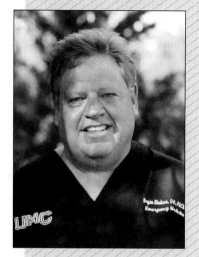

Dr. Bryan Bledsoe is an emergency physician, researcher, and EMS author. Presently he is Professor of Emergency Medicine and Director of the EMS Fellowship program at the University of Nevada School of Medicine and an Attending Emergency Physician at the University Medical Center of Southern Nevada in Las Vegas. He is board-certified in emergency medicine. Prior to attending medical school, Dr. Bledsoe worked as an EMT, a paramedic, and a paramedic instructor. He completed EMT training in 1974 and paramedic training in 1976 and worked for six years as a field paramedic in Fort Worth, Texas. In 1979, he joined the faculty of the University of North Texas Health Sciences Center and served as coordinator of EMT and paramedic education programs at the university.

Dr. Bledsoe is active in emergency medicine and EMS research. He is a popular speaker at state, national, and international seminars and writes regularly for numerous EMS journals. He is active in educational endeavors with the United States Special Operations Command (USSOCOM) and the University of Nevada at Las Vegas. Dr. Bledsoe is the author of numerous EMS textbooks and has in excess of 1 million books in print. Dr. Bledsoe was named a "Hero of Emergency Medicine" in 2008 by the American College of Emergency Physicians as a part of their 40th anniversary celebration and was named a "Hero of Health and Fitness" by *Men's Health* magazine as part of their 20th anniversary edition in November of 2008. He is frequently interviewed in the national media. Dr. Bledsoe is married and divides his time between his residences in Midlothian, TX, and Las Vegas, NV.

ROBERT S. PORTER, MA, EMT-P

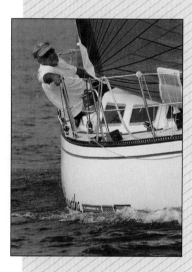

Robert Porter has been teaching in emergency medical services for 38 years and currently serves as the Senior Advanced Life Support Educator for Madison County (New York) Emergency Medical Services. Mr. Porter is a Wisconsin native and received his bachelor's degree in education from the University of Wisconsin. He completed his paramedic training at Northeast Wisconsin Technical Institute in 1978 and earned a master's degree in health education at Central Michigan University in 1990.

Mr. Porter has been an EMT and an EMS educator and administrator since 1973 and obtained his certification and national registration as an EMT-Paramedic in 1978. He has taught both basic and advanced EMS courses in the states of Wisconsin, Michigan, Louisiana, Pennsylvania, and New York. Mr. Porter conducted one of the nation's first rural paramedic programs and developed a university-based, two-year paramedic program. Mr. Porter served for more than ten years as a paramedic program accreditation-site evaluator for the American Medical Association and is a past chair of the National Association of EMTs—Society of EMT Instructor/Coordinators. Mr. Porter also served for 15 years as a flight paramedic with the Onondaga County Sheriff's Department air medical service, AirOne. He has authored Brady's *Paramedic Care: Principles & Practice, Essentials of Paramedic Care, Intermediate Emergency Care: Principles & Practice, Tactical Emergency Care,* and *Weapons of Mass Destruction: Emergency Care,* as well as the workbooks accompanying this text. When not writing or teaching, Mr. Porter enjoys offshore sailboat racing and home restoration.

RICHARD A. CHERRY, MS, EMT-P

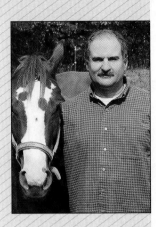

Richard Cherry is the Director of Training for Northern Onondaga Volunteer Ambulance (NOVA) in Liverpool, New York, a suburb of Syracuse. He recently retired from the Department of Emergency Medicine at Upstate Medical University where he held the positions of Director of Paramedic Training, Assistant Emergency Medicine Residency Director, Clinical Assistant Professor of Emergency Medicine, and Technical Director for Medical Simulation. His experience includes years of classroom teaching and emergency fieldwork. A native of Buffalo, Mr. Cherry earned his bachelor's degree at nearby St. Bonaventure University in 1972. He taught high school for the next ten years while he earned his master's degree in education from Oswego State University in 1977. He holds a permanent teaching license in New York State.

Mr. Cherry entered the emergency medical services field in 1974 with the DeWitt Volunteer Fire Department, where he served his community as a firefighter and EMS provider for more than 15 years. He took his first EMT course in 1977 and became an ALS provider two years later. He earned his paramedic certificate in 1985 as a member of the area's first paramedic class.

Mr. Cherry has authored several books for Brady. Most notable are *Paramedic Care: Principles & Practice, Essentials of Paramedic Care, Intermediate Emergency Care: Principles & Practice,* and *EMT Teaching: A Common Sense Approach.* He has made presentations at many state, national, and international EMS conferences on a variety of teaching topics. He and his wife, Sue, run a summer horse-riding camp for children with special needs on their property in West Monroe, New York. He also plays guitar in a Christian band.

Welcome to

PARAMEDIC CARE PRINCIPLES & PRACTICE

FOURTH EDITION

A Guide to Key Features

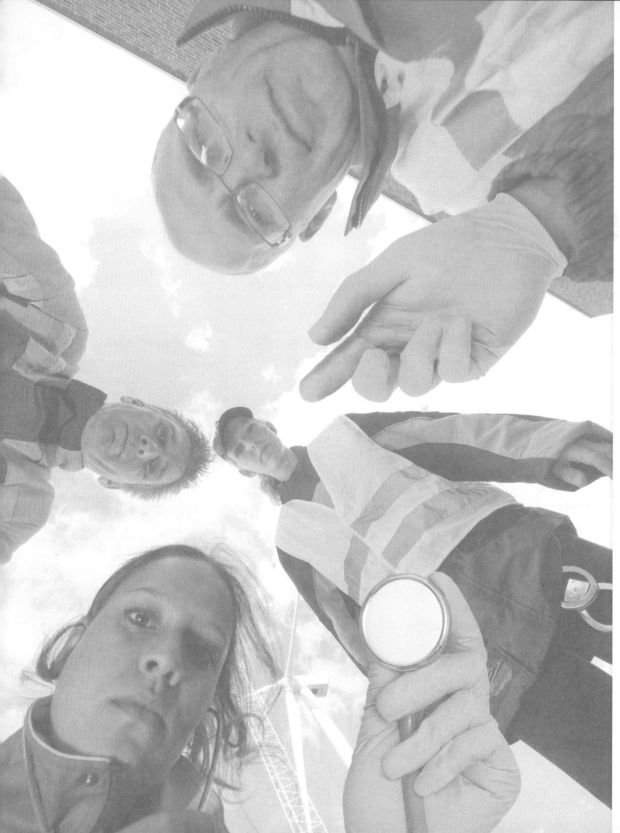

Emphasizing Principles

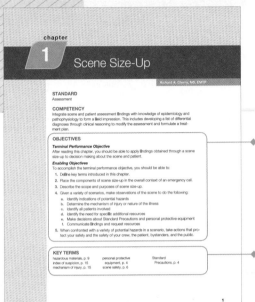

CHAPTER OBJECTIVES

Terminal Performance Objectives and a separate set of Enabling Objectives are provided for each chapter.

KEY TERMS

Page numbers identify where each key term first appears, boldfaced, in the chapter.

TABLES

A wealth of tables offers the opportunity to highlight, summarize, and compare information.

TABLE 4-2	Common Infectious Diseases		
Disease	**Mode of Transmission**	**Incubation Period**
AIDS (acquired immune deficiency syndrome)	AIDS- or HIV-infected blood via intravenous drug use, semen and vaginal fluids, blood transfusions, or (rarely) needlesticks. Mothers also may pass HIV to their unborn children.	Several months or years
Hepatitis B, C	Blood, stool, or other body fluids, or contaminated objects.	Weeks or months
Tuberculosis	Respiratory secretions, airborne or on contaminated objects.	2 to 6 weeks
Meningitis, bacterial	Oral and nasal secretions.	2 to 10 days
Pneumonia, bacterial and viral	Oral and nasal droplets and secretions.	Several days
Influenza	Airborne droplets, or direct contact with body fluids.	1 to 3 days
Staphylococcal skin infections	Contact with open wounds or sores or contaminated objects.	Several days
Chicken pox (varicella)	Airborne droplets, or contact with open sores.	11 to 21 days
German measles (rubella)	Airborne droplets. Mothers may pass it to their unborn children.	10 to 12 days
Whooping cough (pertussis)	Respiratory secretions or airborne droplets.	6 to 20 days
SARS (severe acute respiratory syndrome)	Airborne droplets and personal contact.	4 to 6 days

PHOTOS AND ILLUSTRATIONS

Carefully selected photos and a unique art program reinforce content coverage and add to text explanations.

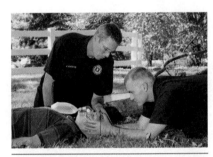

● **Figure 3-3** During the primary assessment of your patient, you will look for and immediately treat any life-threatening conditions.

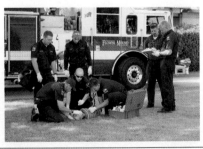

● **Figure 3-7** As leader of the EMS team, the paramedic must interact with patients, bystanders, and other rescue personnel in a professional and efficient manner.

CONTENT REVIEW
▶ Steps of Primary Assessment

- Form a general impression
- Stabilize cervical spine as needed
- Assess baseline mental status
- Assess and manage airway
- Assess and manage breathing
- Assess and manage circulation
- Determine priorities

CONTENT REVIEW

Screened content review boxes set off from the text are interspersed throughout the chapter. They summarize key points and serve as a helpful study guide—in an easy format for quick review.

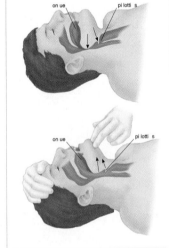

● **Figure 2-4** The head-tilt/chin-lift maneuver in an adult.

SUMMARY

This end-of-chapter feature provides a concise review of chapter information.

SUMMARY

The scene size-up is the initial step in the patient care process. Sizing up the scene and situation begins at your initial dispatch and does not end until you are clear of the call. As the call unfolds, you should be making constant observations and adjustments to your plan of action. Remember that your safety and the safety of your partner are paramount—it is hard to effectively treat both yourself and others.

Scene size-up should be practiced so much that it becomes second nature to you. It is like noticing veins on people in public after you begin starting IVs. (You have all done it—looked across the room at the back of someone's hand and noticed what nice veins they had.) Sizing up a scene is no different. After a while you begin to notice mechanisms of injury and other important details almost subconsciously. But be careful and do not get complacent! Always make it a point to pause for just a few seconds and consciously look around the scene before proceeding into any situation.

Scene size-up is not a step-by-step process, but a series of decisions you make when confronted with a variety of circumstances that are often beyond your control. It is a way to make order out of chaos, keep yourself and your crew safe, and ensure that all necessary resources are focused on patient care and outcomes. With time and experience, you will learn to perform a scene size-up quickly and focus on important issues. Your careful size-up lays the foundation for an organized and timely approach toward patient care and scene management.

REVIEW QUESTIONS

1. Which of the following is *not* a component of the scene size-up?
   a. Standard Precautions
   b. mechanism of injury
   c. primary assessment
   d. location of all patients

2. The HEPA mask is designed to protect you from _____.
   a. tuberculosis
   b. AIDS
   c. hepatitis
   d. meningitis

3. The top priority in any emergency situation is _____.
   a. patient assessment
   b. bystander cooperation
   c. customer service
   d. your personal safety

4. As you approach a scene, something just does not seem right. It is not anything you can put your finger on, just a sense that something is wrong or is about to happen. What should you do about it?
   a. Wait until law enforcement arrives before entering.
   b. Ignore your feelings and enter the scene.
   c. Enter the scene with something with which to protect yourself.
   d. Call out for the patient to come outside.

5. You are responding to a shooting at a well-known bar. How should you approach the scene?
   a. Stage outside the bar until the police arrive.
   b. Wait for another ambulance or rescue crew before entering.
   c. Just enter the scene.
   d. Stage your ambulance a few blocks away until law enforcement arrives.

6. You arrive on the scene and see that a power line lies close to your pediatric patient. You are fairly sure the line is live and decide to move it with a dry piece of equipment. Which of the following should you use?
   a. a wooden-handled ax
   b. a fallen tree branch
   c. a nylon rope
   d. none of the above

7. When you and your partner arrive at a multiple-patient incident, you should _____.
   a. begin assessing and treating the first patient you encounter
   b. establish command and begin triage
   c. provide intensive emergency care to the most critical patient
   d. start at opposite ends and begin assessing patients

REVIEW QUESTIONS

These questions ask students to review and recall key information they have just learned.

REFERENCES

This listing is a compilation of source material providing the basis of updated data and research used in the preparation of each chapter.

REFERENCES

1. U.S. Department of Transportation/National Highway Traffic Safety Administration. *National EMS Scope of Practice Model.* Washington, DC, 2006.
2. National Registry of Emergency Medical Technicians. 2004 National EMS Practice Analysis. Columbus, OH: National Registry of EMTs, 2005.
3. American College of Surgeons. *Verified Trauma Centers.* [Available at: http://www.facs.org/trauma/verified.html]
4. Feldman, M. J., J. L. Lukins, P. R. Verbeek, et al. "Use of Treat-and-Release Directives for Paramedics at a Mass Gathering." *Prehosp Emerg Care* 9 (2005): 213–217.
5. American College of Emergency Physicians. "Interacility Transportation of the Critical Care Patient and Its Medical Direction." *Ann Emerg Med* 47 (2006): 305.
6. Harkins, S. "Documentation: Why Is It So Important?" *Emerg Med Serv* 31 (2002): 93–94.
7. Lerner, E. B., A. R. Fernandez, and M. N. Shah. "Do Emergency Medical Services Professionals Think They Should Participate in Disease Prevention?" *Prehosp Emerg Care* 13 (2009): 64–70.
8. Poliafico, F. "The Role of EMS in Public Access Defibrillation." *Emerg Med Serv* 32 (2003): 73.
9. Streger M. R. "Professionalism." *Emerg Med Serv* 32 (2003): 35.
10. Klugman, C. M. "Why EMS Needs Its Own Ethics. What's Good for Other Areas of Healthcare May Not Be Good for You." *Emerg Med Serv* 36 (2007): 114–122.
11. Touchstone, M. "Professional Development. Part 1: Becoming an EMS Leader." *Emerg Med Serv* 38 (2009): 59–60.
12. Bledsoe, B. E. "EMS Needs a Few More Cowboys." *JEMS* 28 (2003): 112–113.

FURTHER READING

This list features recommendations for books and journal articles that go beyond chapter coverage.

FURTHER READING

Bailey, E. D. and T. Sweeney. "Considerations in Establishing Emergency Medical Services Response Time Goals." *Prehosp Emerg Care* 7 (2003): 397–399.

Bledsoe, B. E. "Searching for the Evidence behind EMS." *Emerg Med Serv* 31 (2003): 63–67.

Heightman, A. J. "EMS Workforce. A Comprehensive Listing of Certified EMS Providers by State and How the Workforce Has Changed Since 1993." *JEMS* 5 (2000): 108–112.

Jaslow, D. J., J. Ufberg, and R. Marsh. "Primary Injury Prevention in an Urban EMS System." *J Emerg Med* 25 (2003): 167–170.

National Academy of Sciences, National Research Council. *Accidental Death and Disability: The Neglected Disease of Modern Society.* Washington, DC:

U.S. Department of Health, Education, and Welfare, 1966.

Page, J. O. *The Magic of 3 AM.* San Diego, CA: JEMS Publishing, 2002.

Page, J. O. *The Paramedics.* Morristown, NJ: Backdraft Publications, 1979. [No longer available for purchase except as a used book. Entire book can be viewed online at www.JEMS.com/Paramedics.]

Page, J. O. *Simple Advice.* San Diego, CA: JEMS Publishing, 2002.

Persse, D. E., C. B. Key, R. N. Bradley, et al. "Cardiac Arrest Survival as a Function of Ambulance Deployment Strategy in a Large Urban Emergency Medical Services System." *Resusc* 59 (2003): 97–104.

CASE STUDY

This feature at the start of each chapter draws students into the reading and creates a link between text content and real-life situations.

CASE STUDY

On a quiet afternoon, paramedic Dean Barker hears the tones for a person slumped over the steering wheel of his car. He and his partner, Kyle Peeper, a new EMT, respond immediately. En route, Dean emphasizes to his rookie partner the need to put safety first and not to rush in without a quick evaluation of the scene. His partner nods agreeably but is obviously both excited and nervous about his first real emergency call.

When they arrive, Dean notices a very unusual and troubling scene. Dean grabs his partner and stops him from jumping out of the vehicle. He asks him to stop and look around. "Tell me what you see," he says. His partner nervously answers, "Right, OK, I see one car parked alongside a cemetery and it looks like someone might be inside. There seems to be a white cloud inside the car and I smell a strong odor of sulfur or rotten eggs. I also see a sign on the driver's side window with what looks like a hazard emblem on it."

"So, is there anything we should do before jumping out and entering this scene? What is our first priority? asks Dean. "Patient care." answers his partner. "No, safety first. We'll park our vehicle upwind from the car and I'll make a quick report to dispatch and call for more help. We already know this is more than we can handle by ourselves."

Dean assumes the role of incident commander; he calls for the fire department's hazmat team, cordons off the area, and alerts all responding personnel that the potential for fire and explosion exists. There also may be a need to evacuate the area. Waiting for the fire department to arrive seems like hours to his energetic partner. Dean asks him what they can do until they arrive. Kyle responds that they can shut down the road and secure the scene from bystanders.

When the hazmat team arrives, they read the signs that someone left on three of the four windows. They appear to be suicide notes and a warning to rescuers of the toxic atmosphere inside the car. The hazmat team begins the arduous process of identifying the toxic substance, containing the exposure, and decontaminating the victim and all rescuers. Dean and his partner are released and head back to the station.

Kyle asks Dean what the substance was inside that car and asks why they didn't try to extricate and resuscitate the driver. Dean calmly explains that the white cloud and rotten-egg odor strongly suggested a deadly asphyxiant, hydrogen sulfide, and if they had opened the door to extricate him, they would have been just as dead as their victim. This day a rookie learned a crucial lesson—on an EMS call, nothing is more important than his safety. Nothing.

YOU MAKE THE CALL

A scenario at the end of each chapter promotes critical thinking by requiring students to apply principles to actual practice.

YOU MAKE THE CALL

On a rainy and windy evening, you hear the tones for a car crash on the interstate highway just five minutes from the station. You are the only ambulance dispatched along with fire department rescue and fire apparatus. On arrival you see three cars smashed up, one on its side, smoke rising from the crash, and what looks like fluid leaking from one vehicle. By the time you arrive, traffic is backed up for three blocks. You realize that the decisions you make in the first few minutes will have a major effect on safety, patient care, and overall operations.

Describe how you would size up this scene. Make sure you cover the following areas:

- Vehicle placement
- Initial radio report
- Assuming incident command
- Safety
- Hazard control
- Standard Precautions
- Location and triaging of patients
- Resource determination
- Mechanisms of injury

See Suggested Responses at the back of this book.

PROCEDURE SCANS

Visual skill summaries provide step-by-step support in skill instruction.

Procedure 5–22 ● Reassessment

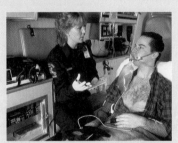

5-22a ● Reevaluate the ABCs.

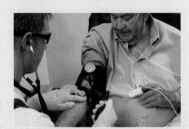

5-22b ● Take all vital signs again.

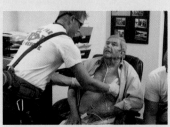

5-22c ● Perform your focused assessment again.

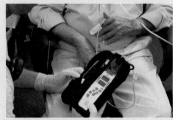

5-22d ● Evaluate your interventions' effects.

Special Features

PATHO PEARLS

Offer a snapshot of pathological considerations students will encounter in the field.

PATHO PEARLS

Patient assessment actually starts as soon as you approach the scene. Clues about the patient's underlying pathophysiology might be evident from such things as positioning of the vehicle, downed power lines, or the appearance and actions of bystanders. However, your safety, and that of your fellow rescuers, is always paramount. Never approach a scene that appears unsafe. With time, you will develop a "sixth sense" about emergency scenes and bystanders.

As you begin the patient encounter, process all that you see into your patient assessment and care. For example, consider this scenario: A car with two 16-year-old girls fails to negotiate a turn on a country road and overturns into a flowing creek adjacent to the road. Although the ambient temperature is in the 60s, you know that the temperature of the water in this area often is in the 40s. Thus, you should immediately suspect the possibility of hypothermia.

As the girls are removed from entrapment, no obvious injuries are noted. Vital signs are normal other than slight tachycardia. However, peripheral pulses are weak and the skin is pale and cool. Is it shock? Is it hypothermia? Is it both? Your index of suspicion is high for both hypothermia and blunt force trauma. You follow local protocols with regard to immobilization, fluid therapy, and monitoring. Once in the ambulance and wrapped in blankets, both girls start to show signs that blood flow to the skin is improving. By the time you reach the hospital, their skin has a normal color and their pulse rates are normal.

Following a comprehensive assessment in the emergency department, the girls are discharged to their parents with no apparent injuries. Thus, your instincts were right. The potential for shock was a greater risk to the girls than the potential for hypothermia, and you had to treat based on this risk. But hypothermia turned out to be the principal problem. Integrating information from the scene size-up, patient history, and patient examination gave you a clear picture of the patients' underlying pathophysiologic process.

CULTURAL CONSIDERATIONS

Provide an awareness of beliefs that might affect patient care.

CULTURAL CONSIDERATIONS

Eye contact is a major form of nonverbal communication. Short eye contact is often seen as friendly, whereas prolonged eye contact may be interpreted as threatening. Thus, timing is an important factor in how a person interprets eye contact.

One's culture also influences how eye contact is interpreted. Eye contact can mean respect in one culture and disrespect in another. Often, Asians will avoid eye contact even when they have nothing to hide. Eye contact between people of different sexes is problematic in Muslim cultures, in which a prolonged look in the face of a member of the opposite sex might be misinterpreted. Because of this, people in Middle Eastern countries might look a person of the same sex in the eye and not look into the eyes of a person of the opposite sex.

If you work in a culturally diverse community, you should learn the customs of eye contact and other forms of nonverbal communication of those you might encounter during the course of your work.

LEGAL NOTES

Present instances in which legal or ethical considerations should be evaluated.

LEGAL CONSIDERATIONS

Gatekeeper to the Health Care System. *The EMS system is often the initial point of contact for a person entering the health care system. Thus, to a certain extent, a paramedic frequently functions as a sort of gatekeeper to the health care system as a whole.*

Part of a paramedic's responsibility is to ensure that a patient is taken to a facility that can appropriately care for the patient's condition. Today, hospitals have become more specialized. That is, some hospitals have chosen to provide certain services and not provide others. For example, one hospital may elect to specialize in cardiac care, another in stroke care, another in burn care, and so on. This is especially true in communities with multiple hospitals. Because of this, it is essential that paramedics understand the capabilities of the hospitals in the system where they work. Also, with overcrowding in modern emergency departments, diversion of ambulances by hospitals whose emergency departments are full has become commonplace.

For all these reasons, local EMS system protocols must be available to guide prehospital personnel in ensuring that each patient is delivered to a facility that can adequately care for the patient's condition.

ASSESSMENT PEARLS

Offer tips, guidance, and information to aid in patient assessment.

ASSESSMENT PEARLS

Chest pain is a common reason that people summon EMS. However, the causes of chest pain are numerous. In emergency medicine or EMS, we often look to exclude the most serious causes before determining whether chest pain is of a benign origin. Internal organs do not have as many pain fibers as do such structures as the skin and other areas. Pain arising from an internal organ tends to be dull and vague. This is because nerves from various spinal levels innervate the organ in question. The heart, for example, is innervated by several thoracic spinal nerve segments. Thus, cardiac pain tends to be dull and is sometimes described as pressure. It also tends to cause referred pain (i.e., pain in an area somewhat distant to the organ), such as pain in the left arm and jaw. Dull pain that is hard to localize (or to reproduce with palpation) may be due to cardiac disease. One sign often seen with patients suffering cardiac disease is Levine's sign. With Levine's sign, the patient will subconsciously cle...
pain. Levine's sign is a...
(e.g., angina or acute c...

ASSESSMENT PEARLS

Assessing skin abnormalities in dark-skinned people can be a challenge. Try the following techniques:

Jaundice Look for a yellow color in the sclera and hard palate.

Erythema Look for an ashen color in the sclera, conjunctiva, mouth, tongue, lips, nail beds, palms, and soles.

Pallor Feel for warmth in the affected area.

Petechiae Look for tiny purplish dots on the abdomen.

Cyanosis Look for a dull, dark coloring in the mouth, tongue, lips, nail beds, palms, and soles.

Rashes Feel for abnormal skin texture.

Edema Look for decreased color and feel for tightness.

Student Workbook

A student workbook with review and practice activities accompanies each volume of the Paramedic Care series. The workbooks include multiple-choice questions, other exercises, case studies, and special projects, along with an answer key with text page references.

REVIEW OF CHAPTER OBJECTIVES

Tied to chapter objectives, content summaries review important information and concepts.

CASE STUDY REVIEW

An in-depth analysis at the start of each chapter highlights essential information and applied principles.

CONTENT SELF-EVALUATION

Multiple-choice, matching, and short-answer questions test reading comprehension.

SPECIAL PROJECTS

Experiences have been designed to help students remember information and principles.

PATIENT SCENARIO FLASHCARDS

Flashcards present scenarios with signs and symptoms and information to make field diagnoses.

DRUG FLASHCARDS

A special set of flashcards represents drugs commonly used in paramedic care.

MyParamedicLab

www.myparamediclab.com

WHAT IS MYPARAMEDICLAB?

MyParamedicLab is a comprehensive online program that gives you the opportunity to test yourself on basic information, concepts, and skills to see how well you know the material. From the test results, the program builds a self-paced, personalized study plan unique to your needs. Remediation in the form of e-text pages, illustrations, animations, exercises, and video clips is provided for those areas in which you may need additional instruction or reinforcement. You can then work through the program until material is learned and mastered. **MyParamedicLab** is available as a standalone program or with an embedded e-text.

MyParamedicLab maps objectives created from the National EMS Education Standards for the Paramedic level to each learning module. With **MyParamedicLab**, you can track your own progress through the entire course. The personalized study plan material supports you as you work to achieve success in the classroom and on certification exams.

HOW DO STUDENTS BENEFIT?

MyParamedicLab helps you:

- Keep up with the new, complex information presented in the text and lectures.
- Save time by focusing study and review on just the content you need.
- Increase understanding of difficult concepts with study material for different learning styles.
- Remediate in areas in which you need additional review.

KEY FEATURES OF MYPARAMEDICLAB

Pre-Tests and Post-Tests Using questions aligned to Paramedic Standards, quizzes measure your understanding of topics and expected learning outcomes.

Personalized Study Material Based on the topic pre-test results, you will receive a personalized study plan highlighting areas where you may need improvement. Study tools include:

- Skills and animation videos
- Links to specific pages in the e-text
- Images for review
- Interactive exercises
- Audio glossary
- Access to full chapters of the e-text

HOW DO INSTRUCTORS BENEFIT?

- Save time by providing students with a comprehensive, media-rich study program
- Track student understanding of course content in the program Gradebook
- Monitor student activity with viewable student assignments

What Resources Are Available to Instructors?

Visit **www.bradybooks.com** to log onto Brady's Resource Central website for the Paramedic Care series. Your Brady sales representative will assist with access codes. At Resource Central instructors will find a wealth of curriculum management material to support class presentations, student assessment, and administrative functions.

Where Do I Get More Information?

Contact your local Brady representative for more information.

chapter

1

Introduction to Paramedicine

Bryan Bledsoe, DO, FACEP, FAAEM, EMT-P

STANDARD
Preparatory (EMS Systems)

COMPETENCY
Integrates comprehensive knowledge of EMS systems, the safety and well-being of the paramedic, and medical-legal and ethical issues, which is intended to improve the health of EMS personnel, patients, and the community.

OBJECTIVES

Terminal Performance Objective
After reading this chapter you should be able to discuss the characteristics of the profession of paramedicine.

Enabling Objectives
To accomplish the terminal performance objective, you should be able to:

1. Define key terms introduced in this chapter.

2. Compare and contrast the roles of emergency medical responders (EMRs), emergency medical technicians (EMTs), and Advanced Emergency Medical Technicians (AEMTs) with the role of paramedics in the emergency medical services system.

3. Describe the requirements that must be met for paramedics to practice the art and science of out-of-hospital medicine.

4. Describe the role of the paramedic in health care, public health, and public safety.

5. Describe the desirable characteristics of paramedics.

6. Explain how paramedicine has made strides toward greater recognition as a health care profession.

7. List settings in which paramedics may work.

KEY TERMS
Advanced Emergency Medical Technician (AEMT), p. 3
critical care transport, p. 6
Emergency Medical Responder (EMR), p. 3
Emergency Medical Services (EMS) system, p. 3

Emergency Medical Technician (EMT), p. 3
National Emergency Medical Services Education Standards: Paramedic Instructional Guidelines, p. 5

Paramedic, p. 3
paramedicine, p. 9

Marcus Ward is a 65-year-old attorney who is celebrating his recent retirement with a weeklong trip to Las Vegas. He has taken in the shows, eaten the fine food, and is spending his last night in town in one of the casinos on the famous Las Vegas strip. He sits down at a Blackjack table and lights a cigarette. As the dealer is shuffling the cards, Marcus starts to feel warm. He turns to his friend Ray and says, "Does it feel warm in here to you?" Then, without another word, Marcus grasps at the collar of his shirt and collapses to the floor. Initially, Ray thinks his friend has slipped on the stool. Quickly, though, he realizes the situation is much worse. He starts screaming for help. The dealer presses a security button and several security officers immediately show up at the table. After a quick exam, the security staff moves Marcus to a beverage area off the casino floor and calls 911. There they start CPR and immediately apply an automated external defibrillator (AED) to Marcus. The AED detects ventricular fibrillation and delivers a shock. Immediately Marcus starts moving and soon opens his eyes. The security staff administers supplemental oxygen, and soon a paramedic fire crew arrives. Shortly thereafter, paramedics from the ambulance service arrive.

The paramedics assess Marcus and obtain a 12-lead ECG. The ECG is consistent with an acute anterior ST-segment elevation myocardial infarction (STEMI). The ECG monitor electronically transmits Marcus's ECG to the hospital emergency department and the on-call STEMI team. The cardiologist reviews the ECG and calls for a "Code STEMI," after which the team is activated. Paramedics insert an IV and administer nitroglycerin and 325 mg of aspirin. He is quickly moved to the ambulance and transported to the designated hospital.

Once Marcus arrives at the emergency department, he is quickly evaluated by the interventional cardiologist and an emergency physician. Finding no contraindications, the cardiologist has Marcus immediately moved to the cardiac catheterization lab. Once he is in the lab, the team goes to work. Marcus is moved to the table. A nurse shaves his groin and applies an antiseptic soap. An anesthesiologist sedates Marcus and monitors his vital signs. The cardiologist quickly inserts a catheter into Marcus's femoral artery and threads it up the aorta to the heart. He injects a dye, and immediately Marcus's coronary arteries can be seen on the monitor. As expected, part of the left anterior descending coronary artery is blocked. The cardiologist then inserts a balloon catheter into the diseased artery and restores blood flow to the affected part of the heart. This is followed by some ventricular irritability and premature ventricular contractions, but these soon abate and the cardiologist then places a stent to keep the artery open. Additional dye is injected, blood flow through the stent looks good, and no other lesions require treatment. Marcus is moved to the coronary care unit, where he ultimately recovers and flies back to Irvine, California, four days later.

Marcus survived because the EMS and emergency health care system worked together cohesively. When he collapsed at the blackjack table, he was defibrillated within 3 minutes of his collapse. His STEMI was promptly identified and treated by prehospital personnel who also notified and activated the STEMI team at the hospital. Once Marcus arrived at the hospital, the time interval from his arrival until blood flow was restored to his diseased artery (door-to-balloon time) was 31 minutes.

Back in Irvine, Marcus has vowed to improve his life and appears to be making important changes. He has quit smoking and has begun an exercise regimen. He now sees a local cardiologist on a regular basis. He and his wife have made major changes in their diet. His prognosis is good, and he should enjoy many more years of his retirement. A month after his cardiac arrest, Marcus purchased an AED and donated it to the fitness center where he now exercises. Moreover, he has developed a whole new understanding and appreciation for the EMS system.

INTRODUCTION

Congratulations on your decision to become a paramedic. Before you begin this long but rewarding endeavor, it is important to understand what the job of a paramedic in the twenty-first century entails. As a member of the allied health professions (ancillary health care professions, apart from physicians and nurses), the paramedic is highly regarded by society (Figure 1-1 ●).

The **Emergency Medical Services (EMS) system** has made significant advances over the last 30 years. Understandably, the paramedic's roles and responsibilities have advanced accordingly. Not that long ago, the ambulance was simply a vehicle that provided rapid, horizontal transportation to the hospital. Today, equipped with the latest in equipment and technology, the modern ambulance is truly a mobile emergency room that brings sophisticated emergency medical care to the patient. The paramedic of the twenty-first century is a highly trained health care professional who provides comprehensive, compassionate, and efficient prehospital emergency medical care.

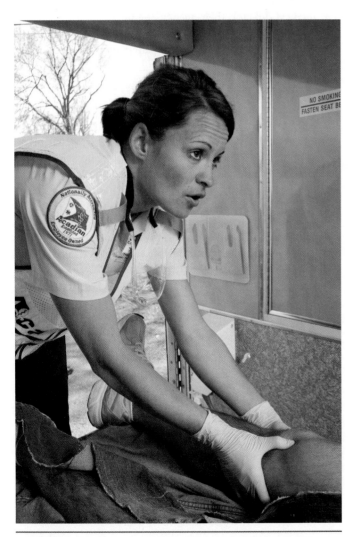

● **Figure 1-1**   The paramedic of the twenty-first century is a highly trained health care professional.

Description of the Profession

The paramedic is the highest level of prehospital care provider and the leader of the prehospital care team.[1] There are four nationally recognized levels of EMS providers in the United States:

● *Emergency Medical Responder (EMR).* The primary focus of the **Emergency Medical Responder (EMR)** is to initiate immediate lifesaving care to critical patients who access the emergency medical system. This individual possesses the basic knowledge and skills necessary to provide lifesaving interventions while awaiting additional EMS response and to assist higher level personnel at the scene and during transport. EMRs must successfully complete an accredited EMR educational program.

● *Emergency Medical Technician (EMT).* The primary focus of the **Emergency Medical Technician (EMT)** is to provide basic emergency medical care and transportation for critical and emergent patients who access the emergency medical system. The EMT possesses the basic knowledge and skills necessary to provide patient care and transportation. EMTs perform interventions with basic equipment and are an essential link in the prehospital emergency care continuum. EMTs must successfully complete an EMT educational program.

● *Advanced EMT (AEMT).* The primary focus of the **Advanced Emergency Medical Technician (AEMT)** is to provide basic and limited advanced emergency medical care and transportation for critical and emergent patients who access the EMS system. The AEMT possesses the basic knowledge and skills necessary to provide patient care and transportation. In addition, AEMTs perform interventions with both basic and advanced equipment. The AEMT must successfully complete an accredited EMT educational program.

● *Paramedic.* The **Paramedic** is an allied health professional whose primary focus is to provide advanced emergency medical care for critical and emergent patients who access the EMS system. The paramedic possesses the complex knowledge and skills necessary to provide patient care and transportation. Paramedics function as part of a comprehensive EMS response under medical oversight. Paramedics perform interventions with both basic and advanced equipment typically found on an ambulance. The paramedic is an essential link in the emergency care system. Because of the amount of complex decision making, paramedics must successfully complete a comprehensive accredited paramedic education program at the certificate or associate's degree level.[2]

CONTENT REVIEW

► Emerging Roles of the Paramedic

- Public education
- Health promotion
- Illness and injury prevention

The Modern Paramedic

The roles and responsibilities of the paramedic are diverse and encompass the disciplines of health care, public health, and public safety. Any of these might come into play on a given day. As EMS research evolves, it is becoming clear that illness and injury prevention are just as important as acute health care and public safety responsibilities (Figure 1-2 ●).

The primary task of the paramedic is to provide emergency medical care in an out-of-hospital setting. As a paramedic, you will use your advanced training and equipment to extend the care of the emergency physician to the patient in the field. However, you must also be able to make accurate independent judgments. The ability to do this in a timely manner is essential, as it can mean the difference between life and death for the patient.

In order to function as a paramedic—to practice the art and science of out-of-hospital medicine in conjunction with medical direction—you must have fulfilled the prescribed requirements of the appropriate licensing or credentialing body. Licensing or credentialing is typically provided by a state or provincial agency. All paramedics must be licensed, registered, or otherwise credentialed by the appropriate agency in the area where they work.

Paramedics may only function under the direction of the EMS system's medical director. Because of this, in addition to being appropriately licensed or credentialed, the system's medical director must also approve the paramedic before being permitted to practice advanced prehospital care. Paramedics must possess knowledge, skills, and attitudes consistent with the expectations of the public and the profession.

As a paramedic, you must recognize that you are an essential component in the continuum of care. Furthermore, paramedics often serve as a link between various health resources in the community. In the future, there will be a continuing demand to control or cut health care costs. As a consequence, paramedics may find themselves in the role of a gatekeeper to the health care system. For example, you may be charged with the responsibility of ensuring that your patient gets to the appropriate health care facility in a timely manner, even though the appropriate health care facility may not be a hospital emergency department.

Paramedics must always strive toward maintaining high-quality health care at a reasonable cost. Nevertheless, you must always be an advocate for your patient and ensure that the patient receives the best possible care—without regard to the patient's ability to pay or insurance status (Figure 1-3 ●).

While paramedics of the twenty-first century will continue to fill the well-defined and traditional role of 911 response, they will also find themselves taking on a wide variety of additional responsibilities. The emerging roles and responsibilities of the paramedic include public education, health promotion, and participation in injury and illness prevention programs. As the scope of paramedic service continues to expand, the paramedic will function as a facilitator of access to care as well as an individual treatment provider.

Paramedics are responsible and accountable to the system medical director, their agency, the public, and their peers. Although this may seem like a difficult standard to meet, if you always act in the best interest of the patient, you will seldom run into problems.

Paramedic Characteristics

There are many different types of EMS system designs and operations. As a paramedic, you may work for a fire department, private ambulance service, third city service, hospital, police department, or other operation. Regardless of the type of service provider you work for, you must be flexible in order to meet the demands of the ever-changing emergency scene.

As a paramedic, you must be a confident leader who can accept the challenge and responsibility of the position. You must have excellent judgment and be able to prioritize decisions so

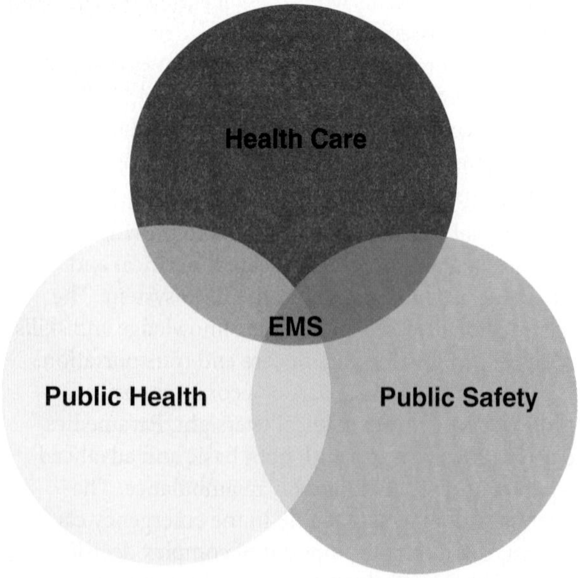

● **Figure 1-2** Modern EMS is a combination of public health, public safety, and health care.

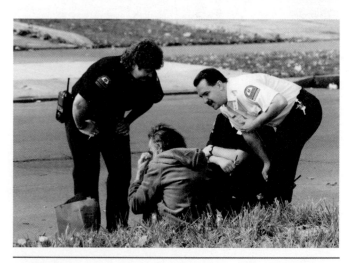

● **Figure 1-3** The paramedic must always be an advocate for the patient. *(© Craig Jackson/In the Dark Photography)*

Which Hat Are You Wearing? *The modern paramedic, whether career or volunteer, must wear several hats. Many paramedics are also cross trained as firefighters or police officers. The role of each of these professions is different, but there is often significant overlapping of duties. Paramedics may participate in rescue operations, directing traffic, firefighting, and other tasks on an emergency scene. However, it is essential that, when functioning in the role of paramedic, you remember that your primary responsibility is the patient and patient care. You must also be an advocate for the patient.*

If you are cross trained, this can cause a certain degree of confusion and conflict. For example, if you are a cross-trained police officer/paramedic who is treating an intoxicated driver, you may have conflicting responsibilities. However, as already noted, when you are functioning as a paramedic your priority should be the patient. Legal issues and other tasks normally addressed by police officers must be handled by other police officers on scene or dealt with after the patient has been treated and transported. Similarly, paramedics who are cross trained may learn information about a patient that is protected from disclosure by the Health Insurance Portability and Accountability Act (HIPAA) and other medical privacy laws and regulations. In a case like this, you may not be able to disclose certain information to your law enforcement colleagues despite the fact that you are also a police officer.

Laws regarding responsibilities of cross-trained individuals vary from state to state. You must be familiar with the laws of the state where you are employed. Remember: When you function as a paramedic, you must put care of the patient above all other tasks—and always remember which hat you are wearing.

as to act quickly in the best interest of the patient. You must be able to develop rapport with a wide variety of patients so that, for example, you can safely interview hostile patients and communicate with members of diverse cultural groups and the various ages within those groups. Overall, you must be able to function independently at an optimum level in a nonstructured, constantly changing environment. The job is never easy and always challenging.

The Paramedic: A True Health Professional

Despite its relative youth as a profession, the field of emergency medical services is now recognized as an important part of the health care system. With this, paramedics are now highly respected members of the health care team. As a paramedic, you must never take this status for granted. Instead, you must always strive to earn your acceptance as a health care professional.

You should consider the completion of your initial paramedic course to be the start of your professional education,

not the end. You should participate in various continuing education programs when they become available. Skills that are infrequently used should be frequently reviewed and practiced to ensure competency when the skill is needed. As a rule, the less a skill or procedure is used, the more frequently you should review that skill or procedure. Most quality continuing education programs acknowledge this by scheduling periodic review and practice of infrequently used skills or procedures. Professional development should be a never-ending, career-long pursuit. Additionally, you should participate in routine peer-evaluation and assume an active role in professional and community organizations (Figure 1-4 ●).

A major step toward the development of EMS as a true health care profession has been to raise the standards of education for prehospital personnel. A significant advance was the 2009 publication by the U.S. Department of Transportation of the ***National Emergency Medical Services Education Standards: Paramedic Instructional Guidelines.***[3] These instructional guidelines have taken paramedic education to a much higher level and were based on a national EMS practice analysis completed by the National Registry of Emergency Medical Technicians in 2004.[4] An anatomy and physiology

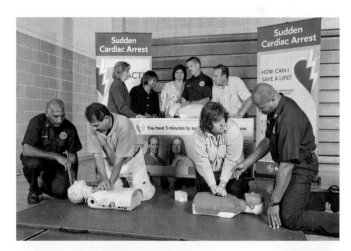

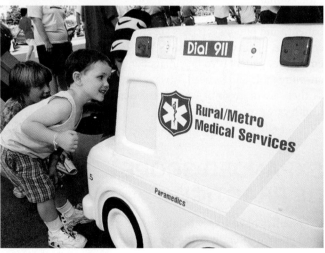

● **Figure 1-4** Public education is an important part of the paramedic's job. *(Bottom Photo: © Craig Jackson/In the Dark Photography)*

CONTENT REVIEW

▶ Out-of-Hospital Paramedic Work Environments

• Critical care transport
• Helicopter EMS
• Tactical EMS
• Primary care
• Industrial medicine
• Sports medicine
• Corrections
• Hospital emergency department

▶ Many aspects of out-of-hospital care now provide opportunities for paramedics to work in environments other than the typical 911 response vehicle.

course is now a prerequisite to the paramedic course. The paramedic course itself requires a far more extensive foundation of medical knowledge to underlie the required skills. In particular, the curriculum provides for an improved understanding of the pathophysiology of the various illness and injury processes paramedics encounter in their work. The materials presented in the 2009 DOT EMS Instructional Guidelines are the foundation for this textbook.

As a paramedic, you must actively participate in the design, development, evaluation, and publication of research on topics relevant to your profession. For years, paramedic practice was based on anecdotal data and tradition. Only during the last two decades did we truly begin applying the scientific method to various aspects of prehospital practice. Surprisingly, we found that there were little or no scientific data to support many of our prehospital practices. As a result of research, many traditional EMS treatments have been abandoned or refined. There are still many unanswered questions about paramedic practice, and these can be answered only by sound scientific research.

An essential aspect of a health professional is acceptance and adherence to a code of professional ethics and etiquette. Ethics are standards of right or honorable behavior, while etiquette refers to good manners. Both can apply to all human relationships. However, you will find that questions of ethics most often arise in relationships with patients and the public, while etiquette more often relates to behavior between health professionals.

The public must feel confident that, for the paramedic, the patient's and public's interests are always placed above personal, corporate, or financial interests. You must never forget that the emergency patient is your primary concern. Emergency patients are vulnerable and in need. Always keep this in mind and serve as their advocate until you turn patient care over to another health care professional.

EXPANDED SCOPE OF PRACTICE

Paramedics have a very bright future. New technologies and therapies can literally bring the emergency department to the patient. Paramedics must be willing to step up to these expanding roles, or persons from other health care disciplines will fill them.[5] There are many aspects of out-of-hospital care that can provide you with the opportunity to work in an environment other than the typical 911 response vehicle. These include:

• Critical care transport
• Helicopter EMS
• Tactical EMS
• Primary care
• Industrial medicine
• Sports medicine
• Corrections medicine
• Hospital emergency department

Paramedics are now stepping into nontraditional roles such as these because of their unique education and ability to think and work independently.[5]

Critical Care Transport

As a result of the specialization of health care facilities that began to occur in the 1990s, an increasing number of patients are being moved from one health care facility to another for specialized care. Many of these patients are critically ill and require equipment and care more sophisticated than that available on standard ambulances. Because of this, many EMS systems have developed specialized **critical care transport** vehicles to move these patients between facilities.

These vehicles include specialized ground ambulances, fixed-wing aircraft, and helicopters. Many services have elected to use large vehicles mounted on a truck chassis to provide the added space needed for critical care transport (Figure 1-5 ●). To staff these vehicles, paramedics have been educated in various aspects of critical care medicine. These include advanced airway management, ventilator management, fluid and electrolyte therapy, advanced pharmacology, specialized monitoring, operation of intraaortic balloon pumps, and other techniques usually found in an intensive care setting. This provides a safe and efficient way to move critical patients between facilities without compromising hospital staffing (Figure 1-6 ●).

Helicopter EMS

Helicopters have been a part of the EMS system for over 30 years and play an important role—especially in rural areas. Most helicopter EMS (HEMS) programs staff the helicopter with two

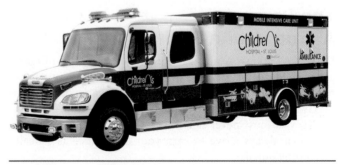

● **Figure 1-5** The modern critical care transport vehicle provides virtually all the capabilities of the hospital intensive care unit.

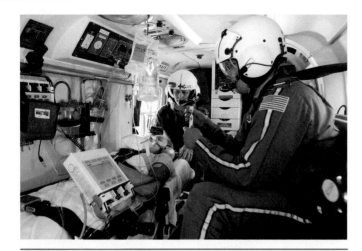

● **Figure 1-6** Critical care transport provides for the safe transfer of critically ill or injured patients between health care facilities.

medical crew members and often include paramedics. The flight paramedic typically will respond to both scene calls and interfacility transfers. The skills of the flight paramedic are very similar to those of a critical care paramedic but must include additional education in flight physiology, aircraft operations, flight safety, and similar areas (Figure 1-7 ●).

Tactical EMS

Over the last decade or so there has been a trend to use EMS personnel in tactical situations. Tactical EMS is designed to enhance the safety of special operations personnel and the public. In some situations, tactical paramedics are cross trained as police officers and carry weapons. The role of the tactical paramedic is to provide lifesaving care, sometimes in dangerous environments, until the patient can be safely evacuated to the general EMS system. Many of the practices and techniques of tactical EMS were drawn from experience with the military—particularly with special operations (Figure 1-8 ●).

Primary Care

Today, many patients can receive primary care outside the hospital at far less cost, for example, in physicians' offices and

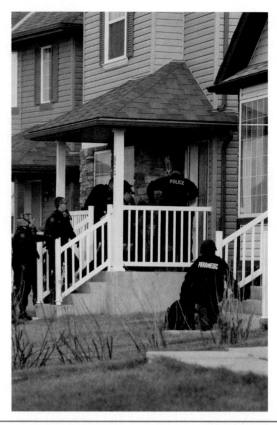

● **Figure 1-8** The tactical paramedic must often provide life-saving care in austere and dangerous situations. *(© Kevin Link)*

minor-care or outpatient clinics.[6] Additionally, many patients can be cared for at home. In certain cases, paramedics, in close contact with medical direction, can provide care at the scene without transport to the hospital (e.g., to treat simple lacerations or to change dressings or gastrostomy tubes). Several EMS systems have designated specialized crews to periodically assess and monitor high-risk patients in their community (Figure 1-9 ●).

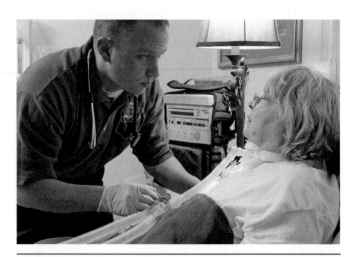

● **Figure 1-9** Paramedics play an important role in ensuring the health of the community they serve—especially high-risk patients.

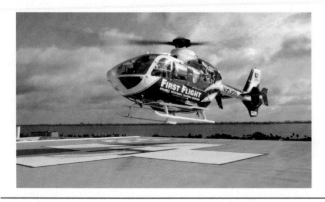

● **Figure 1-7** The helicopter has become an important part of the modern EMS system. *(© REACH Air Medical Services)*

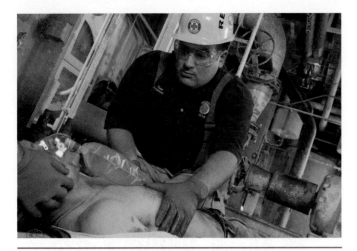

● **Figure 1-10** The industrial paramedic provides several important services in addition to emergency care.

Industrial Medicine

Paramedics have long been the principal health care providers on oil rigs, movie sets, and similar industrial operations. Paramedics are specially trained for the industry in question and often assume additional responsibilities, including safety inspection, accident prevention, medical screening of employees, and vaccinations and immunizations. Many industries use paramedics to assist with sick calls and minor medical care. Having paramedics on site allows for increased employee safety and decreased time lost from work (Figure 1-10 ●).

Sports Medicine

Another area in the expanded scope of paramedic practice is sports medicine. Many teams, including those in professional sports, have found that paramedics complement their athletic trainers. In this role, paramedics assume considerably more responsibility for injury prevention. They are also trained to deal with injuries specific to the sport in question. For example, paramedics working with a football team will assist in pre-game preparation of players. During the game, they provide any needed emergency medical care. They can also advise the staff whether an injured or ill player may return to the game. Paramedics working with hockey teams often learn to perform simple laceration repairs and provide care for orthopedic injuries so as to safely return the players to action as soon as possible (Figure 1-11 ●).

Corrections Medicine

Many states and the federal government have begun to use paramedics as emergency and medical care providers in jails and prisons. In these institutions, paramedics will often do the initial prisoner medical intake assessment and oversee the medical needs of the prison population. They are also responsible for responding to emergencies within the prison. Because of this, they must also have training in correctional operations and similar issues. Paramedics also play a major role in the

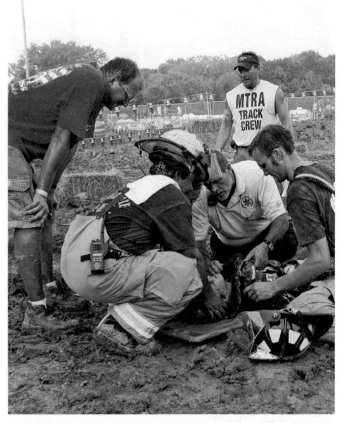

● **Figure 1-11** Injuries and medical emergencies are common at sporting events, and many teams and facilities have paramedics readily available. (© Ray Kemp/Triple Zilch Productions)

U.S. Department of Immigration and Customs Enforcement (ICE). Paramedics often work with Border Patrol agents and Customs agents as they endeavor to maintain homeland security (Figure 1-12 ●).

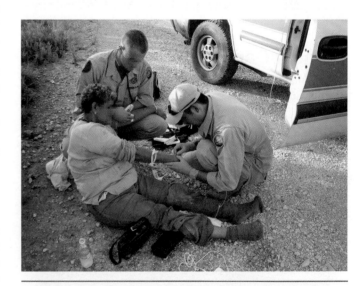

● **Figure 1-12** Paramedics often accompany U.S. Border Patrol agents and provide care to both officers and detainees. *(Photo used by permission. Courtesy of the Office of Border Patrol, Field Communications Branch)*

Hospital Emergency Departments

Faced with a nursing shortage, many hospitals have found paramedics to be very suitable providers for emergency departments and minor care centers. The role of the paramedic in these settings varies significantly from state to state, based on local laws. In some situations paramedics will function in a role comparable to nursing. In others, they will work in a more technical role, assisting the medical and nursing staff with skills and responsibilities within the scope of **paramedicine**. Many paramedics enjoy the diversity and work experience of a busy emergency department (Figure 1-13 ●).

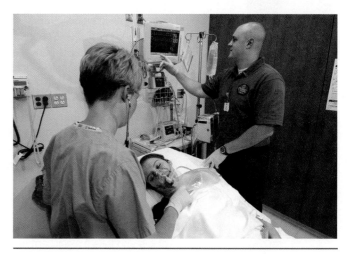

● **Figure 1-13**   Hospitals are increasingly turning to paramedics to help staff at busy emergency departments and trauma centers.

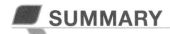 SUMMARY

Even though we are still a young profession, EMS is now recognized as a staple in the health care system. Paramedics have been identified as underutilized medical experts and are being offered opportunities that were unheard-of just a few years ago.

As the scope of practice for paramedicine continues to expand, so will the demand for skilled practitioners. It is truly an exciting time for EMS and paramedicine. The paramedic of the twenty-first century can have a more significant impact on health care than ever before. The paramedic is often the first member of the health care system with whom the patient interacts, and the results of those interactions can affect the patient's opinion of the health care system in general.

EMS is a profession in which you can make a difference. Every call and every patient interaction has the potential to make the difference between life and death for the patient. Few professions carry such awesome responsibility.

YOU MAKE THE CALL

Finally, after two straight years of urban EMS work without a vacation, you and two of your best paramedic friends, Eileen and Dee Dee, are taking the trip you've been planning for some time. The small airplane grinds to a bumpy halt as you land on a tiny speck of land in the midst of a bright turquoise sea. The ride from the mainland was rough, and Eileen has thrown up. To make matters worse, two of your bags didn't make it aboard the plane. You question the ticket agent who says, "Maybe a plane come Monday. No plane Sunday." Your dream vacation is quickly turning into a nightmare.

After standing in the sun for 45 minutes waiting for a taxi, a 1995 Kia shows up. The driver tells you that your hotel is about 45 minutes away. He throws your bags into the trunk, ties the trunk shut with a piece of manila rope, and takes off like a dragster from the starting line. You and your friends hang on for dear life as the cab speeds through the winding streets. You try to remember whether people on this island drive on the left side or the right. You certainly can't tell based on your driver's actions. The driver seems to know everybody and honks accordingly. Loud island music crackles through the small speakers in the cab. Dee Dee, the friend who managed not to vomit on the plane, leans over to you and tells you that she thinks she needs to vomit now.

Suddenly, you see a plume of smoke billowing up on the road ahead. As the cab slows, you spot what appears to be an accident. On closer inspection, you see that another cab has plowed into a station wagon at an intersection. Several people are lying on the ground, and there is the general appearance of pandemonium. Dee Dee throws up.

The three of you, experienced paramedics, get out of the cab to take a look. The scene appears safe to approach. Unfortunately, the accident looks severe, with several persons suffering serious injuries. Bystanders begin to reach inside the station wagon and drag the occupants out to a nearby shade tree. You try to offer some advice on providing cervical spine precautions, but they aren't paying any attention to you. You cringe as you see a patient's head fall back and strike the ground.

Before long, all six victims are spread out under a large magnolia tree. A woman is crying loudly and reciting a prayer. A dog walks among the victims. One of the bystanders says that the police should be there "pretty soon." You ask if anyone has called the fire department. The bystander responds with a confused look on his face. "Why do we call the fire department?" he asks. "I do not see a fire."

One victim is obviously dead of a massive head injury. The others are alive but with various injuries. You and your friends try to provide what care you can with absolutely no medical equipment available. Before long, you hear the shrill siren of an approaching police car. The police officers get out of their vehicle and take a significant amount of time putting their hats on. One officer goes to the vehicles. The other goes to the magnolia tree where he proceeds to get into a heated argument with one of the bystanders. Nobody is paying much attention to the victims except you and your friends.

Before long, there is some excitement as another vehicle pulls up. It seems to be some sort of ambulance. It is an old delivery van painted white with a large orange cross on the side. There are two attendants dressed in white smocks. They carry a canvas litter and, again with no spinal precautions and in no particular order, begin to load up the victims. You and your friends try to relay the results of your assessment and care. The attendants continue with their tasks, both disinterested and unimpressed with your work. From what you can tell, absolutely no medical care is being provided.

When the last victim is loaded with the other five in the van, both attendants take their seats in the front of the van and leave for the hospital. The shrill sound of the siren slowly fades into the distance, and you and your friends go on to the hotel. You look at the local paper each day, hoping to find out something about the crash victims, but you never find a story about the accident.

Although you are still upset about the accident and the unsophisticated level of medical care you witnessed—and after your bags finally arrive—you, Dee Dee, and Eileen have a nice vacation with no further adverse events.

1. Discuss the vast differences between EMS and paramedic care in the United States, Canada, and other economically developed nations compared with those that exist in some less developed countries of the world. How should awareness of such differences affect your attitude about your work?

See Suggested Responses at the back of this book.

 # REVIEW QUESTIONS

1. Paramedics may function only under the direction and license of the EMS system's:
   a. town council.
   b. company owner.
   c. medical director.
   d. Board of Directors.

2. The emerging roles and responsibilities of the paramedic include:
   a. public education.
   b. health promotion.
   c. participation in injury and illness prevention programs.
   d. all of the above.

3. The rules, standards, and expected actions governing the activities of a group or profession are called:
   a. ethics.   c. manners.
   b. morals.   d. etiquette.

4. Which of the following is an aspect of professionalism?
   a. being well groomed
   b. maintaining patient confidentiality
   c. attending continuing education sessions
   d. all of the above

5. All of the following are considered new, nontraditional roles for the paramedic except:
   a. primary care.
   b. sports medicine.
   c. family practitioner.
   d. industrial medicine.

See Answers to Review Questions at the back of this book.

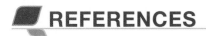

REFERENCES

1. U.S. Department of Transportation/National Highway Traffic Safety Administration. *National EMS Scope of Practice Model*. Washington, DC: 2006.

2. Patterson, P. D., J. C. Probst, K. H. Leith, S. J. Corwin, and M. P. Powell. "Recruitment and Retention of Emergency Medical Technicians: A Qualitative Review." *J Allied Health* 34 (2005): 153–162.

3. U.S. Department of Transportation/National Highway Traffic Safety Administration. *National Emergency Medical Services Educational Standards: Paramedic Instruction Guidelines*. Washington, DC: 2009.

4. National Registry of Emergency Medical Technicians. *2004 National EMS Practice Analysis*. Columbus, OH: 2004.

5. Cooper, S., B. Barrett, and S. Black, et al. "The Emerging Role of the Emergency Care Practitioner." *Emerg Med J* 21 (2004): 614–618.

6. Ball, L. "Setting the Scene for the Paramedic in Primary Care: A Review of the Literature." *Emerg Med J* 22 (2005): 896–900.

FURTHER READING

Bledsoe, B. E. "EMS Needs a Few More Cowboys." *Journal of Emergency Medical Services (JEMS)* 28(12) (2003): 112–113.

Bledsoe, B. E. "Where Are the Wise Men?" *Emergency Medical Services (EMS)* 31(10) (2002): 172.

Bledsoe, B. E. and R. W. Benner,. *Critical Care Paramedic*. Upper Saddle River, NJ: Pearson/Prentice Hall, 2006.

Grayson, S. *En Route: A Paramedic's Stories of Life, Death, and Everything in Between*. New York, NY: Kaplan Publishing, 2009.

Page, J. O. *Simple Advice*. Carlsbad, CA: JEMS Publishing, 2002.

Page, J. O. *The Magic of 3 A.M.: Essays on the Art and Science of Emergency Medical Services*. Carlsbad, CA: JEMS Publishing, 2002.

Page, J. O. *The Paramedics*. Morristown, NJ: Backdraft Publications, 1979.

Perry, M. *Population 485: Meeting Your Neighbors One Siren at a Time*. New York, NY: Harper-Collins, 2002.

2

EMS Systems

Bryan Bledsoe, DO, FACEP, FAAEM, EMT-P
Paul Ganss, MS, NREMT-P

STANDARD
Preparatory (EMS Systems)

COMPETENCY
Integrates comprehensive knowledge of EMS systems, the safety and well-being of the paramedic, and medical-legal and ethical issues, which is intended to improve the health of EMS personnel, patients, and the community.

OBJECTIVES

Terminal Performance Objective
After reading this chapter you should be able to discuss the characteristics, components, and functions of emergency medical services (EMS) systems.

Enabling Objectives
To accomplish the terminal performance objective, you should be able to:

1. Define key terms introduced in this chapter.

2. Describe the out-of-hospital and in-hospital components of EMS systems.

3. Given various scenarios, explain how EMS systems work to respond to out-of-hospital emergencies.

4. Link key events in the history of EMS to the development of the modern EMS system.

5. Describe each of the ten components of EMS systems according to the Statewide EMS Technical Assessment Program.

6. Discuss the vision and documents that are guiding EMS into the future.

7. Discuss the contemporary problems facing EMS as described in the Institute of Medicine document, *Emergency Medical Services: At the Crossroads*.

8. Give examples of various approaches to and configurations of EMS systems in the United States.

9. Explain the role of EMS in the chain of survival from cardiac arrest and in the optimal care of all emergency patients.

10. Describe the purposes of the national documents guiding EMS education and practice.

11. Discuss typical components of local and state-level EMS systems.

12. Explain the purpose and responsibilities of physician medical directors in EMS services.

13. Give examples of on-line medical direction and off-line medical oversight.

14. Describe the purposes of the National Registry of EMTs and the several professional organizations in EMS.

15. Recognize professional journals related to the practice of EMS.

16. Describe the intent of the General Services Administration KKK-A-1822 Federal Specifications for Ambulances.

17. Describe the purpose of categorizing receiving hospital facilities by their capabilities.

18. Explain the purpose and components of an effective continuous quality improvement program.

19. Describe how you can contribute to greater patient safety in emergency medical services.

20. Explain the role of research in EMS.

KEY TERMS

accreditation, p. 27

advanced life support (ALS), p. 15

basic life support (BLS), p. 15

bystander, p. 15

certification, p. 27

chain of survival, p. 22

clinical protocols, p. 24

Department of Homeland Security, p. 20

emergency medical dispatcher (EMD), p. 26

ethics, p. 33

evidence-based medicine (EBM), p. 35

helicopter EMS (HEMS), p. 19

interoperability, p. 26

intervener physician, p. 24

licensure, p. 27

medical director, p. 23

medical oversight, p. 23

National Highway Traffic Safety Administration (NHTSA), p. 20

National Incident Management System (NIMS), p. 20

National Transportation Safety Board (NTSB), p. 22

off-line medical oversight, p. 24

on-line medical direction, p. 23

Ontario Prehospital Advanced Life Support Study (OPALS), p. 20

peer review, p. 24

prearrival instruction, p. 26

profession, p. 27

professionalism, p. 32

prospective medical oversight, p. 24

quality improvement (QI), p. 19

reciprocity, p. 27

registration, p. 27

research, p. 34

retrospective medical oversight, p. 24

rules of evidence, p. 32

scope of practice, p. 23

standing orders, p. 24

teachable moment, p. 24

tiered response, p. 15

trauma, p. 31

trauma centers, p. 19

CASE STUDY

It is a beautiful Fourth of July. You and your family are traveling down the interstate on your way to a concert and fireworks show. Just an hour from your destination, a tire blows out on the BMW ahead of you, and you see it skid into the median and crash into some pine trees. You pull onto the shoulder. As an experienced paramedic, you ensure scene safety before approaching the mangled car. You see no movement inside the passenger compartment.

Your daughter grabs her cell phone and calls 911. The dispatcher asks for the location of the crash and transfers your call to the 911 call center for that area. The emergency medical dispatcher gathers the appropriate information and dispatches the local volunteer fire service and an advanced life support (ALS) ambulance. While you attempt to gain access to the patients, your daughter continues to provide the dispatcher with information that he, in turn, relays to the responding units.

The local volunteer fire and rescue team arrives on scene in about 7 minutes. You provide a verbal report to the arriving rescuers. They do their own scene safety check, approach the car, and determine that there are four patients. Two are priority-1 patients (one of these is a 2-year-old child), and two are priority-3 patients. Based on the primary assessment, Rescuer Lt. C. J. Greenlee requests a medical helicopter and a second ALS unit. Approximately 2 minutes later, a fire truck crew arrives. They reroute traffic and establish a landing zone for the helicopter.

When all EMS personnel summoned are on scene, they decide that the 2-year-old patient will be flown to Children's Hospital, a pediatric specialty center. The other immediate patient will be transported by ground to the closest level-one trauma center. The patients with minor injuries will be taken to the local hospital by ground transport. Working as a team, the fire and ambulance personnel extricate the patients and package them for transport.

Approximately 22 minutes after the arrival of the first ALS unit, all patients are extricated and en route to a receiving facility capable of providing the level of care they need. Within 15 minutes of arrival at the pediatric trauma center and just 31 minutes after the crash, the 2-year-old is moved to surgery for the repair of a ruptured liver and spleen. The other patients are being treated at their destinations as well.

INTRODUCTION

The emergency medical services (EMS) system is a comprehensive network of personnel, equipment, and resources. To meet the needs of the community it serves, an EMS system must function as a unified whole. In general, an EMS system is comprised of both out-of-hospital and in-hospital components. The out-of-hospital component includes:

- Members of the community who are trained in first aid and CPR
- A communications system that allows public access to emergency services dispatch and allows EMS providers to communicate with each other
- EMS providers, including paramedics
- Fire/rescue and hazardous-materials services

- Law enforcement officers
- Public utilities, such as power and gas companies
- Resource centers, such as regional poison control centers

The in-hospital component includes:

- Emergency nurses
- Mid-level practitioners (physicians' assistants and advanced-practice nurses)
- Emergency physicians and specialty physicians
- Ancillary services, such as radiology and respiratory therapy
- Specialty physicians, such as trauma surgeons and cardiologists
- Social workers
- Mental health providers
- Rehabilitation services

Tiered Response

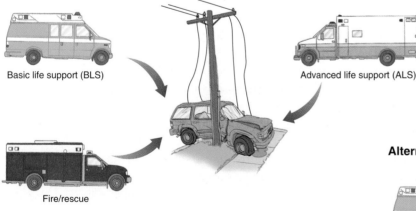

Basic life support (BLS)

Advanced life support (ALS)

Fire/rescue

Alternative Response

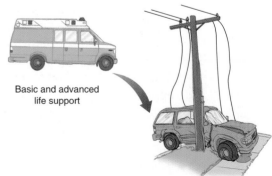

Basic and advanced life support

● **Figure 2-1** Some systems elect to use a tiered response whereby BLS providers provide initial on-scene care while ALS care arrives later. Other systems send an ALS provider to each call.

A typical EMS operation begins with citizen activation. That is, a **bystander**—a family member, friend, or a stranger to the patient—initiates contact with an emergency dispatch center. EMS dispatch is then responsible for collecting essential information and sending out the closest appropriately staffed and equipped unit. In many EMS systems, the dispatcher also provides prearrival instructions.

Usually, the first EMS provider to respond to the scene of an emergency is a police officer, firefighter, lifeguard, teacher, or other community member who has received basic medical training in an Emergency Medical Responder program.

The next EMS provider likely to arrive depends on the type of EMS system involved. In most areas, the dispatcher will send a **basic life support (BLS)** or **advanced life support (ALS)** ambulance. In other areas, EMS uses a **tiered response**, sending multiple levels of emergency care personnel to the same incident.[1] In still other areas, ALS personnel may respond to every incident regardless of the level of care needed (Figure 2-1 ●).

Once emergency care has been initiated, EMS providers must quickly decide on the medical facility to which the patient should be transported. This decision is based on the type of care needed, transport time, and local protocols. In a comprehensive EMS system where specialty centers have been designated (such as pediatric, trauma, and burn centers), it may be necessary to transport the patient to a facility other than the closest hospital.

At the receiving medical facility, an emergency nurse or physician assumes responsibility for the patient. If needed, a surgeon or other specialist will be summoned.

HISTORY OF EMS

To understand EMS today, it is important to know its history. The most significant advances have occurred during the last 40 years (see Table 2-1).

Early Development
Ancient Times

There is evidence that emergency medicine has a very long history. In fact, it may be traced back to biblical times when it was recorded that a "good Samaritan" provided care to a wounded traveler by the side of a road.

Approximately 4,000 to 5,000 years ago, scribes in Sumer, a civilization in Mesopotamia (southwest Asia), inscribed clay tablets with some of the earliest medical records. Similar to protocols that EMS uses today, the ancient tablets provided healers with step-by-step instructions for patient care based on the patient's description of symptoms. The tablets also included instructions on how to create the medications needed to cure the patient and explained how and when to administer them. The most striking difference between these first "protocols" and EMS today is the absence of a physical exam.

In 1862, the Egyptologist Edwin Smith purchased a papyrus scroll dating back to about 1500 B.C.E. It contained 48 medical case histories with data arranged in head-to-toe order and in order of severity, an arrangement very similar

TABLE 2-1	An EMS Timeline	
1797	Napoleon's chief physician implements a prehospital system designed to triage and transport the injured from the field to aid stations.
1860s	Civilian ambulance services begin in Cincinnati and New York City.
1891	Dr. Friedrich Maass performs the first equivocally documented chest compression in humans.
1915	First-known air medical transport occurs during the retreat of the Serbian army from Albania.
1920	First volunteer rescue squads organize in Roanoke, Virginia, and along the New Jersey coast.
1947	Claude Beck develops first defibrillator and first human saved with defibrillation.
1958	Dr. Peter Safar demonstrates the efficacy of mouth-to-mouth ventilation.
1960	Cardiopulmonary resuscitation (CPR) is shown to be efficacious.
1965	J. Frank Pantridge converts an ambulance into a mobile coronary care unit with a portable defibrillator and recorded ten prehospital resuscitations with a 50% long-term survival rate.
1966	The National Academy of Sciences, National Research Council publishes *Accidental Death and Disability: The Neglected Disease of Modern Society*.
1966	Highway Safety Act of 1966 establishes the Emergency Medical Services Program in the Department of Transportation.
1967	Star of Life is patented by the American Medical Association.
1968	AT&T designates 911 as its new national emergency number.
1970	National Registry of EMTs is founded.

(Continued)

TABLE 2-1 | An EMS Timeline *Continued*

1972	Television show *Emergency!* debuts on NBC.
1972	Department of Health, Education, and Welfare allocates $16 million to EMS demonstration programs in five states.
1973	The Emergency Medical Services Systems (EMSS) Act provides additional federal guidelines and funding for the development of regional EMS systems; the law establishes 15 components of EMS systems.
1975	National Association of Emergency Medical Technicians (NAEMT) is organized.
1979	Field automated external defibrillators (AEDs) become available.
1981	The Omnibus Budget Reconciliation Act consolidates EMS funding into state preventive health and health services block grants, and eliminates funding under the EMSS Act.
1981	Prehospital Trauma Life Support (PHTLS) is developed.
1981	International Trauma Life Support (ITLS), formerly basic trauma life support (BTLS), is developed.
1984	The EMS for Children (EMSC) program, under the Public Health Act, provides funds for enhancing the EMS system to better serve pediatric patients.
1985	National Research Council publishes *Injury in America: A Continuing Public Health Problem* describing deficiencies in the progress of addressing the problem of accidental death and disability.
1988	The National Highway Traffic Safety Administration initiates the Statewide EMS Technical Assessment program based on ten key components of EMS systems.
1990	The Trauma Care Systems and Development Act encourages development of inclusive trauma systems and provides funding to states for trauma system planning, implementation, and evaluation.
1993	The Institute of Medicine publishes *Emergency Medical Services for Children*, which points out deficiencies in our health care system's ability to address the emergency medical needs of pediatric patients.
1995	Congress does not reauthorize funding under the Trauma Care Systems and Development Act.
1999	President Clinton signs bill designating 911 as national emergency number.
2003	Health Insurance Portability and Accountability Act (HIPAA) becomes effective, strictly regulating the flow of confidential information.
2006	The National Highway Traffic Safety Administration publishes *Emergency Medical Services: Agenda for the Future* to guide the development of EMS in the United States in the twenty-first century.

to today's patient assessment. Each case also had a particular format, including a title, specific instructions to the healer, and a projection of possible outcomes. One section, called the "Book of Wounds," explains the treatment of injuries such as fractures and dislocations. It includes descriptions of the materials needed for making bandages and splints as well as information about sutures and solutions that may be used to clean wounds.

At about the same time, in another civilization in the Mesopotamian region, King Hammurabi of Babylon commissioned a large painting of 282 case laws known today as the "Code of Hammurabi." That code governed criminal and civil matters, and it established strict penalties for violations, a concept called *lex talionis* or "law of the claw" (very similar to the idea of "an eye for an eye").

One section of the code was devoted to the regulation of medical fees and penalties, which were based on the social class of the patient. For example, if a surgeon operated successfully on a commoner, he would be paid only half of what his fee would be if he had operated on a rich man. Social class was also the basis for penalties. If a surgeon caused the death of a rich man, the surgeon's hand would be cut off. But if a slave died under his care, he only had to replace the slave.

EMS came from humble beginnings. Initially, out-of-hospital care involved nothing more than transport. Around 900 C.E., the Anglo-Saxons used a hammock suspended across a horse-drawn wagon. In 1100, the Normans devised a litter that was carried between two horses to transport patients. The first recorded use of an ambulance was in the Siege of Malaga in 1487. Queen Isabella of Spain designated certain wagons for the transport of injured soldiers. Her grandson, King Charles V, reportedly again used field ambulances in 1553 in the Siege of Metz.

The Napoleonic Wars

In the wars between Napoleon's French Empire and other European countries from 1803 to 1815, ambulances were often used to evacuate the wounded. Military surgeon Dominique-Jean Larrey, one of Napoleon's chief surgeons, devised this idea. Larrey became distressed to see that many of the wounded were neglected for a long period of time and that most died before reaching a hospital. He subsequently developed a light carriage that allowed the movement of injured soldiers from the battlefield. These carriages came to be called *ambulance volante* or "Larrey's Flying Ambulances" because they were positioned with the French "flying artillery" on the battlefield. Though the *ambulance volante* was little more than a covered horse-drawn cart, Larrey is credited with the development of the first prehospital system that used both triage and transport. Larrey was also credited with being the first to place a medical attendant in an ambulance.[2]

Although the first use of aircraft for medical evacuation is lost to history, there are records of hot air balloons being used to evacuate wounded from the Prussian Siege of Paris in 1870. During the retreat of the Serbian Army from Albania in 1915, unmodified French fighter aircraft were used to ferry the injured.

The United States in the Nineteenth Century

The development of ambulances in the United States occurred in the first part of the nineteenth century. In 1861, during the Civil War, surgeon Jonathan Letterman reorganized battlefield medical care and initiated the use of ambulances for the evacuation of battlefield casualties. In 1864, President Abraham Lincoln signed into law an act that firmly established a uniform army ambulance plan. This act separated ambulance transport from all other transport services in the Army and placed it under the medical command.

Between 1861 and 1865, a nurse named Clara Barton coordinated care for the sick and injured at Civil War battlefield sites along the East coast. Defying army leaders, she persisted in going to the front, where wounded men suffered and often died from lack of the simplest medical attention. She continued the concept of the *ambulance volante* by organizing the triage and transport of injured soldiers to improvised hospitals in nearby houses, barns, and churches away from the battlefield.[3]

Following the success of ambulances in the Civil War, several communities and hospitals began to develop civilian ambulance services. The first civilian ambulance was established in 1860 in Cincinnati, Ohio, by Commercial Hospital (actually before the Civil War). In 1869, Bellevue Hospital, on the island of Manhattan in New York City, began to operate an ambulance service. The ambulances of both services were specially designed horse-drawn carts that were staffed with physician interns from the various hospital wards. By 1899, Michael Reese Hospital in Chicago began to operate a motorized ambulance.[4]

The Twentieth Century

From World War I to World War II

During World War I, a high mortality rate of soldiers was associated with an average evacuation time of 18 hours. As a result, in World War II a system of transportation to increasing echelons (levels) of care was created. Battlefield ambulance corps transported wounded soldiers from the front lines to the echelons of care. However, many of the echelons were so far from the battlefield and from each other that there were huge delays in patient care. In many cases, it was often days from the injury itself to definitive surgery.

There were some developments in American civilian ambulance services after World War I. Some hospitals experimented with placing physician interns on ambulances. In 1926, the Phoenix Fire Department began providing "inhalator" service and officially entered into the realm of medical care. In 1928, the first bona fide rescue squad, called the Roanoke Life Saving Crew, was started in Roanoke, Virginia. However, in 1929, the United States entered the severe economic crisis known as the Great Depression, which lasted until the start of American involvement in World War II in 1941. Little changed in the civilian ambulance service during this period.

Effects of World War II

Following the bombing of Pearl Harbor on December 7, 1941, the United States entered into World War II. Because of the demands of war, many hospital-based ambulance services shut down. Many city governments turned ambulance services over to local police and fire departments. Unfortunately, there were no requirements for minimal training or care. In fact, ambulance work was often seen as a punishment, and many departments were quick to eliminate ambulance service as soon as they could.

Post-World War II

The end of World War II brought prosperity to the United States. Several medical advances occurred subsequently, improving the lives of the public. But not long after World War II, the United States found itself at war again—this time on the Korean peninsula.

The 1950s

Korea is a mountainous country that lacked an organized system of highways and roads. Because of this, the U.S. Army began using helicopters to move the injured from the front lines to Mobile Army Surgical Hospitals (MASH) located fairly close to the front lines. Thus, injured soldiers were being promptly evacuated to a surgical center and were receiving emergency care and surgery shortly after their injury. This practice resulted in significant improvements in battlefield mortality.[5]

Similarly, in the late 1950s the United States entered into the Vietnam War. This time the battles took place in the jungles of Southeast Asia. As in Korea, there were few roads, and jungles slowed movement of the injured. Again, helicopters were called on to evacuate the wounded to forward-placed surgical hospitals. In Vietnam, in many cases, evacuation occurred within 10 to 20 minutes of injury (Figure 2-2 ●). Once stabilized and able to be moved (generally within 24 to 48 hours), the patients would be flown by jet to Clark Air Force Base in the Philippines, where they would receive any necessary further treatment. The decrease in the amount of time to definitive care plus advances in medical procedures significantly reduced mortality rates. This strategy also set the stage for trauma system development in the United States.[6]

Several significant medical developments occurred in the 1950s. In 1956, physicians Peter Safar and James Elam pioneered the use of mouth-to-mouth resuscitation. In 1959, the first portable defibrillator was used at Johns Hopkins Hospital in Baltimore.[7] In 1960, cardiopulmonary resuscitation (CPR)

▶ 1973 EMSS Act: 15 Components of EMS Systems

- Manpower
- Training
- Communications
- Transportation
- Emergency facilities
- Critical care units
- Public safety agencies
- Consumer participation
- Access to care
- Patient transfer
- Standardized record keeping
- Public information and education
- System review and evaluation
- Disaster management plans
- Mutual aid

was refined and deemed to be effective for human resuscitation.[8]

The 1960s

Throughout history, significant advances in trauma care occurred during wartime. However, until the late 1960s, few areas of the United States provided adequate civilian prehospital emergency care similar to what was provided to soldiers and sailors during war. The prevailing thought was that medical care began in the hospital emergency department. Rescue techniques were crude, ambulance attendants poorly educated, and equipment minimal. Police, fire, and EMS personnel often had no radio communication. Proper medical direction was not available, and the only interaction between physicians and EMS personnel was at the receiving facility.

Eventually, as costs and demand for additional services forced many rural mortician-operated ambulances to withdraw, local police and fire departments found that they had to provide the ambulance service. In many areas, volunteer ambulance services made up of local, independent EMS provider agencies proliferated. In urban settings, the increased demand on hospital-based EMS systems resulted in the development of municipal services, which were operated on city, county, or regional levels. However, because they could not communicate with each other, it was impossible to coordinate a response to any but the simplest local calls.

In 1966 the publication of *Accidental Death and Disability: The Neglected Disease of Modern Society* by the National Academy of Sciences, National Research Council, focused attention on the problem. "The White Paper," as the report was called, spelled out the deficiencies in prehospital emergency care.[9] It suggested guidelines for the development of EMS systems, the training of prehospital emergency medical providers, and the upgrading of ambulances and their equipment. The problems identified in the study included:

- Lack of uniform laws and standards for prehospital care
- Poorly equipped ambulances
- Poor quality ambulances
- Lack of communications between the ambulance and the hospital
- Inadequate training of ambulance personnel
- Inadequate physician and nursing staffing of hospital emergency departments

Civilian EMS, as we know it today, started to evolve significantly in the 1960s. In 1960, the Los Angeles Fire Department placed medical personnel with every engine, ladder, and rescue company. It was one of the first large fire departments to embrace the concept of emergency medical care.

In 1966, the Highway Safety Act promulgated initial EMS guidelines for the United States. The same year, Dr. J. Frank Pantridge developed a mobile coronary response unit in Belfast, Northern Ireland. Using a portable defibrillator, he treated ten cardiac arrest patients, five of whom enjoyed long-term survival.[10] In 1969, the first paramedic program began in Miami, Florida, by Dr. Eugene Nagel.[11]

The 1970s

The 1970s were the decade when EMS truly came into its own. The National Registry of Emergency Medical Technicians was established in 1970. Interestingly, EMS got one of its biggest boosts from Hollywood. On January 15, 1972, the television show *Emergency!* made its debut on NBC. The show, produced by Hollywood legend Jack Webb, featured two Los Angeles County Fire Department paramedics and the new paramedic program in southern California (Figure 2-3 ●). The show brought public attention to the concept of prehospital care and provided considerable encouragement for development of the modern EMS system.[12]

Then, in 1973, Congress passed the Emergency Medical Services Systems Act, which provided funding for a series of projects related to the delivery of trauma care. This enabled the development of regional EMS systems that took place from 1974 through 1981. A total of $300 million was allocated to study the feasibility of EMS planning, operations, expansion, and research.[13]

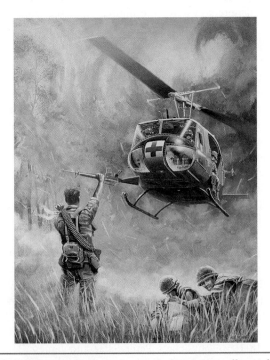

● **Figure 2-2** Medical evacuation helicopters, colloquially called "Dustoff," saved many lives during the Vietnam War. (*Dust off © Joe Kline Aviation Art*)

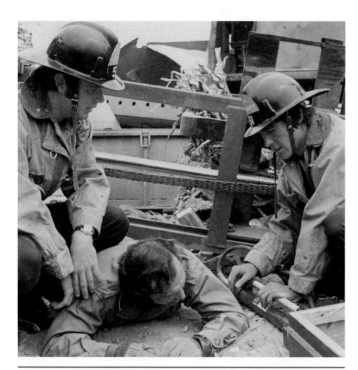

● **Figure 2-3** The television show *Emergency!* played a major role in bringing the world of EMS into the public spotlight. *(Larry Barbier/NBCU Photo Bank via AP Images)*

In order to be eligible for this funding, an EMS system had to include the following 15 components: manpower, training, communications, transportation, emergency facilities, critical care units, public safety agencies, consumer participation, access to care, patient transfer, standardized record keeping, public information and education, system review and evaluation, disaster management plans, and mutual aid. As farsighted as these criteria were, the designers of the legislation unfortunately omitted two key components: system financing and medical direction.

When federal funding was significantly reduced in the early 1980s, many EMS systems faced economic disaster. Subsequently, the Emergency Medical Services Systems Act was amended in 1976 and again in 1979, and a total of $215 million was appropriated over a seven-year period toward the establishment of regional EMS systems. However, many systems were still operating without medical direction.

The 1980s

In 1981, the passage of the Consolidated Omnibus Budget Reconciliation Act (COBRA) essentially wiped out federal funding for EMS. The small amount of funding that remained was placed into state preventive-health and health-services block grants. The National Highway Traffic Safety Administration (NHTSA) attempted to sustain the efforts of the Department of Health and Human Services, but with its other EMS responsibilities and no additional funding, the momentum for continued development was lost.

In 1988, the Statewide EMS Technical Assessment Program was established by the NHTSA. It defines elements necessary to all EMS systems. Briefly, they are:

- *Regulation and policy.* Each state must have laws, regulations, policies, and procedures that govern its EMS system. It also is required to provide leadership to local jurisdictions.

- *Resources management.* Each state must have central control of EMS resources so all patients have equal access to acceptable emergency care.

- *Human resources and training.* Qualified instructors should teach a standardized EMS curriculum, and all personnel who transport patients in the prehospital setting should be adequately trained.

- *Transportation.* Patients must be safely and reliably transported by ground or air ambulance.

- *Facilities.* Every seriously ill or injured patient must be delivered in a timely manner to an appropriate medical facility.

- *Communications.* A system for public access to the EMS system must be in place. Communication among dispatchers, the ambulance crew, and hospital personnel must also be possible.

- *Trauma systems.* Each state should develop a system of specialized care for trauma patients, including one or more **trauma centers** and rehabilitation programs. It also must develop systems for assigning and transporting patients to those facilities.

- *Public information and education.* EMS personnel should participate in programs designed to educate the public. The programs are to focus on the prevention of injuries and how to properly access the EMS system.

- *Medical direction.* Each EMS system must have a physician as its medical director. This physician delegates medical practice to nonphysician caregivers and oversees all aspects of patient care.

- *Evaluation.* Each state must have a **quality improvement (QI)** system in place for continuing evaluation and upgrading of its EMS system.

Helicopter EMS (HEMS) began to develop in the early 1980s. A hospital or consortium of hospitals operated most helicopter programs. These services initially used all-nurse crews. However, as the operations matured, a paramedic was often used in place of one of the nurses on the flight. HEMS is primarily used for both scene-to-hospital and interhospital transfer of critically ill or injured patients.

CONTENT REVIEW

▶ 1988 NHTSA: "Ten System Elements"

- Regulation and policy
- Resources management
- Human resources and training
- Transportation
- Facilities
- Communications
- Trauma systems
- Public information and education
- Medical direction
- Evaluation

The 1990s

Further improvements were made to EMS during the 1990s. In 1990, Congress passed the Trauma Care Systems and Development Act. This Act provided funding to states for trauma system planning, development, implementation, and evaluation.

In 1993, the Institute of Medicine published *Emergency Medical Services for Children*. This document pointed out the deficiencies in pediatric emergency care in the United States. A small amount of federal funding subsequently financed the Emergency Medical Services for Children (EMSC) program.

In 1995, Congress did not reauthorize the Trauma Care Systems and Development Act, and the funding for trauma systems fell back on the states. This resulted in significant variability in trauma system care across the United States.

By the late 1990s, EMS systems and EMS practice had started to mature. It was at this point that self-assessment of EMS began to occur. Researchers and systems began to link patient outcomes (morbidity and mortality—illness and death) with various EMS practices. Surprisingly, some practices that had seemed intuitive did not hold up to the test of science. One of the largest studies of prehospital practices and outcomes was the **Ontario Prehospital Advanced Life Support (OPALS) study** that was conducted in various regions of the province of Ontario, Canada. The study has provided significant information about early defibrillation, response times, advanced life support procedures, and much more.[14]

EMS Agenda for the Future

The **National Highway Traffic Safety Administration (NHTSA)** published the *EMS Agenda for the Future* in 1996.[15] This document examined what had been learned during the prior three decades of EMS and endeavored to create a vision for the future of EMS in the United States. It was published at an important time, when those agencies, organizations, and individuals that affect EMS were evaluating their respective roles in the context of a rapidly evolving health care system—a process of evaluation that is ongoing.

NHTSA is a division of the U.S. Department of Transportation (DOT) and the Health Resources and Services Administration (HRSA), Maternal and Child Health Bureau. *The EMS Agenda for the Future* focused on aspects of EMS related to emergency care outside traditional health care facilities. It recognized the changes that occurred in the health care system of which EMS is a part. The document recommended that EMS of the future would be a community-based health management system that would be fully integrated into the overall health care system. EMS of the future would have the ability to identify and modify illness and injury risks, provide acute illness and injury care and follow-up, and contribute to the treatment of chronic conditions and to community health monitoring. EMS would be integrated with other health care providers and public health and public safety agencies in the effort to improve community health, which would result in more appropriate use of acute health care resources. Overall, EMS would remain the public's emergency medical safety net.

To realize this vision, *The EMS Agenda for the Future* proposed continued development of 14 core EMS attributes. They were:

- Integration of health services
- EMS research
- Legislation and regulation
- System finance
- Human resources
- Medical direction
- Education systems
- Public education
- Prevention
- Public access
- Communication systems
- Clinical care
- Information systems
- Evaluation

While many of the recommendations proposed by the *EMS Agenda for the Future* have been realized, many have not. Despite this, this document continues to serve as a guide for EMS providers, health care organizations and institutions, governmental agencies, and policy makers who must be committed to improving the health of their communities and to ensuring that EMS efficiently contributes to that goal. They must invest the resources necessary to provide the nation's population with emergency health care that is reliably accessible, effective, subject to continuous evaluation, and integrated with the remainder of the health care system.

The Twenty-First Century

The United States has changed significantly following the terrorist attacks of September 11, 2001 (Figure 2-4 ●). Among other things that occurred as a result of 9/11, review of the public safety system found numerous flaws. President George W. Bush established the **Department of Homeland Security** to coordinate the various agencies responsible for protecting the country. With this came a **National Incident Management System (NIMS)** and other strategies to prepare the country for terrorist attacks and other threats.[16]

In 2005, two devastating hurricanes (Katrina and Rita) hit several Gulf Coast states causing massive damage and loss of life. The emergency response, in some cases, was less than ideal. Additional changes were made to improve the Federal Emergency Management Agency (FEMA) and other governmental agencies following these disasters. A significant economic downturn in 2008 forced many cities to cut back on EMS and fire operations. As in most times of economic distress, EMS and hospital emergency departments were faced with less funding and more patients.

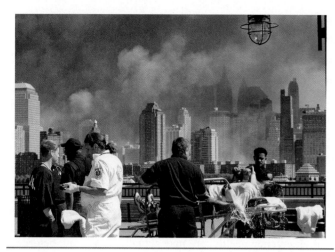

● **Figure 2-4** The attacks on New York City and Washington, DC on September 11, 2001, forever changed the face of EMS. (© Reuters)

EMS at the Crossroads

In 2006, the National Academies Institute of Medicine published another evaluation of the status of emergency services in the United States. This document, entitled *Emergency Medical Services: At the Crossroads,* was critical of many EMS practices. The study found that there were significant problems at the federal level. Despite the advances made in EMS, sizable challenges remained. At the federal policy level, government leadership in emergency care was found to be fragmented and inconsistent. As it is currently organized, responsibility for prehospital and hospital-based emergency and trauma care is scattered across multiple agencies and departments. Similar divisions are evident at the state and local levels. In addition, the current delivery system suffers in a number of key areas:

- **Insufficient coordination.** EMS care is highly fragmented, and often uncoordinated among providers. Multiple EMS agencies serving within a single population center do not operate cohesively. Agencies in adjacent jurisdictions often are unable to communicate with each other. In many cases, EMS and other public safety agencies cannot talk to one another because they operate with incompatible communications equipment or on different frequencies.

- *Coordination of transport within regions is limited.* The management of the regional flow of patients is poor, and patients may not be transported to facilities that are optimal and ready to receive them. Communications and hand-offs between EMS and hospital personnel are frequently ineffective and often omit important clinical information.

- *Disparities in response times.* The speed with which ambulances respond to emergency calls is highly variable. In some cases this variability is related to geography. In dense population centers, for example, the distances ambulances must travel are small,

but traffic and other problems can cause delays. In contrast, rural areas involve longer travel times, sometimes over difficult terrain. This is further worsened by problems in the organization and management of EMS services, the communications and coordination between 911 dispatch and EMS responders, and the priority placed on response time given the resources available.

- *Uncertain quality of care.* There is very little known about the quality of care delivered by EMS services in the United States because there are no standardized measures of EMS quality, no nationwide standards for the training and certification of EMS personnel, no accreditation of institutions that educate EMS personnel, and virtually no accountability for the performance of EMS systems. While most Americans assume that their communities are served by competent EMS services, the public has no idea whether this is true, and no way to know.

- *Lack of readiness for disasters.* Although EMS personnel are among the first to respond in the event of a disaster, they are the least prepared component of community response teams. Most EMS personnel have received little or no disaster response training for terrorist attacks, natural disasters, or other public health emergencies. Despite the massive amounts of federal funding directed to homeland security, only a tiny proportion of those funds have been directed to medical response. Furthermore, EMS representation in disaster planning at the federal level has been highly limited.

- *Divided professional identity.* EMS is a unique profession, one that straddles both medical care and public safety. Among public safety agencies, however, EMS is often regarded as a secondary service, with police and fire taking more prominent roles; within medicine, EMS personnel often lack the respect afforded to other professionals, such as physicians and nurses. Despite significant investments in education and training, salaries for EMS personnel are often well below those for comparable positions, such as police officers, firefighters, and nurses. In addition, there is a cultural divide among EMS, public safety, and medical care workers that contributes to the fragmentation of these services.

- *Limited evidence base.* The evidence base for many practices routinely used in EMS is limited. Strategies for EMS have often been adapted from settings that differ substantially from the prehospital environment and, consequently, their value in the field is questionable, and some may even be harmful. For example, field intubation of children, still widely practiced, has been found to do more harm than good in many situations.[17] While some recent research has added to the EMS evidence base, a host of critical

CONTENT REVIEW

▶ Types of EMS Services

• Fire-based
• Third service
• Private
• Hospital-based
• Volunteer

▶ Regardless of the delivery type, all emergency operations must be closely integrated and work together.

clinical questions remain unanswered because of limited federal research support, as well as inherent difficulties associated with prehospital research due to its sporadic nature and the difficulty of obtaining informed consent for the research.[18]

National Report on the State of Emergency Medicine

The American College of Emergency Physicians (ACEP) in 2006 published a study similar to EMS at the Crossroads. The paper, entitled *The National Report Card on the State of Emergency Medicine: Evaluating the Environment of Emergency Care Systems State by State,* pointed out the significant problems that existed in all aspects of emergency care.[19] This paper primarily addressed problems in hospital emergency departments but also addressed EMS issues. Overall, the report detailed that emergency services in the United States are so overstressed that the quality of care has been compromised. Multiple causes were indentified and included such things as inadequate funding, patient overcrowding, lack of alternate care facilities, problems with medical liability, the effect of illegal immigration, and many other factors. Each state was given a letter grade that reflected the reported standard of emergency care in that state.

Helicopter EMS

In 2001 federal reimbursement for medical helicopters improved, and the national medical helicopter fleet expanded from 300 aircraft to almost 900 in a matter of years. With the increase in helicopters came an increase in accidents and overutilization. In 2008, there were a record number of helicopter EMS crashes with related fatalities. As a result, the **National Transportation Safety Board (NTSB)** held hearings in 2009 and later recommended sweeping improvements for the helicopter EMS industry.

TODAY'S EMS SYSTEMS

The EMS system of today remains a mixture of various types of operations. The modern EMS system is now fairly well integrated with the health care system and, to a lesser degree, with the public safety system. Despite some federal oversight, the provision of EMS is still primarily a local government responsibility. Because of the differences across the United States, there are significantly different approaches to the provision of EMS across the United States. Government entities have elected to operate EMS in various service types. These include:

• Fire-based
• Third service
• Private (profit or nonprofit)
• Hospital-based
• Volunteer
• Hybrid (combination of any of these)

Regardless of the delivery type, the lessons of 9/11 have shown that all emergency operations must be closely integrated and work together. An explosion in EMS technology is making this possible and has simplified many aspects of EMS.

Chain of Survival

Generally speaking, emergency health care begins at the time of the emergency. More recently, however, it has been shown that emergency health care may actually begin long before an emergency occurs. In this regard, EMS and emergency medicine practitioners are embracing preventive health care measures that may help to reduce emergency illnesses and accidents. It also now includes such innovative measures as EMS personnel periodically visiting high-risk and homebound citizens and assessing their health status and needs.

Aside from such preventive activities, the EMS system is part of a continuum of care that begins once an emergency occurs and ends when the patient completes care and returns to his normal activities of daily living. This continuum is often referred to as the **chain of survival**. As defined by the American Heart Association (AHA), the chain of survival consists of the five most important factors affecting survival of a cardiac arrest patient: (1) immediate recognition and activation of EMS; (2) early CPR; (3) rapid defibrillation; (4) effective advanced life support; and (5) integrated post–cardiac arrest care. A similar continuum of events, essential to the optimal care of any emergency patient, might include, but would not be limited to, the following:

• Bystander care
• Dispatch
• Response
• Prehospital care
• Transportation
• Emergency department care
• Definitive care
• Rehabilitation

To achieve this continuum, several components of the EMS system must be in place.

Levels of Licensure/Certification

As noted in the preceding chapter, the *National EMS Scope of Practice Model* defines and describes four levels of EMS licensure:

• Emergency Medical Responder (EMR)
• Emergency Medical Technician (EMT)
• Advanced EMT (AEMT)
• Paramedic

Each level represents a unique role, set of skills, and knowledge base.[20] In 2009, *National EMS Education Instructional Guidelines* were developed and published for each of these four levels.[21] These instructional guidelines replace the various curricula that had been previously published to guide EMS education. The use of instructional guidelines, as opposed to a rote curriculum, allows EMS educators to adapt their educational strategies to the specific student population they serve. When used in conjunction with the *National EMS Core Content*, national EMS certification, and national EMS Education program accreditation, the *National EMS Scope of Practice Model* and the *National EMS Education Standards* create a strong and interdependent system that provides the foundation to ensure the competency of out-of-hospital emergency medical personnel throughout the United States.

Education

One of the fundamental principles of quality EMS is a solid education program for providers. EMS education has evolved significantly in the last two decades. Now, there are more educators with advanced degrees and EMS is being recognized in the academic community. Despite the advances, there remains considerable variation in EMS educational programs across the country.

In response to *The EMS Agenda for the Future*, several documents have been prepared to guide EMS education. The first of these was the *National EMS Core Content* published by NHTSA in 2005.[22] This document defined the body of knowledge, skills, and abilities desired in EMS personnel. It was followed shortly thereafter by the *National EMS Scope of Practice*, also published in 2005, which helped to define the future roles of EMS providers. This consensus document supported a system of EMS personnel licensure that was common in other allied health professions and was designed to serve as a guide for states and territories in developing their **scope of practice** legislation, rules, and regulations. States following the *National EMS Scope of Practice Model* as closely as possible would increase the consistency of the nomenclature and competencies of EMS personnel nationwide, facilitate reciprocity, improve professional mobility, and enhance the name recognition and public understanding of EMS. Some states have adopted the *National EMS Scope of Practice* model in its entirety while others have adopted only parts of it.

Local- and State-Level Agencies

The efficient delivery of emergency medical care requires a systematic approach and team effort to make the best use of existing resources. That means each community must develop an EMS system that best meets its needs. Though EMS systems across the country and the world will vary, certain elements are essential to ensure the best possible patient care.

At the municipal and regional levels, the first step in developing a comprehensive EMS system is to establish an administrative oversight agency. This agency is responsible for managing the local system's resources, developing operational protocols, and establishing standards and guidelines. Within the agency, a planning board is often formed. The planning board should be composed of community representatives, including emergency physicians, the emergency nurse association, the firefighter association, state and local police, and consumers. The planning board develops a budget and selects a qualified administrative staff capable of managing an EMS agency.

Once established, the agency designates who may function within the system and develops policies consistent with existing state requirements. It also creates a quality assurance or quality improvement program to evaluate the system's effectiveness and to ensure that the best interests of the patient are always a top priority. State EMS agencies are typically responsible for allocating funds to local systems, enacting legislation concerning the prehospital practice of medicine, licensing and certification of field providers, enforcing all state EMS regulations, and appointing regional advisory councils.

In essence, EMS is made up of a series of systems within a system. The integration of these systems and the cooperation of all participants help to result in the best quality of emergency care.

Medical Oversight

An EMS system must retain a **medical director**—a physician who is legally responsible for all clinical and patient-care aspects of the system. The medical director serves as the *de facto* conscience of the EMS system and must first be an advocate for quality patient care. Prehospital medical care provided by nonphysicians is considered a delegated practice of the system medical director; that is, prehospital care providers are the medical director's designated agents, regardless of who their employers may be.

The medical director's roles in an EMS system are to:

- Educate and train personnel
- Participate in personnel and equipment selection
- Develop clinical protocols in cooperation with expert EMS personnel
- Participate in quality improvement and problem resolution
- Provide direct input into patient care
- Interface between the EMS system and other health care agencies
- Advocate within the medical community
- Serve as the "medical conscience" of the EMS system, including advocating for quality patient care

In addition to the responsibilities just listed, the medical director is the ultimate authority for all medical issues within the system. Traditionally, **medical oversight** has been divided into an on-line (direct) component and an off-line (indirect) component. The trend has been to decrease on-line activities and to bolster the off-line component.[23]

On-line Medical Direction

On-line medical direction occurs when a qualified physician gives direct orders to a prehospital care provider by either radio or telephone (Figure 2-5 ●). Medical direction may be delegated to a mobile intensive care nurse (MICN), a physician assistant

CONTENT REVIEW

► Four "Ts" of Emergency Care

• Triage
• Treatment
• Transport
• Transfer

(PA), or a paramedic. In all circumstances, ultimate on-line responsibility remains with the medical director.

On-line medical direction offers several benefits to the patient. It gives the EMS provider direct and immediate access to medical consultation for specific patient care. It also allows for the transmission of essential data such as 12-lead ECGs. The transmission of physiologic data provides the on-line physician with diagnostic information that can be used to make critical decisions while the patient is still on scene or en route. Most EMS systems have the equipment to record on-line consultations. Those recordings can then be used for **peer review** and other continuous quality improvement activities.

When at the scene of an emergency, the health care provider with the most knowledge and experience in the delivery of prehospital emergency care should be in charge. When a nonaffiliated physician or **intervener physician** is on scene and on-line medical direction may not exist, the paramedic should relinquish responsibility to the physician. However, the intervener physician must first identify himself, demonstrate a willingness to accept responsibility, and document the intervention as required by the local EMS system. If his treatment differs from established protocols, the intervener physician must accompany the patient in the ambulance to the hospital.

If an intervener physician is on scene and on-line medical direction does exist, the on-line physician is ultimately responsible. In case of a disagreement, the paramedic must take orders from the on-line physician.

Off-Line Medical Oversight

Off-line medical oversight refers to medical policies, procedures, and practices that a system medical director has established in advance of a call. It includes **prospective medical oversight** such as guidelines on the selection of personnel and

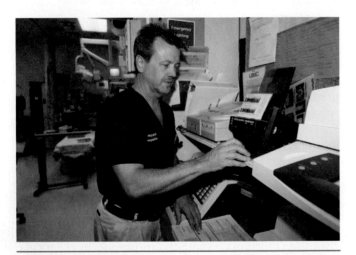

● **Figure 2-5** The medical director can provide on-line guidance to EMS personnel in the field. (© *Dr. Bryan E. Bledsoe*)

supplies, training and education, and protocol development. An important part of medical oversight is participation in the selection of medical equipment. Off-line medical oversight also includes **retrospective medical oversight**, such as auditing, peer review, conflict resolution, and other quality assurance processes.

Clinical protocols are the policies and procedures of all medical components of an EMS system and are the responsibility of the medical director. Many EMS systems use committees, often made up of physicians within the community, to develop medical treatment protocols. EMS protocols provide a standardized approach to common patient problems and a consistent level of medical care as well as a standard for accountability. When treatment is undertaken based on such protocols, the on-line physician, if needed, can assist prehospital personnel in interpreting the patient's complaint, understanding the findings of their evaluations, and providing the appropriate treatment.[24] Protocols are designed around the four "Ts" of emergency care:

● *Triage.* Guidelines that address patient flow through an EMS system, including how system resources are allocated to meet the needs of patients.

● *Treatment.* Guidelines that identify procedures to be performed upon direct order from medical direction and procedures that are preauthorized protocols called **standing orders**.

● *Transport.* Guidelines that address the mode of travel (air vs. ground) based on the nature of the patient's injury or illness, the condition of the patient, the level of care required, and estimated transport time.

● *Transfer.* Guidelines that address receiving facilities to ensure that the patient is admitted to the one most appropriate for definitive care.

Protocols also are established for special circumstances, such as the proper handling of "Do Not Resuscitate" orders, patients who refuse treatment, sexual abuse, abuse of children or elderly people, termination of CPR, and intervener physicians. Although protocols standardize field procedures, they should allow the paramedic the flexibility necessary to improvise and adapt to special circumstances.

Public Information and Education

The public is an essential, yet often overlooked, component of an EMS system. EMS should have a plan to educate the public on recognizing an emergency, accessing the system, and initiating basic life support procedures. Because of this, public education has become an increasingly important role for EMS. As already noted, patient education can occur before the emergency occurs (prevention) through activities such as bicycle safety programs, infant car seat programs, and similar strategies (Figure 2-6 ●). In addition, it has been found that patients are more likely to listen to advice and consider lifestyle changes following an emergency. This is often referred to as a **teachable moment**. A teachable moment is an unplanned opportunity to present information when the circumstances are such that a person is likely to understand and accept the information. EMS

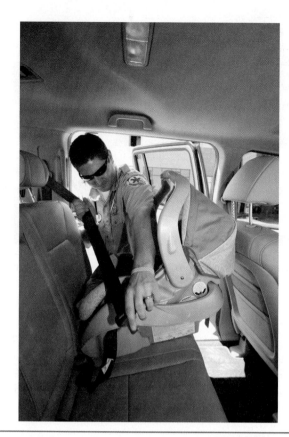

● **Figure 2-6** Providing disease and injury prevention education to the public has become an important role of EMS in the twenty-first century. (© *Dr. Bryan E. Bledsoe*)

public education can take several forms including role modeling, community involvement, leadership, and prevention.

One of the most fundamental components of EMS public education is to help members of the public to recognize an emergency when it occurs and to learn how to access the EMS system. Prompt recognition of an emergency can save lives. For example, the American Heart Association estimates that over 300,000 cardiac arrests per year occur before the patient reaches the hospital. Such arrests are called "sudden death" because most happen within 2 hours of the onset of cardiac symptoms. Many patients delay calling for help when symptoms occur. If the patient and bystanders are taught to recognize the emergency and call for help in time, many cases of sudden death could be prevented.

The second aspect of public education is system access. Citizens must know how to activate EMS in an emergency to avoid life-threatening delays. Whether access is by way of 911 or a local seven-digit phone number, the number should

be well publicized, and citizens should be taught how to give the necessary information to the Emergency Medical Dispatcher.

Finally, after recognizing an emergency and activating EMS, citizens must know how to provide basic life support assistance, such as cardiopulmonary resuscitation (CPR) and bleeding control after major trauma. Abundant research indicates that a relationship exists between rapid emergency care and mortality (death) rates of patients—especially cardiac arrest. Communities have proven that when many citizens are trained in basic life support and early defibrillation—and there is a rapid advanced life support (ALS) response—a larger number of patients can be successfully resuscitated. The American Heart Association (AHA) estimates that thousands of lives could be saved each year with implementation of bystander CPR programs and rapid ALS response. Because of the widespread availability of automated external defibrillators (AEDs) in private homes and public places, early defibrillation has become more commonplace and more successful. Cardiac arrest survival takes a fully engaged public and an effective EMS system.

Communications

The communications network is the heart of a regional EMS system (Figure 2-7 ●). Coordinating the components into an organized response to urgent medical situations requires a comprehensive, flexible communications plan. Such a plan should include:

● *Citizen access.* A well-publicized universal number, such as 911, provides direct citizen access to emergency services. Multiple community numbers only add life-threatening minutes to emergency response times. Enhanced 911, or E911, gives automatic location of the caller, instant routing of the call to the appropriate emergency service (fire, police, or EMS), and instant callback capability. The proliferation of cell telephone and Internet-based phone lines (voice over Internet protocol, or VOIP) has made caller location more difficult, although strategies have been developed to address these issues.

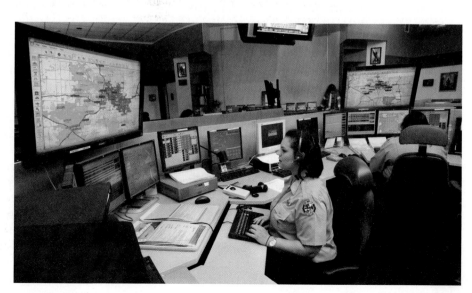

● **Figure 2-7** The EMS communications center is truly the heart of the modern EMS system.

- *Single control center.* One control center that can communicate with and direct all emergency vehicles within a large geographical area is best. Ideally, all public service agencies should be dispatched from the same communications center in order to ensure the best use of resources in an emergency response.

- *Operational communications capabilities.* With these, EMS dispatch can manage all aspects of system response and assess the system's readiness for the next response. Emergency units can communicate with each other and with other agencies during mutual aid and disaster operations. Hospitals also can communicate with other hospitals in the region to assess specialty capabilities.

- *Medical communications capabilities.* EMS providers can communicate with the receiving facility and, in many areas, transmit ECG and other patient information to the hospital or a physician's office. Newer technologies can send patient information to designated sites at the same time the information is attained. The growth in communications technology has been one of the biggest advances in EMS in recent years.

- *Communications hardware.* The North American communications infrastructure has changed drastically. The utility of the Internet has changed the way we send and receive information. The massive development of the cell telephone network has impacted this as well. EMS communications uses all these technologies as well as more typical radio communications systems. Most ambulances now have notebook computers and global positioning system (GPS) and vehicle tracking system capabilities. As a result of the terrorist attacks of 2001, there has been considerable federal emphasis on updating and improving the national emergency and public safety communications system. An important related directive has been to ensure **interoperability**—a feature that allows personnel from different jurisdictions and systems to communicate with one another effectively.

- *Communications software.* This includes the radio frequencies needed for in-system communication and, in many systems, the satellite and high-tech computer programs that track ambulances. Radio procedures, policies consistent with FCC standards and local protocols, and back-up communication plans for disaster operations are essential to the modern EMS operation.

An EMS system must have an effective and efficient communications network in place. Because no single design will meet the needs of all communities, each system should design a network that is simple, flexible, and practical.

Emergency Medical Dispatcher

The activities of the **Emergency Medical Dispatcher (EMD)** are crucial to the efficient operation of EMS (Figure 2-8 ●). EMDs not only send ambulances to the scene, they also make sure that system resources are in constant readiness to respond.

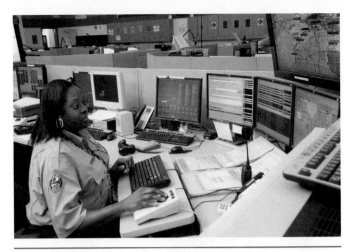

● **Figure 2-8** The modern EMS dispatcher plays a major role in EMS system operations and can impact the quality of emergency care provided.

EMDs must be both medically and technically trained. Their training should cover basic telecommunication skills, medical interrogation (questioning), giving prearrival instructions, and dispatch prioritization. The course should be standardized, and it should include certification by a government agency.

EMS Dispatch

Emergency medical dispatching is the nerve center of an EMS system. It is the means of assigning and directing appropriate medical care to patients and should be under the full control of the medical director and the EMS agency. An emergency medical dispatch plan should include interrogation protocols, response configurations, system status management, and prearrival caller instructions.

Another management method is called "priority dispatching," which was first used by the Salt Lake City Fire Department. Using a set of medically approved protocols, EMDs are trained to medically interrogate a distressed caller, prioritize symptoms, select an appropriate response, and give lifesaving prearrival instructions.[25]

In 1974, the Phoenix Fire Department introduced a **prearrival instruction** program developed by medically trained dispatchers. In that program, callers initiate lifesaving first aid with the dispatcher's help while they wait for emergency units to arrive on scene. In 1985, the Seattle EMS system initiated a successful program of instructing callers in CPR. Critics point out that prearrival instruction programs may result in increased liability. Even so, the increased liability of *not* providing such a service may far outweigh the risk of providing it.

An effective EMS dispatch system places the first responding units on scene within minutes of the onset of the emergency. The American Heart Association reports that brain resuscitation will not be successful if response time exceeds 4 minutes unless there was proper BLS intervention (CPR). Many studies have shown that defibrillation is most effective when delivered in 4 minutes or less after patient collapse. If EMS responders arrive more than 4 minutes after patient collapse, patient outcomes are better if the patient receives at least 90 seconds of

CPR prior to defibrillation. For many years the desired EMS response time was established at 8 minutes, but recent studies have shown that a response time of 8 minutes has not been associated with improved outcomes. A response time of 4 minutes or less has been highly associated with improved outcomes in cardiac arrest. However, few EMS systems can routinely deliver response times of 4 minutes or less. Further research is needed in order to determine the best desired response times for a specific EMS system[26, 27] and how to achieve them.

Education and Certification

The two kinds of EMS education programs for EMS personnel are initial education and continuing education. *Initial education* programs are the original courses for prehospital providers. They involve the completion of a standardized course that meets or exceeds recommended standards. (As noted earlier, instead of various curricula for the various levels of EMS, the *National EMS Instructional Guidelines* now allow instructors more latitude in instructional strategies.) *Continuing education* programs include refresher courses for recertification and periodic in-service training sessions. All education programs should have medical oversight and a medical director who is involved in the process. The EMS agency is responsible for ensuring funding for its education programs.

Initial Education

A paramedic's initial education is accomplished by successfully completing a course following the most recent *National EMS Education Instructional Guidelines* published by the U.S. DOT. The Guidelines establish the minimum content for the course and set a standard for paramedic programs across the country. The Instructional Guidelines offer guidance of three specific learning domains:

- *Cognitive,* which consists of facts, or information knowledge
- *Affective,* which requires students to assign emotions, values, and attitudes to that information
- *Psychomotor,* which consists of hands-on skills students learn while in laboratory and clinical settings

There is a national effort to have all paramedic education programs accredited. The **accreditation** process ensures that all paramedic education programs meet minimal guidelines in regard to faculty, facilities, equipment, medical oversight, clinical affiliations, and financial stability.[28] The primary accrediting organization in EMS is the *Committee on Accreditation of Educational Programs for the Emergency Medical Services Professions (CoAEMSP),* an entity of the *Commission on Accreditation of Allied Health Programs (CAAHEP).* Some states have their own program accreditation process.

Continuing Education

Once a paramedic has completed the initial education program, he must remain current on changes in EMS care. To achieve this, a continuing education program is essential. There are various methods available for a paramedic to attain necessary continuing education. These include traditional lectures and prepackaged programs but also include innovative strategies such as web-based programs, podcasts, videos, and similar alternative delivery models. Most continuing education programs must be accredited or approved by an oversight body. The *Continuing Education Coordinating Board for Emergency Medical Services (CECBEMS)* is a national continuing education certifying body although some states provide their own continuing education certifying process.

Continuing education is mandatory and is just as important as the initial paramedic education program. EMS is a relatively young **profession** and information and technology changes rapidly. More important, continuing education allows you to stay abreast of the changes in emergency care procedures to ensure that you are providing the best patient care possible. The best paramedics are those who seek and complete quality continuing education.

Licensure/Certification

Once initial education is completed, the paramedic will become either certified or licensed, depending on the laws governing EMS in the particular state. **Certification** is the process by which an agency or association grants recognition to an individual who has met its qualifications. Many states certify paramedics. After attaining state certification, paramedics are permitted to work within an established EMS system under the direct supervision of a physician medical director.

Licensure is a process of occupational regulation. Through licensure, a governmental agency (usually a state agency) grants permission to engage in a given trade or profession to an applicant who has attained the degree of competency required to ensure the public's protection. Some states choose to license paramedics instead of certifying them. (Note that there is an unfounded general belief that a licensed professional has greater status than one who is certified or registered. However, a certification granted by a state, conferring a right to engage in a trade or profession, is in fact a license.)

Regardless of what it is called, the paramedic must realize that the authority granted to him by the state is a privilege and his personal responsibility. He must take a proactive role in maintaining his good standing through continuing education, conduct his practice in a manner to uphold the public trust he has been given, and protect this privilege. The paramedic should never assume that anyone else would take over this responsibility for him.

Registration is accomplished by entering your name and essential information within a particular record. Paramedics are registered so that the state can verify the provider's initial certification and monitor recertification. Almost every state has an EMS office that tracks the registration of emergency care providers. While some states track only ALS providers, others maintain registers on the certifications of emergency medical responders, EMTs, advanced EMTs, and paramedics.

Reciprocity is the process by which an agency grants automatic certification or licensure to an individual who has comparable certification or licensure from another agency. For example, some states grant reciprocity to paramedics who are certified in another state. In some states, certification or licensure is not automatic. In these cases, the state may grant certification or licensure through Equivalence or Legal Recognition. This is when the state determines the out-of-state paramedic's initial education meets the requirements of the state, and the paramedic is then allowed to participate in a licensure examination or other activity to gain licensure or certification.

National Registry of EMTs

The National Registry of Emergency Medical Technicians (NREMT) is a nonprofit entity based in Columbus, Ohio. It prepares and administers standardized tests for the various EMS provider levels. The National Registry establishes the qualifications for registration and biennial reregistration and serves as a vehicle for establishing a national minimum standard of competency. Through these services, the National Registry serves as a major tool for reciprocity by providing a process for paramedics to become certified when moving from one state to another. The National Registry also supports the development and evaluation of EMS education programs with the goal of developing nationwide professional standards for EMS providers.

Currently, in the majority of states, National Registry examinations are being used at some level by EMS regulators. Several states offer locally developed examinations because their levels of certification or licensure differ from those recognized by the National Registry. The states that use the National Registry examinations benefit from savings that result from spreading exam development costs over a large user base as well as from the assurance that the examinations are widely recognized as providing a national standard.

Professional Organizations

The public image of EMS is often shaped by the professional organizations that represent that profession. Membership in professional organizations is a great way to stay abreast of changes in the profession and to interact with members from other parts of the country. It also provides an excellent opportunity to share ideas. National EMS organizations include the following:

- National Association of Emergency Medical Technicians (NAEMT)
- National Association of Search and Rescue (NASAR)
- National Association of EMS Educators (NAEMSE)
- National Association of EMS Physicians (NAEMSP)
- International Association of Flight and Critical Care Paramedics (IAFCCP)
- National EMS Management Association (NEMSMA)
- National Council of State EMS Training Coordinators (NCSEMSTC)

In addition to these, most states have EMS organizations that provide information and assistance at a state or local level.

These are just some examples of organizations through which paramedics, emergency physicians, and nurses can enrich themselves and pursue their particular interests. Such organizations assist in the development of educational programs, operational policies and procedures, and the implementation of EMS. They establish guidelines with input from the public and the profession, which ensure that the public interest is served in the delivery of emergency medical services. They also provide a means to promote and enhance the status of EMS within the health care community, and their efforts help to create a unified voice for EMS providers.

Professional Journals and Magazines

A variety of journals are available to keep the paramedic aware of the latest changes in this ever-changing industry. These journals provide an abundant source of continuing-education material, as well as an excellent opportunity for EMS professionals to write and publish articles. The following is just a partial list of journals that routinely publish articles relating to the medical care of patients in EMS:

- *Academic Emergency Medicine*
- *American Journal of Emergency Medicine*
- *Annals of Emergency Medicine*
- *Emergency Medical Services*
- *EMS World*
- *Journal of Emergency Medical Services (JEMS)*
- *Journal of Pediatric Emergency Medicine*
- *Journal of Trauma: Injury, Infection and Critical Care*
- *Prehospital Emergency Care*

The Internet

The Internet has changed the world and certainly has changed EMS. There are now numerous websites designed for EMS providers. Many of the trade magazines and similar entities offer websites with constantly updated content and news. There are numerous websites that provide quality, accredited continuing education programs. There has been a similar trend in placing much of the didactic portion of initial EMS education on the Internet. This allows students to receive initial and continuing education in their local communities. Interestingly, several EMS-oriented social communities have been developed. These have allowed international EMS discussions and networking and have a considerable following among EMS providers (Figure 2-9 ●).

Patient Transportation

Patients who are transported under the direction of an EMS system should be taken to the nearest appropriate medical facility whenever possible. Medical oversight should designate that facility, based on the needs of the patient and the availability of services. In some cases, the patient's need for special services (such as care for burns) means designating a facility that is not nearby. At other times, the closest facility will be designated for stabilization of the patient while transfer is arranged. The ultimate authority for this decision remains with on-line medical direction.

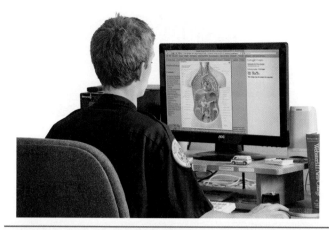

● **Figure 2-9** The Internet has allowed paramedics, regardless of their location, to obtain quality continuing education.

Patients may be transported by ground or air (Figure 2-10 ●). As noted earlier, use of helicopters for medical transport was introduced during the Korean War and expanded in Vietnam, and success of military evacuation procedures led to their use in civilian ambulance systems. In 1970, the Military Assistance to Safety and Traffic (MAST) program was established. This demonstration project set up 35 helicopter transportation programs nationwide to test the feasibility of using military helicopters and paramedics in civilian medical emergencies.[29]

Today, trauma care systems use law enforcement, municipal, hospital-based, private, and military helicopter transport services to transfer patients. Fixed-wing aircraft also are used when patients must be transported long distances, usually more than 200 miles (Figure 2-11 ●).

All transport vehicles must be licensed and meet local and state EMS requirements. Equipment lists should be consistent with system-wide standards. There are various national and regional standards regarding what equipment and technologies should be available on both emergency and nonemergency ambulances. Regional standardization of equipment and supplies is most effective in facilitating interagency efforts during disaster operations.

In 1974, in response to a request from the DOT, the General Services Administration (GSA) developed the "KKK-A-1822 Federal Specifications for Ambulances." This was the first attempt at standardizing ambulance design to permit intensive life support for patients en route to a definitive care facility. The act defined the following basic types of ambulance:

- *Type I (Figure 2-12 ●).* This is a conventional cab and chassis on which a module ambulance body is mounted, with no passageway between the driver and patient's compartments.

- *Type II (Figure 2-13 ●).* A standard van, body, and cab form an integral unit. Most have a raised roof.

- *Type III (Figure 2-14 ●).* This is a specialty van with forward cab and integral body. It has a passageway from the driver's compartment to the patient's compartment.

Only these certified ambulances may display the registered "Star of Life" symbol as defined by the National Highway Traffic Safety Administration (NHTSA). The word *ambulance* should appear in mirror image on the front of the vehicle so that other drivers can identify the ambulance in their rear-view mirrors.

Many services now place a variety of specialized equipment on board ambulances, including specialty rescue, hazmat, and additional advanced life support equipment. This has often meant exceeding the gross vehicle weight and has resulted in introduction of a medium-duty truck chassis built for rugged durability and large storage and work areas (Figure 2-15 ●). Another newer type of ambulance, developed for fuel economy

LEGAL CONSIDERATIONS

Emergency Department Closures. *Numerous factors have resulted in emergency department closures and ambulance diversions. This can significantly impact the EMS system. All systems must address this situation so that patient care does not suffer.*

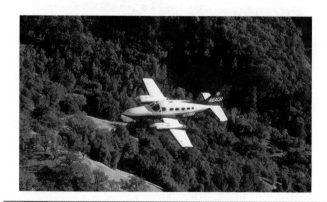

● **Figure 2-10** Patients may be transported by ground or air. Medical helicopter transport was introduced in the 1950s during the Korean War. (© *REACH Air Medical Services*)

● **Figure 2-11** Fixed wing aircraft, as well as helicopters, have become an important part of patient transport in the modern EMS system. (© *REACH Air Medical Services*)

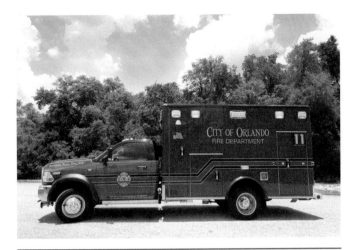

● **Figure 2-12** Type I ambulance.

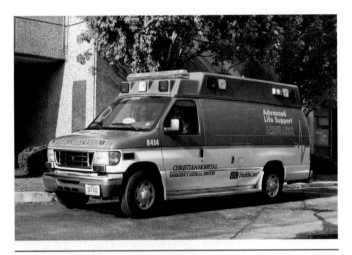

● **Figure 2-13** Type II ambulance.

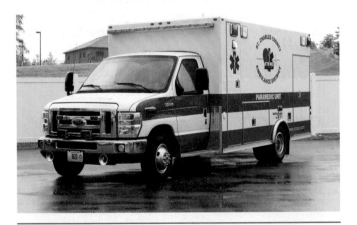

● **Figure 2-14** Type III ambulance.

and enhanced safety, is the diesel ambulance (Figure 2-16 ●). Ambulance standards will continue to evolve. Concerns about the future of the environment have led to a trend to consider vehicle emissions (exhaust and carbon footprint) in ambulance design.

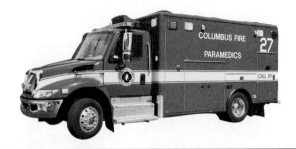

● **Figure 2-15** Some EMS systems have elected to use medium-duty ambulances that are built on a commercial truck chassis.

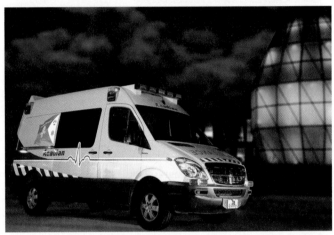

● **Figure 2-16** The diesel, unibody ambulance is becoming increasingly popular because of cost, fuel economy, and safety. (© *Acadian Ambulance Services*)

In 1980, the revision "KKK-A-1822A" aimed at improving ambulance electrical systems by designing a low-amp lighting system to replace antiquated light bars and beacons. This standard helped to reduce electrical system overloads. In 1985, another revision, "KKK-A-1822B," specified changes based on the National Institute for Occupational Safety and Health (NIOSH) standards. These include reduced internal siren noise, high engine temperatures, and exhaust emissions; safer cot-retention systems; wider axles; handheld spotlights; battery conditioners for longer life; and venting systems for oxygen compartments. In 2002, revision "KKK-A-1822E" provided guidelines to improve occupant protection in the patient compartment including additional occupant restraints, more rounded interior corners, and more secure locations of the sharps container for needles and other potentially dangerous items. "KKK-A-1822F" was published in 2007 and primarily addressed electrical systems, signage, and safety.[30]

All ambulances purchased with federal funds during the 1970s were required to comply with the KKK criteria. Since then, however, some states have adopted their own criteria.

Receiving Facilities

Not all hospitals are equal in emergency and support service capabilities. So how do you get the right patient to the right facility in an appropriate amount of time? EMS systems organize

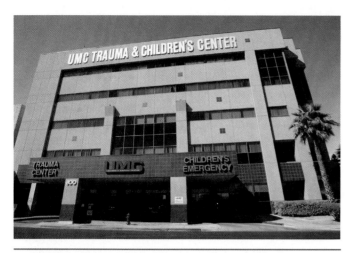

● **Figure 2-17** The development of specialized trauma centers has resulted in significant improvements in trauma morbidity and mortality. (© Dr. Bryan E. Bledsoe)

hospitals into categories that identify the readiness and capability of each hospital and its staff to receive and effectively treat emergency patients. EMS coordinators can use these categories to quickly recognize the most appropriate medical facility for definitive treatment or lifesaving stabilization.

Categorization was initially designed to identify **trauma** care capabilities for hospitals. The hospitals that made a commitment to providing accredited trauma care were designated as trauma centers. As the system has evolved, other categorizations have been developed including various categories of chest pain centers, stroke centers, and other specialzed care capabilities.[31]

Once categorization has been established, regionalizing available services helps give all patients reasonable access to the appropriate facility. Burn, trauma, pediatric, psychiatric, perinatal, cardiac, spinal, and poison centers are examples of specialty service facilities that offer high-level care for specific groups of patients (Figure 2-17 ●). Large EMS systems should designate a resource hospital that will coordinate specialty resources and ensure appropriate patient distribution.

Ideally, all receiving facilities should have the following capabilities: an emergency department with an emergency physician on duty at all times, surgical facilities, a lab and blood bank, medical imaging capabilities available around the clock, and critical and intensive care units. They should have a documented commitment to participate in the EMS system, a willingness to receive all emergency patients in transport regardless of their ability to pay, and medical audit procedures to ensure quality care and medical accountability. Finally, receiving facilities should exhibit a desire to participate in multiple-casualty preparedness plans.

Mutual Aid and Mass-Casualty Preparation

The resources of any one EMS system can be overwhelmed. A mutual-aid agreement ensures that help is available when needed. Such agreements may be between neighboring departments, municipalities, systems, or states. Cooperation among EMS agencies must transcend geographical, political, and historical boundaries.

Each EMS system should put a disaster plan in place for catastrophes that can overwhelm available resources. There should be a coordinated central management agency that identifies commanders within the framework of the incident command system and an existing mutual-aid agreement. The plan should integrate all EMS system components and have a flexible communications system. Frequent drills should test the plan's effectiveness and practicality. The communications and control systems should be capable of coordinating a systemwide response to a major medical incident without a major change in personnel, equipment, or operating protocol.

Quality Assurance and Improvement

An EMS system must be designed with the needs of the patient as its chief concern. The only acceptable level of quality is excellence, and systems should take the approach that they will never fully attain total excellence. For quality assurance and improvement programs to be effective, they must be dynamic and comprehensive. The EMS system must constantly monitor the community's expectations and standards of practice, and be willing to initiate, change, or eliminate its practices accordingly.

In 1997, the National Highway Traffic Safety Administration (NHTSA) released a manual called *A Leadership Guide to Quality Improvement for Emergency Medical Services Systems*. Its guidelines are based on the following components:

- Leadership
- Information and analysis
- Strategic quality planning

- Human resources development and management
- EMS process management
- EMS system results
- Satisfaction of patients and other stakeholders

Many EMS systems have developed ongoing quality assurance programs, while others have gone a step further with quality improvement programs. A quality assurance (QA) program is primarily designed to maintain continuous monitoring and measurement of the clinical care delivered to patients. It is in essence a problem-identifying mechanism. QA programs tend to look at the results, or the outputs of the EMS system, much like a manufacturer looks at the finished product coming off the assembly line. QA programs document the effectiveness of the care provided after the fact. They help to identify problems and selected areas that need improvement. The limitation with QA is that it tends to address the actions of individuals within the system, and looks at established performance measurements. These performance measurements are often based on criteria that are set in an arbitrary manner. These criteria—for example, that an IV success rate will be greater than 80 percent—tend to become a ceiling. As long as the paramedics in the system are establishing 8 of 10 IV starts successfully, no one looks any further. Yet if the success rate drops below 80 percent, the QA process may look at the individuals and miss that a change to new IV catheters has caused the decline. Furthermore, the QA system will probably not look at future improvements that could increase the success rate to 85 percent, 90 percent, or higher. A common complaint about QA programs is that they tend to identify only the problems and therefore focus only on punitive corrective action. Thus, prehospital personnel often view QA programs negatively.

As a result, many EMS systems have taken the quality process a step further with continuous quality improvement (CQI). In a CQI program, there is an ongoing effort to refine and improve the system in order to provide the highest level of service possible. CQI can be thought of as a problem-solving methodology. CQI programs are based on facts, data, and specifications, or management by fact. By its very nature, the statistical approach of CQI looks at the group as a whole, looking at the processes in an EMS system instead of the individual provider. In short, CQI is development of the "best possible" system whereas the QA approach accepts a system that is "good enough."[32]

A CQI program emphasizes the improvement of the overall process that will in turn lead to improved patient care. The dynamic process of CQI includes a four-step cycle known as plan, do, check, and act. In this process, data is analyzed and a *plan* of action developed. In the *do* phase, the plan is implemented, and further data is collected in the *check* phase to assess the viability of the changes. Finally action is taken in the *act* phase to address the findings of the previous step, and the process repeats itself. This process helps to ensure the improvement in the system is ongoing and does not stall.

In general, EMS quality can be divided into two categories: "good enough" quality and "best possible" quality.

LEGAL CONSIDERATIONS

QI: A Risk Management Strategy. *A good EMS Quality Improvement (QI) program is also an excellent risk management strategy. Problems in the system or with individual EMS providers can often be identified early through the QI program and remedied before patient care is harmed. Experience has shown that EMS services with an ongoing QI program have a decreased incidence of being sued. EMS cases can be divided into four areas of risk: high frequency/low risk; high frequency/high risk; low frequency/low risk; and low frequency/high risk. A good QI program should continuously monitor all high-risk cases and procedures, especially those that fall into the low-frequency category.*

High-risk cases in EMS include cardiac arrest patients, patients who must be restrained, patients who refuse EMS care, those who later file a complaint about care, and others. High-risk procedures include endotracheal intubation, medication administration, and others. A good QI program will continuously monitor high-risk cases and procedures such as these at both a system and provider level. If a provider is determined not to be managing these cases appropriately, that provider can be referred for additional education. Similarly, if it is learned that the system is not managing these cases appropriately, then changes must be made in the system to ensure that the problems are corrected.

So never look at an EMS QI program as punishment; look at it instead as an educational opportunity. If properly used, it will make you a better paramedic and your system a better EMS system.

"Take-It-for-Granted" Quality

People take it for granted that EMS will respond quickly to a 911 call. Because patients do not usually have medical training, they must assume that we are always acting in their best interests and at the highest level of **professionalism**. Thus, they also take it for granted that the care they receive from us is safe, appropriate, and the best that is available.

Quality improvement in this area is accomplished through continuous evaluation. Such clinical evaluation and improvement should be subject to rigorous examination prior to implementation and periodically thereafter. When considering a new medication, process, or procedure, for example, we must follow set rules before permitting its use in EMS. These rules are often called **rules of evidence**. Joseph P. Ornato, MD, PhD, developed them. They include the following guidelines:

- *There must be a theoretical basis for the change.* That is, the change must make sense based on relevant anatomy, physiology, biochemistry, and other basic medical sciences.
- *There must be ample scientific human research to support the idea.* Any device or medication used in patient care

must have adequate scientific human research to justify its use.

- *It must be clinically important.* The device, medication, or procedure must make a significant clinical difference to the patient. For example, a device such as an automated external defibrillator (AED) may mean the difference between living and dying for some patients, while color-coordinated stretcher linen has little clinical significance.

- *It must be practical, affordable, and teachable.* Some medical devices remain too expensive and too impractical for use in routine prehospital emergency care.

If a clinical innovation or improvement meets all these guidelines, then the change should be made. Only devices, medications, and procedures that pass these rigorous tests should be implemented.

Another way to accomplish "take-it-for-granted" quality improvement is through the ongoing education of personnel. Paramedics can improve their skills by reading, taking classes, soliciting feedback on clinical performance from receiving hospitals, and following up on patients. Peer review—the process of EMS personnel reviewing each other's patient reports, emergency care, and interactions with patients and families—is another way for paramedics to improve their knowledge and skills.

Ethics are the rules or standards that govern the conduct of members of a particular group or profession. Prehospital providers at all levels have an ethical responsibility to their patients and to the public. (See Chapter 8 for a detailed discussion of professional ethics.) The public expects excellence from the EMS system, and we should accept no less than excellence from ourselves.

Service Quality

In the business world, service quality is called "customer satisfaction." This is the kind of quality that individual customers get excited about, feel good about, and tell stories about. These are the little extras that exceed a customer's expectations and elicit thank-you letters. Prime examples of customer satisfaction include patient statements such as: "You fed my cat before we left." "You remembered my name and introduced me to the nurse." "You held my hand." "You seemed like a friend when I needed one."

Customer satisfaction can be created or destroyed with a simple word or deed. A significant part of the way we communicate with one another is through body language and tone of voice. Paramedics who genuinely care about their patients communicate it in many subtle ways. From the patient's perspective this is much more important than IVs, backboards, and ECGs. It is essential to remember the ultimate reason for our existence: to serve the patient by providing the highest quality service and care available (Figure 2-18 ●).

Patient Safety

The primary tenet of medicine is *primum non nocere* (first, do no harm). The safety of the patient must be considered in any medical endeavor. This holds true for EMS. As the health care

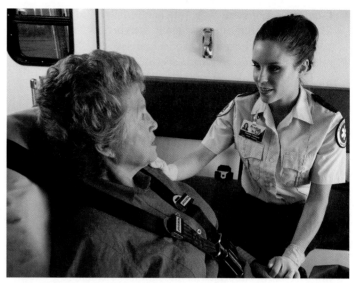

● **Figure 2-18** Our patients are our customers. We must strive to provide them with service that is compassionate and kind.

system becomes more complicated, the chances for errors and accidents increase. In 2000 the Institute of Medicine of the National Academies of Sciences published *To Err Is Human: Building a Safer Health System.* In this document the Institute estimated that between 44,000 and 98,000 Americans die annually because of medical errors. EMS is a part of the health care system and medical errors occur.[33] Three areas have been identified as causes for medical errors:

- *Skills-based failures.* Skills-based failures occur because a health care worker failed to perform a skill or procedure properly. These often occur in a skill that is almost automatic to a provider and can occur when the provider's "routine" is interrupted.

- *Rules-based failures.* All health care systems, including EMS, have rules in place to ensure safety and prevent medical errors. Rules-based failures occur when a provider fails to follow the relevant rule, misapplies a good rule, or applies a bad rule.

- *Knowledge-based failures.* Knowledge-based failures are the most complex of the three causes of medical errors. They primarily result from insufficient information or misinterpreting the situation. They tend to occur when the provider is stressed or pressured. They can also occur when a provider thinks his judgment is "error proof"—a narcissistic trait.[34]

Although medical errors can occur at any time, some high-risk areas of EMS practice have been identified. These include:

- *Hand-off.* The transfer of patient care and the patient from an EMS crew to hospital staff is called the hand-off. During this time essential information about the patient must be communicated. The failure to provide information by the EMS crew and the failure to receive (or ask for) information by the hospital staff can lead to misunderstanding and possible errors.[35]

- **Communications issues.** As with hand-off, the failure to communicate with family members, other responders, and hospital personnel can lead to misunderstandings and medical errors.

- **Medication issues.** Medications can heal, but they can also kill. Because of the large number of medications used in EMS, there is always the potential for error. Common errors include administering the wrong medication, administering the wrong dose of the right medication, or failing to administer a medication. Every paramedic must understand his responsibilities when given the authority to administer medications and treatment.

- **Airway issues.** Prehospital airway management has come under increased scrutiny following several studies that showed that patient outcomes are often not improved with endotracheal intubation.[36] The failure to recognize improper placement of an endotracheal tube (e.g., esophageal intubation) has been an ongoing issue in EMS and a source of malpractice litigation. Airway management is a skill that must be mastered, performed flawlessly, and carefully documented. Airway errors are often fatal and can be prevented.

- **Dropping patients.** Physically dropping a patient is not uncommon and not limited to emergency responses. There are several occasions in emergency care when patients are dropped—the most common being loading and unloading the patient into and out of the ambulance.

- **Ambulance crashes.** There has been an alarming increase in ambulance crashes in the last decade and the causes appear multifactorial. We are learning that most modern American ambulances are not particularly crashworthy, and there are strategies being developed to address this. Most ambulance crashes can be avoided by following established guidelines and procedures.

- **Spinal immobilization.** Spinal immobilization is often considered a high-risk endeavor because the consequences of spinal injury are life changing for the victim. Various spinal immobilization protocols and practices have been put in place to help address this issue.

- **Death Pronouncements.** It is not uncommon for paramedics to encounter a patient who is clearly dead or who has what appears to be obviously mortal injuries. However, EMS personnel often arrive minutes after the onset of the problem and initial findings may not accurately indicate what will eventually happen to the patient. There have been many reports where paramedics have declared a patient dead and the patient was later found to be alive. Such an error is fodder for the media. EMS systems should have a protocol and practices to ensure that death pronouncement is accurate.

Medical error prevention is an important part of EMS. There are several practices that will help with this. One is to address possible EMS environmental issues that can lead to errors. In order to minimize these, an EMS system must have clear protocols and they must be fully understood by all providers. When procedures are performed there must be adequate lighting to ensure the procedure can be carried out safely. There should be minimal interruptions (to the degree possible). Standardization and organization of drugs and their packaging can help to minimize medication errors—a major problem in EMS and health care.

Besides environmental strategies, the individual provider must also address medical error prevention. Medical errors can be minimized if the provider always reflects on what they are planning to do. They should also constantly question assumptions. Often initial assumptions as to patient condition and needed treatment change as more is learned about the patient and his condition. Tools to help in decision making and prompts (checklists, electronic reminders) can help reduce medical errors (a strategy gleaned from the aviation industry). Also, simply asking for help when a question arises can effectively reduce medical errors. While there has been a decrease in the routine use of on-line medical oversight, virtually all EMS systems have a medical director available to answer questions. A practice called "time outs" is now routinely used in the operating room to help minimize errors—particularly when medical procedures are involved. Before beginning the actual procedure, all involved take a "time out" and ensure that everything is in order—the right patient, the correct supplies, the correct personnel, and so on. This methodology can be applied to certain aspects of EMS, particularly high-risk procedures.

Medical errors are common and pose a clear and present danger for our patients. Just as airline pilots use strategies to maximize safety, EMS providers should also actively employ strategies and procedures that will help to minimize medical errors. One of the best strategies is simply: when in doubt, ask for help!

Research

A formal, ongoing **research** program is an essential component of the EMS system for moral, educational, medical, financial, and practical reasons. The future enhancement of EMS is strongly dependent on the availability of quality research.[37] Future changes in EMS procedures, techniques, and equipment must be evaluated to prove they make a positive difference prior to implementation. The current trend of introducing "new and improved" ideas or new "high-tech" equipment to existing procedures must be evaluated scientifically. Unfortunately, many EMS protocols and procedures in use today have evolved without clinical evidence of usefulness, safety, or benefit to the patient.

One particular area that will rely heavily on research is funding. As managed care increases its influence on the delivery of emergency care, EMS systems will be forced to scientifically validate their effectiveness and necessity. The restrictions on reimbursement by managed care organizations and governmental agencies will drive the need for quality EMS research. Outcome studies will also be required to justify funding and ensure the future of EMS (Figure 2-19 ●).

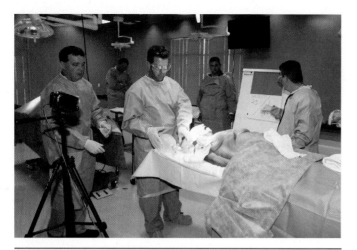

● **Figure 2-19** The future of EMS will be driven by research and paramedics should try to participate in research projects when possible. (© *Dr. Bryan E. Bledsoe*)

Future EMS research must address the following issues: Which prehospital interventions actually reduce morbidity and mortality? Are the benefits of certain field procedures worth the potential risks? What is the cost-benefit ratio of sophisticated prehospital equipment and procedures? Is field stabilization possible, or should paramedics begin immediate transport in every case?

Paramedics can play a valuable role in data collection, evaluation, and interpretation of research. The components of a research project include the following:

● Identify a problem, explain the reason for the proposed study, and state the hypothesis or a precise question.

● Identify the body of published knowledge on the subject.

● Select the best design for the study, clearly outline all logistics, examine all patient-consent issues, and get them approved through the appropriate investigational review process.

● Begin the study, and collect raw data.

● Analyze and correlate your data in a statistical application.

● Assess and evaluate the results against the original hypothesis or question.

● Write a concise, comprehensive description of the study for publication in a medical journal.

Current EMS practice must be justified by hard clinical data derived from an objective, valid program of ongoing research. EMS providers at all levels share the responsibility for identifying research opportunities, conducting peer review programs, and publishing the results of their projects. As leaders in the prehospital care environment, paramedics should set an example in the development of and participation in research projects.[37] For a more detailed discussion of research in EMS, see Chapter 5.

Evidence-Based Medicine

A movement has been building in the house of medicine called **evidence-based medicine (EBM)**. This movement has been widely embraced by those in emergency medicine. It is only logical that the principles of EBM be applied to EMS. After all, EMS is an extension of the practice of emergency medicine. There is really nothing all that new about EBM. Its roots can be traced back to the mid-nineteenth century and beyond. The current resurgence of EBM began in Great Britain and has spread throughout the medical world.

EBM is the conscientious, explicit, and judicious use of the current best scientific evidence in making decisions about the care of individual patients. It requires combining clinical expertise with the best available clinical evidence from systematic research. Thus, to practice effective EBM, EMS personnel must first be proficient in prehospital care and exercise sound clinical judgment. These traits can be developed only by following a comprehensive initial education program, followed by clinical experience and practice.

To move to the next level, prehospital personnel must be familiar with the current and past research pertinent to prehospital care and be able to integrate that knowledge into the care of individual patients. An essential skill is knowing how to read and interpret the scientific literature and to determine whether the information is sound. (Again, refer to Chapter 5, which discusses how to read and evaluate research.)

External clinical evidence can invalidate previously accepted treatments and procedures and replace them with new ones that are more powerful, more effective, and safer. Good paramedics can become excellent paramedics by using both their clinical expertise and the best available external evidence. In today's medical setting, neither clinical experience nor external evidence alone is enough; there must always be a balance between the two.

Some might say that EBM is simply "cookbook" medicine. This is simply not true. As previously noted, EBM requires paramedics to be, first, clinically proficient. Anybody can follow simple "cookbook" directions and provide some level of patient care. But to achieve excellent patient care, external evidence can inform but never replace the individual paramedic's clinical expertise. Clinical expertise is required to form the best determination of the optimum treatment for each individual patient.

There has been a trend in EMS over the last decade or so to study the various practices and procedures of prehospital care. When studied, some treatments, such as pneumatic anti-shock garments (PASG), did not stand up to the test. Likewise, some treatments, such as early defibrillation, were found to have a significant positive impact on survival following out-of-hospital cardiac arrest. Looking at this from a different perspective, by using the best research data available, we were able to abandon a practice (PASG) that helped few if any patients. Later, we were able to embrace a practice (early defibrillation) that has saved countless lives through diverse programs that include bystander defibrillation.

Practicing EBM helps to ensure that we are providing our patients the best possible care at the lowest possible price.

System Financing

At present in the United States, there are a wide variety of EMS system designs. EMS can be hospital–based, fire or police department–based, a municipal service, a private commercial business, a volunteer service, or some combination. Major differences exist in methods of EMS system finance, too. They range from fully tax-subsidized municipal systems to all-volunteer squads supported solely by contributions.

EMS funding can come from many sources. However, the most common is fee-for-service revenue, which may be generated from Medicare, Medicaid, private insurance companies, specialty service contracts, or private paying patients. Most of these sources of revenue are referred to as "third-party payers," because payment comes from someone other than the patient. To date, almost all third-party payers require the patient to be transported or the EMS service will not be compensated for a response. Reimbursement may also be based on the level of care the patient receives during transport. For the most part, third-party reimbursement rarely covers the expenses of operating an EMS system. Because of this, many EMS systems are subsidized by local taxing entities (e.g., city or county government) to remain operational. For the most part, funding has been, and remains, one of the biggest problems faced by EMS systems.

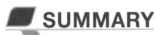 SUMMARY

The evolution of EMS has occurred over thousands of years. Many of its innovations are the result of lessons learned from military conflicts. EMS today is also largely the result of federal legislation and investment from private foundations.

A comprehensive EMS system has many components. EMS provides a continuum of care that extends from the EMT who conducts public education classes to the mechanic who keeps the ambulance fleet running; from the Emergency Medical Dispatcher who calms a distressed caller to the emergency department physician, surgeon, and physical therapist who see the patient through to definitive care and rehabilitation. No one component, no one person, is more important than another. EMS is a total team effort.

EMS systems are designed with the patient as the highest priority. Each system has an administrative agency, which structures the system around the community's needs and grants the medical director ultimate authority in all issues of patient care.

Most EMS systems may be activated by way of a single, universal number (911). They rely on a centralized communications center, which handles all medical emergencies in the area and coordinates all levels of communication—operational and medical—within a region. The goal of an emergency response is BLS care in less than 4 minutes and ALS care in less than 8 minutes after the onset of an event. Coordination of ground and air transport follows established protocols at the communications center.

Mutual-aid agreements ensure a continuum of care during multiple-casualty incidents. Disaster plans are formalized, rehearsed regularly, continuously evaluated, and revised when necessary. Hospitals are categorized according to their readiness to provide essential and specialty services within a region. EMS providers are trained according to U.S. DOT Instructional Guidelines. Continuing education programs encourage providers to achieve excellence.

A continuous quality improvement program documents the EMS system's performance. Ongoing research validates the actions of prehospital providers through scientific evaluation. Finally, EMS systems flourish because of strong, stable financial plans that ensure consistent development on a regional, state, and national basis.

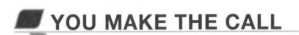 YOU MAKE THE CALL

While you and your family are watching the fireworks display, one of the rockets tips over, shoots into the air, and explodes just above the crowd. There is a mad rush of people, and moments later everyone has scattered, leaving 11 injured people lying on the ground. You and your family are unhurt and move to a safe distance from the scene.

Luckily, the local fire and ambulance service has units on standby at the show. The crews immediately call dispatch and request additional ground and air transport units. The 911 dispatcher puts the region's mass-casualty plan into effect and dispatches the appropriate law enforcement and fire personnel.

Meanwhile, the EMS crews on scene are triaging the patients. Five minutes after the incident, a breakdown of patients is reported to the incident commander. There are seven injured adults: one immediate, three delayed, and three minor. There are four injured children: one delayed and three minor.

It isn't long before the top-priority patient is transported by helicopter to a regional burn center, which is 80 miles from the scene. As the ambulances arrive on scene, the remaining patients are loaded and transported to appropriate receiving facilities. During transport, EMS providers follow local protocols for patient care. One EMS provider radios medical direction for guidance in the care of the youngest injured child. All units radio the receiving facility to provide updated patient information and an estimated time of arrival.

1. Which of the "ten system elements" identified by NHTSA are mentioned in this scenario?

2. For what possible reason was the top-priority patient sent so far from the scene?

3. How important was the role played by the Emergency Medical Dispatcher in this scenario? Explain.

4. How might the EMS system benefit from an evaluation of this incident?

See Suggested Responses at the back of this book.

REVIEW QUESTIONS

1. EMS trauma care generally evolves following:
   a. studies and scientific reviews.
   b. conflicts.
   c. medical consortiums.
   d. quality improvement reviews.

2. Which document published in 1966 outlined the deficiencies in prehospital emergency care?
   a. National Standard Curriculum
   b. Accidental Death and Disability: The Neglected Disease of Modern Society
   c. EMS Agenda for the Future
   d. Consolidated Omnibus Budget Reconciliation Act

3. _____ is a project published in 1996 and supported by the National Highway Traffic Safety Administration.
   a. Emergency Medical Services for Children (EMS-C)
   b. EMS Agenda for the Future
   c. White Paper
   d. OPALS

4. The _____ was established following the terrorist attacks of September 11, 2001.
   a. National Highway Transportation and Safety Act
   b. Department of Homeland Security
   c. National Incident Improvement and Mitigation
   d. Federal Emergency Management Agency

5. An essential, yet often overlooked, component of an EMS system is:
   a. the QI process.
   b. the public.
   c. the medical director.
   d. the training officer.

6. All of the following are components of the communications network of a regional EMS system except:
   a. citizen access.
   b. single control center.
   c. operational communications capabilities.
   d. medical direction.
   e. communications hardware and software.

7. Crucial to the efficient operations of EMS, _____ are responsible for sending ambulances to the scene and ensuring that system resources are in constant readiness.
   a. Emergency Medical Radio Technicians
   b. Emergency Telecommunications Operators
   c. Emergency Medical Dispatchers
   d. Paramedical Telecommunications

8. There are two types of education in EMS: _____ and _____ education.
   a. prehospital, hospital
   b. initial, continuing
   c. clinical, field
   d. initial, hospital

9. The act of receiving a comparable certification or licensure from another state or agency is known as _____.
   a. registration   c. regulation
   b. reciprocity   d. reciprocation

10. Professional organizations that help shape the public perception of EMS include all of the following except:
   a. NASAR.   c. NAEMSP.
   b. NAEMSE.   d. NFPA.

See Answers to Review Questions at the back of this book.

REFERENCES

1. Stout, J., P. E. Pepe, and V. N. Mosesso, Jr. "All Advanced-Life Support vs. Tiered Response Ambulance Systems." *Prehosp Emerg Care* 4 (2000): 1–6.

2. Skandalakis, P. N., P. Lainas, O. Zoras, et al. "To Afford the Wounded Speedy Assistance": Dominique Jean Larrey and Napoleon. *World J Surg* 30 (2006): 1392–1399.

3. Evans, G. D. "Clara Barton: Teacher, Nurse, Civil War Heroine, Founder of the American Red Cross." *Int Hist Nurs J* 7 (2003): 75–82.

4. Barkley, K. T. *The Ambulance*. Kiamisha Lake, NY: Load N Go Press, 1978.

5. Apel, O. F., Jr. and P. Apel. *MASH: An Army Surgeon in Korea*. Lexington, KY: University of Kentucky Press, 1998.

6. Allison, C. E. and D. D. Trunkey. "Battlefield Trauma, Traumatic Shock and Consequences: War-Related Advances in Critical Care." *Crit Care Clin* 25 (2009): 31–45, vii.

7. Elam, J. O., E. S. Brown, and J. D. Elder, Jr. "Artificial Respiration by Mouth-to-Mask Method: A Study of the Respiratory Gas Exchange of Paralyzed Patients Ventilated by Operator's Expired Air." *NEJM* 250 (1954): 749–754.

8. Safer, P., T. C. Brown, W. J. Holtey, and J. Wilder. "Ventilation and Circulation with Closed-Chest Cardiac Massage in Man." *JAMA* 176 (1961): 574–576.

9. National Academy of Sciences, National Research Council. *Accidental Death and Disability: The Neglected Disease of Modern Society*. Washington, DC: U.S. Department of Health, Education, and Welfare, 1966.

10. Pantridge, J. F. and J. F. Geddes. "A Mobile Intensive Care Unit in the Management of Myocardial Infarction." *Lancet* 290 (1967): 271–273.

11. Hirschman, J. C., S. R. Nussenfeld, and E. L. Nagel. "Mobile Physician Command: A New Dimension in Civilian Telemetry-Rescue Systems." *JAMA* 230 (1974): 255–258.

12. Page, J. O. *The Paramedics*. Morristown, NJ: Backdraft Publications, 1979.

13. Harvey, J. C. "The Emergency Medical Services Act of 1973." *JAMA* 230 (1974): 1139–1140.

14. Stiell, I. G., D. W. Spaite, G. A. Wells, et al. "The OPALS Study: Rationale and Methodology for Cardiac Arrest Patients." *Ann Emerg Med* 32 (1998): 180–190.

15. National Highway Traffic Safety Administration. *The EMS Agenda for the Future*. Washington, DC: National Highway Traffic Safety Administration, 1996. [Available at http://www.nhtsa.dot.gov/people/injury/ems/agenda/emsman.html]

16. Department of Homeland Security, Federal Emergency Management Agency (FEMA). *About the National Incident Management System (NIMS)*. [Available at: http://www.fema.gov/emergency/nims/AboutNIMS.shtm]

17. Gausche, M., R. J. Lewis, S. J. Stratton, et al. "Effect of Out-of-Hospital Pediatric Endotracheal Intubation on Survival and Neurological Outcome: A Controlled Clinical Trial." *JAMA* 283 (2000): 783–790.

18. Institute of Medicine of the National Academies. *Emergency Medical Services at the Crossroads.* Washington, DC: National Academies Press, 2006.

19. American College of Emergency Physicians. *The National Report Card on the State of Emergency Medicine.* Irving, TX: American College of Emergency Physicians, 2006.

20. U.S. Department of Transportation/National Highway Traffic Safety Administration. *National EMS Scope of Practice Model*. Washington, DC, 2006.

21. U.S. Department of Transportation/National Highway Traffic Safety Administration. *National Emergency Medical Services Educational Standards: Paramedic Instruction Guidelines*. Washington, DC, 2009.

22. U.S. Department of Transportation/National Highway Traffic Safety Administration. *National EMS Core Content*. Washington, DC, 2005.

23. Munk, M. D., S. D. White, M. L. Perry, et al. "Physician Medical Direction and Clinical Performance at an Established Emergency Medical Services System." *Prehosp Emerg Care* 13 (2009): 185–192.

24. Jensen, J. L., D. A. Petrie, A. H. Travers, and PEP Project Team. "The Canadian Prehospital Evidence-Based Protocols Project: Knowledge Translation in Emergency Medical Services Care." *Acad Emerg Med* 16 (2009): 668–673.

25. Wilson, S., M. Cook, R. Morrell, et al. "Systematic Review of the Evidence Supporting the Use of Priority Dispatch of Emergency Ambulances." *Prehosp Emerg Care* 6 (2002): 42–49.

26. Pons, P. T., J. S. Haukoos, W. Bloodworth, et al. "Paramedic Response Time: Does It Affect Patient Survival?" *Acad Emerg Med* 12 (2005): 594–600.

27. Blackwell, T. H., J. A. Kline, J. J. Willis, and J. M. Hicks. "Lack of Association between Prehospital Response Times and Patient Outcomes." *Prehosp Emerg Care* 13 (2009): 144–150.

28. Dickinson, P., D. Hostler, T. E. Platt, and H. E. Wang. "Program Accreditation Effect on Paramedic Credentialing Examination Success Rate." *Prehosp Emerg Care* 10 (2006): 224–228.

29. Schneider, C., M. Gomez, and R. Lee. "Evaluation of Ground Ambulance, Rotor-Wing and Fixed-Wing Aircraft Services." *Crit Care Clin* 8 (1992): 533–564.

30. United States General Services Administration. *Federal Specification for the Star-of-Life Ambulance: KKK-A-1822F*. Washington, DC: General Services Administration, 2007.

31. Demetriades, D., M. Martin, A. Salim, et al. "Relationship between American College of Surgeons Trauma Center Designation and Mortality in Patients with Severe Trauma (Injury Severity Score >15)." *J Am Coll Surg* 202 (2006): 212–215.

32. Goldstone, J. "The Role of Quality Assurance versus Continuous Quality Improvement." *J Vasc Surg* 28 (1998): 378–380.

33. National Academies of Science, Institute of Medicine. *To Err Is Human: Building a Safer Health System*. Washington, DC: National Academies Press, 2000.

34. Banja, J. *Medical Errors and Medical Narcissism*. Sudbury, MA: Jones and Bartlett, 2005.

35. Yong, G., A. W. Dent, and T. J. Welland. "Handover from Paramedics: Observations and Emergency

Department Clinical Perceptions." *Emerg Med Australas* 20 (2008): 149–155.

36. Davis, D. P., J. Peay, M. J. Sise, et al. "The Impact of Prehospital Endotracheal Intubation on Outcome in Moderate to Severe Traumatic Brain Injury." *J Trauma* 58 (2005): 933–939.

37. Sayre, M. R., L. J. White, L. H. Brown, et al. National EMS Research Agenda. *Prehosp Emerg Care* 6 (2002): S1–S43.

 FURTHER READING

Bledsoe, B. E. "The Golden Hour: Fact or Fiction?" *Emergency Medical Services (EMS)* 31 (2002): 105.

Bledsoe, B. E. "Searching for the Evidence behind EMS." *Emergency Medical Services (EMS)* 31 (2003): 63–67.

National Academies of Emergency Dispatch. *Emergency Telecommunicator Course Manual.* Sudbury, MA: Jones and Bartlett Publishers, 2001.

Walz, B. *Introduction to EMS Systems*. Albany, NY: Delmar/Thompson Learning, 2002.

3 Roles and Responsibilities of the Paramedic

Bryan Bledsoe, DO, FACEP, FAAEM, EMT-P

STANDARD
Preparatory (EMS Systems)

COMPETENCY
Integrates comprehensive knowledge of EMS systems, the safety and well-being of the paramedic, and medical-legal and ethical issues, which is intended to improve the health of EMS personnel, patients, and the community.

OBJECTIVES

Terminal Performance Objective
After reading this chapter you should be able to explain the roles and responsibilities of paramedics.

Enabling Objectives
To accomplish the terminal performance objective, you should be able to:

1. Define key terms introduced in this chapter.
2. Discuss each of the primary responsibilities of paramedics.
3. Give examples of additional responsibilities of paramedics.
4. Integrate expected characteristics of professionalism into all facets of your practice of paramedicine.
5. Given a variety of EMS scenarios, identify and resolve ethical issues.
6. Give examples of behaviors that demonstrate the expected professional attitudes and attributes of paramedics.
7. Advocate for high standards of professionalism in EMS.

KEY TERMS
allied health professions, p. 48   nature of the illness (NOI), p. 43   pathophysiology, p. 41
mechanism of injury (MOI), p. 43   paramedicine, p. 41   primary care, p. 45

CASE STUDY

The central dispatch center for your city receives a call for a medical emergency. The patient's name, address, and street number appear on the computer monitor, so the dispatcher clicks a mouse and a map of the city appears on screen. In this EMS system, satellites are used continuously to track and monitor the location and availability of emergency vehicles using Automatic Vehicle Location (AVL). The dispatcher selects Medic 49, the unit closest to the scene, and, by way of the computer-aided dispatch (CAD) system, gives them specific directions and patient information.

While the ambulance is responding, the dispatcher talks to the caller and provides him with emotional support and prearrival instructions for immediate patient care.

On arrival, the ambulance personnel find a 66-year-old female patient lying in bed, unable to speak clearly or move the right side of her body. The primary assessment reveals her to be disoriented. It also finds that she has an open airway, a normal rate of breathing, and strong radial and carotid pulses.

Paramedic Bobby Moore directs his partner to place the patient on oxygen and prepare for transport. Then he performs a rapid stroke assessment scoring system, after which he determines that the patient has had a stroke. She is immediately moved to the stretcher and placed into the ambulance. Paramedics determine that the onset of the stroke was probably within the last 45 minutes and the patient is well within the stroke interventional window of 4½ hours.

In the ambulance, the paramedics complete a more detailed assessment and determine that the patient requires transport to a hospital that is an accredited stroke center. During transport, they radio the hospital and report the patient's condition and estimated time of arrival. The hospital activates their "Code Gray" team to await the patient's arrival. Vital signs and pulse oximetry are continuously monitored and an ECG is performed.

After approximately 18 minutes en route, the patient is delivered to the emergency department where the stroke team—the emergency physician and a neuologist—is waiting for her. Forty-five minutes later, after an emergency CT scan of the brain, the patient is receiving interventional therapy to help minimize the size of the injury in her brain. One week later, the patient is discharged to her home with a schedule of appointments for rehabilitation. She has minimal residual deficits. A home health nurse is also scheduled to perform follow-up assessments twice each week.

INTRODUCTION

In the past several years, the United States has seen dramatic changes in the health care delivery system. EMS has not been immune to these changes. Driving forces such as technology, cost, and trends in patient population are forcing change. One such change involves the paramedic, whose roles and responsibilities are dramatically different than they were 10 or 15 years ago.

Today, **paramedicine** is an enormous responsibility for which you must be mentally, physically, and emotionally prepared. You will be required to have a strong knowledge of **pathophysiology** and of the most current medical technology. You will have to be capable of maintaining a professional attitude while making medical and ethical decisions about severely injured and critically ill patients. You will be required to provide not only competent emergency care but also emotional support to your patients and their families.

As a paramedic, the most highly trained prehospital emergency care provider in the EMS system, you will often serve people who are unaware of your knowledge and skills. However, if self-satisfaction and pride in a job well done are rewards enough—and if you have a genuine desire to help people in need—then being a paramedic will be a very fulfilling career.

PRIMARY RESPONSIBILITIES

A paramedic's responsibilities are diverse. They include emergency medical care for the patient (Figure 3-1 ●) and a variety of other responsibilities that are attended to before, during, and after a call.[1, 2]

Preparation

Prior to responding to a call, you must be mentally, physically, and emotionally able to meet the demands of the patient, his family, and other health care providers. Your ongoing training should include aerobics for cardiovascular fitness, exercises for muscle strength and endurance, stretching for increased flexibility, and an understanding of the biomechanics of lifting for prevention of lower-back injuries. Other keys to a successful career are recognizing the effects of stress and practicing ways to alleviate it.

CONTENT REVIEW

▶ Primary Responsibilities

- Preparation
- Response
- Scene size-up
- Patient assessment
- Treatment and management
- Disposition and transfer
- Documentation
- Clean-up, maintenance, and review

You must be prepared. This means making sure that inspection and routine maintenance have been completed on your emergency vehicle and on all equipment. It means restocking medications and intravenous solutions and checking their expiration dates. In addition, you must be very familiar with:

- All local EMS protocols, policies, and procedures
- Communications system hardware (radios) and software (frequency utilization and communication protocols)
- Local geography, including populations during peak utilization times, and alternative routes during rush hours
- Support agencies, including services available from neighboring EMS systems, and the methods by which efforts and resources are coordinated

Response

During an emergency response, remember that personal safety is your number one priority. If your ambulance crashes en route to an incident because of speeding or running red traffic lights, you will be of no benefit to the patient. Responding safely to an emergency will reduce the risk to you, your partners, and other agencies responding to the same incident. Always follow basic safety precautions en route to an incident. Wear a seat belt, obey posted speed limits, and monitor the road for potential hazards.

Just as important as getting to the scene safely is getting to the scene in a timely manner. Make certain you know the correct location of the incident and that the appropriate equipment is en route. Also while you are en route, request any additional personnel or services that you think may be needed; for example, with alcohol- or drug-related issues. Waiting to ask for such assistance until you get to a chaotic scene can only delay the appropriate response. Learn to anticipate potential high-risk situations based on dispatch information and experience. For example, if any of the following is reported, you may need to call for assistance:

- Multiple patients
- Motor-vehicle collisions
- Hazardous materials
- Rescue situations
- Violent individuals (patients or bystanders)
- Use of a weapon
- Knowledge of previous violence

Scene Size-Up

Your primary concern during scene size-up is the safety of your crew, the patient, and bystanders. Identify all potential hazards such as fire, smoke, traffic, bystanders, angry or distraught family members, unstable structures or vehicles, and hazardous materials (Figure 3-2 ●). Never enter an unsafe scene until the hazards have been dealt with. Remember that any scene has the potential to deteriorate, so learn to anticipate problems and be prepared for anything.

When the scene is safe to enter, determine the number of patients. In medical emergencies, there usually is only one. However, in some cases—such as carbon monoxide poisoning or exposure to other toxic substances—it may be necessary to

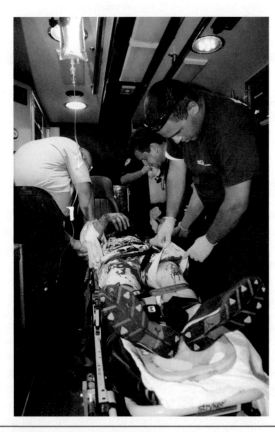

● **Figure 3-1** A paramedic provides emergency care to ill and injured patients—at the scene and in the ambulance. *(© Craig Jackson/In the Dark Photography)*

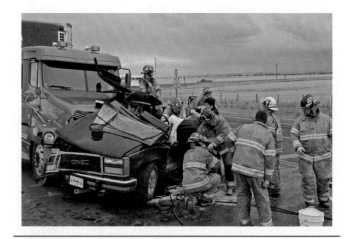

● **Figure 3-2** Always assess the scene for potential hazards as you approach. *(© Kevin Link)*

search the entire area for patients. Once the number of patients and the severity of their illnesses or injuries are determined, quickly request any additional or specialized services required to manage the incident.

The **mechanism of injury (MOI)** or the **nature of the illness (NOI)** also must be identified. For a trauma patient, some mechanisms of injury can be a cause for alarm. For example, a child struck by a fast-moving car is likely to have serious, multiple injuries. Knife and gunshot wounds suggest severe injury to internal organs and life-threatening internal bleeding. How far a patient is found from a collision or explosion, or how far a patient fell from a height, will also indicate how severe an injury may be. For a medical patient, clues identified at the scene can provide important insights into the nature of the illness. Identifying medications, such as insulin, or devices, such as an inhaler, may prevent misdiagnosis and speed the proper treatment of the patient.

Patient Assessment

One of the most critical skills you will learn is patient assessment. Though the order of the steps may vary for trauma and medical patients, the basic components are the same: primary assessment, patient history, secondary assessment, and ongoing assessment. (Volume 3 deals with patient assessment in detail.)

The primary assessment of a patient is usually performed in a scant minute or so. During this assessment, you must note your general impression of the patient's appearance. Then assess the patient's responsiveness; that is, determine if the patient is alert, responding to verbal or painful stimuli, or not responding at all. Finally, you will assess the patient's airway, breathing, and circulation (Figure 3-3 ●). If the patient is in cardiac arrest, circulation takes priority over airway and breathing. If you discover any life threats, you will treat them immediately.

As part of the primary assessment, you will decide whether to continue the assessment on scene or immediately transport the patient to a medical facility. The next step of assessment is gathering the facts of the patient's medical history from the

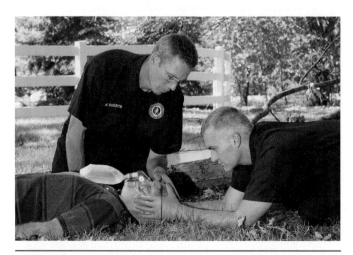

● **Figure 3-3** During the primary assessment of your patient, you will look for and immediately treat any life-threatening conditions.

patient and/or bystanders and performing a physical examination of the patient, with all information recorded and reported to the hospital. It is also the paramedic's responsibility to continuously monitor the patient and provide any additional emergency care needed until the patient is transferred to the care of the hospital's emergency department staff.

Recognition of Illness or Injury

Recognizing the nature of the illness or severity of injury, accomplished during the scene size-up and the primary assessment, is the first aspect of patient prioritization. Most commonly, patient priority is based on the urgency for transport. No matter what method of prioritization your EMS system uses, it is essential that you learn and practice it. Note that the method should be standardized so that all health care professionals within your system understand each other and can respond appropriately.

Patient Management

Almost all EMS systems have a set of protocols that providers follow. As a paramedic, you must always follow your system's protocols. They ensure that various personnel, when presented with the same emergency, will respond in the same manner. Protocols related to patient care also specify when it is necessary for you to communicate with medical oversight. In response, medical direction will give you instructions on how to proceed with emergency care, permission to perform certain procedures, or alternatives to the standard care.

Patient management includes the task of moving the patient from one location to another. In order to do so, you must make sure that the proper equipment is used and that there are adequate personnel available. Remember, back injury is the number one career injury in EMS. Ensure your own safety, and call dispatch for any additional assistance needed whenever you must lift or move a patient.

Appropriate Disposition

The paramedic must ensure, within the constraints of the EMS system and local protocols, that the patient gets to the appropriate facility by the appropriate mechanism of transport. With emergency department crowding on the increase, many EMS systems are looking at strategies to route patients to facilities that may be more appropriate for the patient's specific condition. In some situations, these facilities may not be traditional hospital emergency departments. There are many factors that affect ultimate patient disposition including hospital capabilities, medical staffing, technology, transfer agreements, and reimbursement issues.

Transportation

A critical decision to be made is the mode of transportation for your patient. Time and distance are key factors to consider. For example, if an unstable patient needs to be taken to a facility that is far from the scene, an air medical service—helicopter or fixed-wing aircraft—rather than ground transport may be the best choice. However, there may be only a single receiving facility option if you practice in a rural setting. Know the resources available in your EMS system. Follow all local protocols on their use.

Receiving Facilities

Selecting the appropriate receiving facility for your patient is your responsibility. In order to do so, it is important for you to know which medical facilities in your area offer the following services:

- Fully staffed and equipped emergency department
- Trauma care capabilities
- Operating suites available 24 hours a day and 7 days a week

- Critical care units, such as postanesthesia recovery rooms and surgical intensive care units
- Cardiac facilities with on-staff cardiologists (chest pain centers)
- Designated stroke center
- Acute hemodialysis capability
- Pediatric capabilities, including pediatric and neonatal intensive care units
- Obstetric capabilities, including facilities for high-risk delivery
- Radiological specialty capabilities, such as angiography, computerized tomography (CT), and magnetic resonance imaging (MRI)
- Burn specialization for infants, children, and adults
- Acute spinal cord and head injury management capability
- Rehabilitation staff and facilities
- Clinical laboratory services
- Toxicology, including hazmat decontamination facilities
- Hyperbaric oxygen therapy capability
- Microvascular surgical capabilities for replants
- Psychiatric facilities

Receiving facilities are categorized based on the level of care they can provide. For example, the American College of Surgeons categorizes trauma centers by levels:

Level I The Level I facility is a regional resource trauma center and serves as a tertiary care facility for the trauma care system. Ultimately, all patients who require the resources of the Level I center should have access to it. This facility must have the capability of providing leadership and total care for every aspect of injury, from prevention through rehabilitation. In its central role, the Level I center must have adequate depth of resources and personnel.

A Level I trauma center requires a large number of personnel and an adequate facility for patient care, education, and research. Most Level I trauma centers are university-based teaching hospitals. Other hospitals willing to commit these resources, however, may meet the criteria for Level I recognition.

In addition to patient care responsibilities, Level I trauma centers have the major responsibility of providing leadership in education, research, and system planning. This responsibility extends to all hospitals caring for injured patients in their regions.

Medical education programs include residency program support and postgraduate training in trauma for physicians, nurses, and prehospital providers. Education can be accomplished through a variety of mechanisms, including classic continuing medical, trauma, and critical care fellowships, preceptorships, personnel exchanges, and other approaches appropriate to the local situation. Research and prevention programs, as defined in this document, are essential for a Level I trauma center.

Level II The Level II trauma center is a hospital that also is expected to provide initial definitive trauma care, regardless of the severity of injury. Depending on geographic location, patient volume, personnel, and resources, the Level II trauma center may not be able to provide the same comprehensive care as a Level I trauma center. Therefore, patients with more complex injuries may have to be transferred to a Level I center (for example, patients requiring advanced and extended surgical critical care). Level II trauma centers may be the most prevalent facilities in a community, managing the majority of trauma patients.

The Level II trauma center can be an academic institution or a public or private community hospital located in an urban, suburban, or rural area. In some areas where a Level I center does not exist, the Level II center should take on the responsibility for education and system leadership.

Level III The Level III trauma center serves communities that do not have immediate access to a Level I or II institution. Level III trauma centers can provide prompt assessment, resuscitation, emergency operations, and stabilization and also arrange for possible transfer to a facility that can provide definitive trauma care. General surgeons are required in a Level III facility. Planning for care of injured patients in these hospitals requires transfer agreements and standardized treatment protocols. Level III trauma centers are generally not appropriate in an urban or suburban area where Level I and/or Level II resources are available.

Level IV Level IV trauma facilities provide advanced trauma life support before patient transfer in remote areas where no higher level of care is available. Such a facility may be a clinic rather than a hospital and may or may not have a physician available. Because of geographic isolation, however, the Level IV trauma facility is often the *de facto* primary care provider. If willing to make the commitment to provide optimal care, given its resources, the Level IV trauma facility should be an integral part of the inclusive trauma care system. As at Level III trauma centers, treatment protocols for resuscitation, transfer protocols, data reporting, and participation in system performance improvement are essential.

A Level IV trauma facility must have a good working relationship with the nearest Level I, II, or III trauma center. This relationship is vital to the development of a rural trauma system in which realistic standards must be based on available resources. Optimal care in rural areas can be provided by skillful use of existing professional and institutional resources supplemented by guidelines that result in enhanced education, resource allocation, and appropriate designation for all levels of providers. Also, it is essential for the Level IV facility to have the involvement of a committed health care provider who can provide leadership and sustain the affiliation with other centers.[3]

In addition to designated trauma centers, there may be other facilities that offer unique services. They include burn, pediatric, psychiatric, perinatal, cardiac, spinal, and poison centers.

The best receiving facility is the one best able to care for your patient. Most patients request transportation to the nearest medical facility. However, patients enrolled in managed-care programs, such as health maintenance organizations (HMOs) or designated provider groups, may request transport to a facility approved by their group, which may be a facility other than the nearest hospital. Other patients may ask you to transport them to a facility outside your run area. Even though the requested facility may be appropriate for the patient, there may be an equally appropriate hospital that is closer. Remember, you are responsible for patient care and therefore ultimately responsible for selecting the transport destination. When in doubt, contact on-line medical direction for advice and support.

Other Types of Disposition

In some areas, paramedics provide **primary care**. They have well-defined protocols that allow them to treat patients at the scene and transfer them to facilities other than a hospital. For example, consider a child who cuts his arm on a rusty nail. The father activates EMS by calling 911. When the paramedics arrive, they control the bleeding and perform a patient assessment. They find a simple 2-inch laceration on the child's forearm. Instead of transporting the patient to the hospital and using resources that are not needed for the treatment of this patient, the paramedics contact medical direction and request permission to transport the child to a local outpatient center for treatment. This decision saves the family from paying a costly emergency department fee, and it keeps the emergency department available for a more serious emergency.

Another type of disposition is called "treat and release." In this type of program, paramedics arrive on scene, assess the patient, and provide emergency care. If they determine that there is no need for further medical attention, they contact medical direction and request orders not to transport. In some systems, paramedics may then contact a specialized dispatch center where an office appointment is made with a physician in the patient's area.[4]

While disposition systems such as these are not widely accepted, the increasing numbers of people in managed-care programs (which generally attempt to achieve optimum care while finding ways to control costs) may change that. Innovative programs such as these are setting standards for the future of EMS.

Patient Transfer

The managed-care environment has caused many people—both laypersons and health care providers—to occasionally question whether certain actions that are intended to reduce the cost of medical care are actually in the patient's best interest. For example, to avoid the cost of duplicating equipment and services in a number of facilities that serve the same geographic area, managed-care systems have encouraged facilities to specialize and, often, to transfer patients to a facility that can provide the specific care needed.

Occasionally, there may be a question as to whether the transfer of a patient from one facility to another has been approved for cost reasons but may not actually be in the patient's best interest. When you are assigned to transport a patient, you share responsibility—with the receiving and accepting physician—for the treatment and care of the patient. When you are in doubt about the patient's stability for the duration of transport, or about the capabilities of the receiving facility, contact medical direction.

Prior to removing the patient from a hospital, request a verbal report from the primary-care provider (usually a registered nurse or a physician). This report is often called the "hand-off." Also request a copy of essential parts of the patient's chart, including a summary of the patient's past and present medical history. However, if the results of diagnostic tests taken at the facility are not ready when you are prepared to leave, do not delay patient transport. The data can be faxed, e-mailed, or telephoned to the receiving facility.

Your first priority during transport is the patient. While en route, contact the receiving facility and provide them with an estimated time of arrival (ETA) and an update on the patient's condition. On arrival at your destination, seek out the contact person (usually a registered nurse or physician). Provide that person with an updated patient report, including any treatment or changes in status while en route. All documents provided by the sending facility should be turned over to the receiving care provider along with a copy of your run report. If required by your service, obtain appropriate billing/insurance information at this time.[5]

Documentation

Maintaining a complete and accurate written patient care report is essential to the flow of patient information, to research efforts, and to the quality improvement of your EMS system. The patient care report should be completed in its entirety as soon as emergency care has been completed—no later. Any brief notes that were taken during patient assessment—vital signs, for example—should be copied into the report.

The importance of accurate and complete documentation cannot be overemphasized. Proper recordkeeping helps to ensure continuity of patient care from the emergency scene to the hospital setting. To avoid potential legal problems and embarrassing court situations, record only your observations, not your opinions. For example, do record "patient has an odor of alcohol on his breath." Do not record "patient is drunk." The former cannot be disputed, and the latter cannot be proved. Your final report should be complete, neat in appearance, and written legibly with no spelling errors. This ensures that other health care providers can readily understand your assessment and interventions as well as the patient's responses to your treatment. It is important to note that your patient care report will be a reflection of the emergency care you provided if a lawsuit is filed in the future.[6]

Returning to Service

Once you have completed patient care, turned the patient over to the hospital staff, and completed all documentation, immediately prepare to return to service (Figure 3-4 ●). Clean and decontaminate the unit, properly discard disposable materials, restock supplies, and replace and stow away equipment. If necessary, refuel the unit on the way back to your station or post. Review the call with crew members, including any problems that may have occurred. Such a dialogue can lead to solutions that enhance the delivery of quality patient care. Finally, the paramedic team leader should check crew members for signs of critical incident stress and assist anyone who needs help.

ADDITIONAL RESPONSIBILITIES

The role of the paramedic involves duties in addition to those associated with emergency response. They may include training civilians in CPR, EMS demonstrations and seminars, teaching

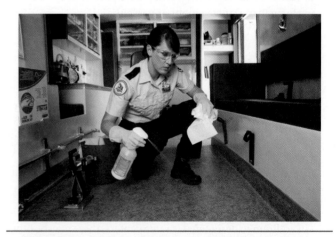

● **Figure 3-4** A paramedic's responsibility does not end with providing patient care. Documentation, restocking, and cleaning of the ambulance and emergency equipment are equally important.

first aid classes, organizing prevention programs, and engaging in professional development activities. All involve taking an active role in promoting positive health practices in your community.

Administration

The paramedic has administrative duties that ensure that the EMS system operates as efficiently as possible. These include such things as station duties, recordkeeping and reporting, special projects, and developing interagency relationships. Station duties include such things as stocking the ambulance, washing and cleaning the ambulance, and general housekeeping. EMS and fire stations are, in essence, a small community, and all members of that community must share housekeeping responsibilities. Recordkeeping is also extremely important to ensure that the system operates cohesively. Much of the necessary EMS system recordkeeping and documentation is electronic and this allows easier data entry and faster sharing of information. Regardless of the type of recordkeeping used, it is an essential part of the job.

Community Involvement

Prehospital providers should take the lead in helping the public learn how to recognize an emergency, how to provide basic life support (BLS), and how to properly access the EMS system. A successful effort can save lives. Providing educational programs can also encourage positive health practices in the community, such as the American Heart Association's "prudent heart living" campaign. EMS injury prevention projects, such as seat belt awareness and the proper use of child safety seats, are essential to the reduction of long-term disability and accidental death.

In order to decide what injury prevention projects need to be developed in a community, EMS systems often conduct illness and injury risk surveys, both formally and informally. For example, consider an EMS service that reviews run reports for a six-month period. They might find that for a single county they responded to ten vehicle collisions at various railroad crossings. A public safety campaign directed at the safe crossing of railroad tracks may be appropriate. Once an EMS service has identified a problem and the target audience, EMS personnel should seek out community agencies—including the local political structure—to assist in the development, promotion, and delivery of the campaign.

Among the benefits of community involvement are the following: It enhances the visibility of EMS, promotes a positive image, and puts forth EMS personnel as positive role models. It also creates opportunities to improve the integration of EMS with other health care and public safety agencies through cooperative programs.

Support for Primary Care

Promoting wellness and preventing illness and injury will be important components of EMS in the future. Some systems have already begun to direct resources toward the development of prevention and wellness programs that decrease the need for emergency services. The theory is to reduce the cost of the services provided to the community by decreasing the burden on the system.[7]

One strategy is to establish protocols that specify the mode of transportation for nonemergency patients. Some systems already operate vans rather than ambulances to transport such patients to and from nursing facilities or from their residences to a doctor's office. Although it is an additional expense to the system, this service reduces emergency equipment costs and the demand for emergency personnel. The result is a decrease in the overall operating expense, which results in an increase in revenue.

Another strategy being used in many areas of the country is having EMS and hospitals team up to provide an alternative to the emergency department. They transport patients to freestanding outpatient centers or clinics, which ultimately reduces the cost of care to the patient and the system. The development of such alliances will undoubtedly continue. However, caution should be taken to ensure that the patient always receives the appropriate emergency care based on need, not cost.

Citizen Involvement in EMS

Citizen involvement in EMS helps to give "insiders" an outside, objective view of quality improvement and problem resolution. Whenever possible, members of the community should be used in the development, evaluation, and regulation of the EMS system. When considering the addition of a new service or the enhancement of an existing one, community members should help to establish what is needed. After all, they are your "customers," and their needs are your priority.[8]

Personal and Professional Development

Only through continuing education and recertification can the public be assured that quality patient care is being delivered consistently. Therefore, after you are certified and/or licensed, you have an important responsibility to continue your personal and professional development. Remember, everyone is subject to the decay of knowledge and skills over time. Use this as a rule of thumb: As the volume of calls decreases, training should correspondingly increase. Refresher requirements and courses vary from state to state, but the goal is the same: to review previously learned materials and to receive new information.

Since EMS is a relatively young industry, new technology and data emerge rapidly. Make a conscious effort to keep up. A variety of journals, seminars, computer news groups, and

CONTENT REVIEW

► Additional Responsibilities

• Community involvement
• Support for primary care
• Citizen involvement
• Personal and professional development

learning experiences are available to help. So are professional EMS organizations, which exist at the local, state, and national levels.

There are other options for keeping up your interest and staying informed, too. By participating in activities designed to address work-related issues—such as case reviews and other quality improvement activities, mentoring programs, research projects, multiple-casualty incident drills, in-hospital rotations, equipment in-services, refresher courses, and self-study exercises—you can expect substantial career growth.

Alternative career paths may be open to you as well. For example, a career paramedic may decide to explore management by applying for a supervisory position or may take a critical care class to prepare for a job on a transport unit. Nontraditional careers for paramedics include working in the primary care setting, providing emergency care on offshore oil rigs, and taking on the occupational-safety role in an industrial setting.

PROFESSIONALISM

A paramedic is a member of the health care professions. Note that the word *profession* refers to the existence of a specialized body of knowledge or skills. Generally self-regulating, a profession will have recognized standards, including requirements for initial and ongoing education. When you have satisfied the initial education requirements for your training as a paramedic, you may then be either certified or licensed. The EMS profession has regulations that ensure that members maintain standards. For the paramedic, these regulations come in the form of periodic recertification with a specified amount of continuing education time.

In addition, the term *professionalism* refers to the conduct or qualities that characterize a practitioner in a particular field or occupation. Health care professionals promote quality patient care and generate pride in their profession. They set and strive for the highest standards. They earn the respect and confidence of team members and the public by performing their duties to the best of their ability. Attaining professionalism is not easy.

It requires an understanding of what distinguishes the professional from the nonprofessional.[9]

Professional Ethics

Ethics are the rules or standards that govern the conduct of members of a particular group or profession. Physicians have long subscribed to a body of ethical standards developed primarily for the benefit of the patient. These standards cover the allied health professions, such as paramedic, respiratory therapist, and physical therapist. Ethics are not laws, but they are standards for honorable behavior. Conformity to ethical standards is expected. As members of an allied health profession, paramedics must recognize a responsibility not only to patients, but also to society, to other health professionals, and to themselves.[10]

In 1948, the World Medical Association adopted the "Oath of Geneva" (Figure 3-5 ●). In 1978, the National Association of Emergency Medical Technicians adopted the "EMT Code of Ethics" (Figure 3-6 ●). These documents detail the guiding principles for professional EMT service.

Professional Attitudes

A commitment to excellence is a daily activity. While on duty, health care professionals place their patients first; nonprofessionals place their egos first. True professionals establish excellence as their goal and never allow themselves to become complacent about their performance. They practice their skills to the point of mastery and then keep practicing them to stay sharp and improve. They also take refresher courses seriously, because they know they have forgotten a lot and because they are eager for new information. Nonprofessionals believe their skills will never fade.

Professionals set high standards for themselves, their crew, their agency, and their system. Nonprofessionals aim for the minimum standard and can be counted on to take the path of least resistance. Professionals critically review their performance, always seeking ways to improve. Nonprofessionals look to protect themselves, hide their inadequacies, and place blame on others. Professionals check out all equipment prior to the emergency response. Nonprofessionals hope that everything

---

OATH OF GENEVA

I solemnly pledge myself to consecrate my life to the service of humanity; I will give to my teachers the respect and gratitude which is their due; I will practice my profession with conscience and dignity; the health of my patient will be my first consideration; I will respect the secrets which are confided in me; I will maintain by all the means in my power the honor and noble traditions of the medical profession; my colleagues will be my brothers; I will not permit considerations of religion, nationality, race, party, politics, or social standing to intervene between my duty and my patient; I will maintain the utmost respect for human life from the time of conception; even under threat, I will not make use of my medical knowledge contrary to the laws of humanity. I make these promises solemnly, freely and upon my honor.

● **Figure 3-5** The Oath of Geneva.

EMT CODE OF ETHICS

Professional status as an Emergency Medical Technician-Paramedic is maintained and enriched by the willingness of the individual practitioner to accept and fulfill obligations to society, other medical professionals, and the profession of Emergency Medical Technician. As an Emergency Medical Technician at the basic level or an Emergency Medical Technician-Paramedic, I solemnly pledge myself to the following code of professional ethics:

A fundamental responsibility to the Emergency Medical Technician is to conserve life, to alleviate suffering, to promote health, to do no harm, and to encourage the quality and equal availability of emergency medical care.

The Emergency Medical Technician provides services based on human need, with respect for human dignity, unrestricted by consideration of nationality, race, creed, color, or status.

The Emergency Medical Technician does not use professional knowledge and skills in any enterprise detrimental to the public well being. The Emergency Medical Technician respects and holds in confidence all information of a confidential nature obtained in the course of professional work unless required by law to divulge such information.

The Emergency Medical Technician, as a citizen, understands and upholds the law and performs the duties of citizenship; as a professional, the Emergency Medical Technician has the never-ending responsibility to work with concerned citizens and other health care professionals in promoting a high standard of emergency medical care to all people.

The Emergency Medical Technician shall maintain professional competence and demonstrate concern for the competence of other members of the Emergency Medical Services health care team. An Emergency Medical Technician assumes responsibility in defining and upholding standards of professional practice and education.

The Emergency Medical Technician assumes responsibility for individual professional actions and judgement, both in dependent and independent emergency functions, and knows and upholds the laws which affect the practice of the Emergency Medical Technician.

The Emergency Medical Technician has the responsibility to be aware of and participate in matters of legislation affecting the Emergency Medical Technician and the Emergency Medical Services System.

The Emergency Medical Technician adheres to standards of personal ethics which reflect credit upon the profession.

Emergency Medical Technicians, or groups of Emergency Medical Technicians, who advertise professional services, do so in conformity with the dignity of the profession.

The Emergency Medical Technician has an obligation to protect the public by not delegating to a person less qualified, any service which requires the professional competence of an Emergency Medical Technician.

The Emergency Medical Technician will work harmoniously with and sustain confidence in Emergency Medical Technician associates, the nurse, the physician, and other members of the Emergency Medical Services health care team.

The Emergency Medical Technician refuses to participate in unethical procedures, and assumes the responsibility to expose incompetence or unethical conduct of others to the appropriate authority in a proper and professional manner.

National Association of Emergency Medical Technicians

● **Figure 3-6**   The EMT Code of Ethics. *(Written by: Charles B. Gillespie, M.D. Adopted by the National Association of Emergency Medical Technicians (NAEMT), 1978. Reprinted with permission by NAEMT)*

will work, supplies will be in place, batteries will be charged, and oxygen levels will be adequate.

A professional paramedic is responsible for acting in a professional manner both on and off duty. Remember, the community you serve will judge other EMS providers, the service you work for, and the EMS profession as a whole by your actions.

Professionalism is an attitude, not a matter of pay. It cannot be bought, rented, or faked. Although it is a young industry, EMS has achieved recognition as a bona fide allied health profession. Gaining professional stature is the result of many hard-working, caring individuals who refused to compromise their standards. Always strive to maintain that level of performance and commitment.

Professional Attributes

There are several traits and attitudes that characterize a professional. True EMS professionals exemplify the traits detailed in the following table (Table 3-1).

CONTENT REVIEW

▶ Professional Attributes

- Leadership
- Integrity
- Empathy
- Self-motivation
- Professional appearance and hygiene
- Self-confidence
- Communication skills
- Time-management skills
- Diplomacy in teamwork
- Respect
- Patient advocacy
- Careful delivery of service

TABLE 3-1 | Attributes of a Health Care Professional
Respects the patient
Provides quality patient care
Advocates for the patient (and his family)
Instills pride in the profession
Strives for high standards and has a commitment to excellence
Earns respect of others
Minimizes pain and suffering
Places patient safety above all but personal safety
Maintains a professional image and behavior
Excellent time manager
Works well with other team members

Leadership

Leadership is an important but often forgotten aspect of paramedic training. Paramedics are the prehospital team leaders (Figure 3-7 ●). They must develop a leadership style that suits their personalities and gets the job done. Although there are many successful styles of leadership, certain characteristics are common to all great leaders. They include:

- Self-confidence
- Established credibility
- Inner strength
- Ability to remain in control
- Ability to communicate
- Willingness to make a decision
- Willingness to accept responsibility for the consequences of the team's actions

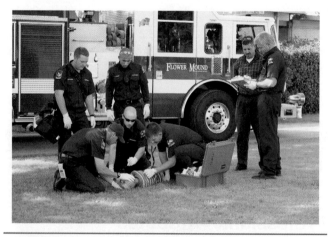

● **Figure 3-7** As leader of the EMS team, the paramedic must interact with patients, bystanders, and other rescue personnel in a professional and efficient manner.

The successful team leader knows the members of the crew, including each one's capabilities and limitations. Ask crew members to do something beyond their capabilities and they will question your ability to lead, not their ability to perform.[11]

Integrity

Paramedics assume the leadership role for patient care in the prehospital setting. As a paramedic, you represent the EMS service and the health care system. The patient and other members of the health care team assume you are sincere and trustworthy. The single most important behavior that you will be judged by is honesty. The environment you work in will often put you in the patient's home or in charge of the patient's wallet and other personal possessions, such as jewelry and items left in a vehicle. You must be trustworthy. The easiest way for a paramedic to lose respect is to be dishonest.[12]

A paramedic functions as an extension of the system's medical director, with authority delegated by the medical director. Because you may be practicing in an area that is remote from your medical director, you will be depended on to follow protocols and accurately document all patient care.

Empathy

Successfully interacting with a patient and family is a challenging skill to master. One of the most important components is empathy. To have empathy is to identify with and understand the circumstances, feelings, and motives of others. To be considered a professional, you will often have to place your own feelings aside to deal with others, even when you are having a bad day. Paramedics who act in a professional manner can show empathy by:

- Being supportive and reassuring
- Demonstrating an understanding of the patient's feelings and the feelings of the family
- Demonstrating respect for others
- Having a calm, compassionate, and helpful demeanor

Self-Motivation

The environment in which you work is often unsupervised, so it is up to you to be able to motivate yourself and establish a positive work ethic. Examples of a positive work ethic are:

- Completing assigned duties without being asked or told to do so
- Completing all duties and assignments without the need for direct supervision
- Correctly completing all paperwork in a timely manner
- Demonstrating a commitment to continuous quality improvement
- Accepting constructive feedback in a positive manner
- Taking advantage of learning opportunities

Self-motivation is an internal drive for excellence. Remember, providing adequate patient care is not enough. You must strive for excellence in the care that you provide.

Appearance and Personal Hygiene

Society has high expectations for everyone in the allied health professions. From the moment you arrive at the scene of an emergency, you are being judged by the way you present yourself. Good appearance and personal hygiene are critical. If you do not look like a health care provider, then your patient may feel you must not be one. If you have a sloppy appearance, your patient may suspect that your medical care will be sloppy, too. Using slang, foul, abusive, or off-color language is not acceptable and will alienate you from your patients. Your appearance, as well as your behavior, is vital to establishing credibility and instilling confidence.

A paramedic should always wear a clean, pressed uniform and should always be well groomed. Hair should be kept off the collar. If facial hair is allowed, it should be kept neat and trimmed. A light-colored tee shirt may be worn under your uniform shirt, which should be buttoned up, with only the top collar button open. Jewelry, other than a wedding ring, a watch, or small plain earrings, is unprofessional. Long fingernails that have the potential to puncture protective gloves also should be avoided.

Self-Confidence

Having confidence in yourself and your abilities is very important. The patient and family will not trust you if they sense you do not trust yourself. A lack of self-confidence shows and is the basis of many lawsuits. The easiest way to gain self-confidence is to accurately assess your strengths and limitations, and then seek every opportunity to improve any weaknesses. Also, keep in mind that self-confidence does not equal cockiness. When a self-confident paramedic is presented with a complex situation, he will ask for assistance.

Communication

Communication is a skill often underestimated in EMS services. Providing emergency care in the prehospital environment requires constant communication with the patient, family, and bystanders, as well as with other EMS providers and rescuers from other public agencies.

To be an effective communicator, the paramedic should remember to gather all patient information and present it in a clear and concise format. Speaking clearly, listening actively, and writing legibly are obviously very important skills. Remember, too, to speak in a way that is appropriate for your audience. For example, just as you would not refer to a laceration as a "booboo" when consulting with a physician, you should not use complicated medical terminology to explain a procedure to an injured child.

Being able to adjust your communication strategies to various situations is also an important skill. For example, learning a manual alphabet (sign language) or learning simple medical questions in foreign languages common in your area are just two ways to prepare yourself.

Time Management

Good time-management skills are important to the paramedic. The experienced paramedic who plans ahead, prioritizes tasks, and organizes them to make maximum use of time will generally be more effective in the field. A paramedic with good time-management skills is punctual for shifts and meetings and completes tasks such as paperwork and maintenance duties on or ahead of schedule.

Some simple time-management techniques that you can use are making lists, prioritizing tasks, arriving at meetings or appointments early, and keeping a personal calendar. By implementing just one or two of these techniques, you may find your schedule to be more manageable and less stressful.

Teamwork and Diplomacy

The paramedic is a leader. Leadership implies the ability to work with other people—to foster teamwork. Teamwork requires diplomacy, or tact and skill, in dealing with people, even when you are under siege from the patient or family.

Diplomacy requires the paramedic to place the interest of the patient or team ahead of his own interests. It means listening to others, respecting their opinions, and being open-minded and flexible when it comes to change. A strong leader of any team realizes that he will be successful only if he has the support of all team members. A confident leader will:

- Place the success of the team ahead of personal self-interests
- Never undermine the role or opinion of another team member
- Provide support for members of the team, both on and off duty
- Remain open to suggestions from team members and be willing to change for the benefit of the patient
- Openly communicate with everyone
- Above all, respect the patient, other care providers, and the community you serve

Respect

To respect others is to show—and feel—deferential regard, consideration, and appreciation for others. A paramedic respects all patients, and provides the best possible care to each and every one of them, no matter what their race, religion, sex, age, or economic condition. Showing that you care for a patient's or family member's feelings, being polite, and avoiding the use of demeaning or derogatory language toward even the most difficult patients are simple ways to demonstrate respect. By demonstrating respect, you will earn credit for yourself, your service, and the EMS profession.

Patient Advocacy

A paramedic is also an advocate for patients, defending them, protecting them, and acting in their best interests. For example, as a paramedic you should not allow your personal biases (religious, ethical, political, social, or legal) to interfere with proper emergency care of your patients. Except when your safety is threatened, you should always place the needs of your patient above your own self-interests. In addition, always keep a patient's health care information confidential. (Refer to Chapter 7, "Medical/Legal Aspects of Prehospital Care," and Chapter 8, "Ethics in Paramedicine," for details about patient confidentiality.)

Careful Delivery of Service

Professionalism requires the paramedic to deliver the highest quality of patient care with very close attention to detail. Examples of behaviors that demonstrate a careful delivery of service include:

- Mastering and refreshing skills
- Performing complete equipment checks
- Careful and safe ambulance operations
- Following policies, procedures, and protocols

Review of individual performance—and attitude—is also important in ensuring that all patients are receiving the proper care in the proper setting. Most EMS agencies have adopted or developed continuous quality improvement (CQI) programs to identify and correct substandard patient care.

Continuing Education

Maintaining certification is the responsibility of the paramedic. Most paramedics use continuing education programs to develop further knowledge or skills in a particular area of emergency health services. This type of education is most often acquired by attending lectures, seminars, conferences, and demonstrations. Each state, region, and local system may have its own policies, regulations, and procedures for recertification. Paramedics cannot work without satisfying those requirements.

There are many benefits to participating in as much continuing education as possible. The most obvious is the expansion of the paramedic's own personal knowledge and skills. Another important reason is to keep up with an emergency health care delivery system that is constantly being updated with more technologically advanced equipment and procedures.

Finally, the skills you learn in this course will need to be practiced. Continuing education programs provide the opportunity to review material and address weak points in patient care.

 CHAPTER REVIEW

SUMMARY

To become a paramedic, you must be willing to accept the responsibility of being a leader in the prehospital phase of emergency medical care. Your responsibilities include on-call emergency duties and off-duty preparation. When the emergency call comes in, you must already be prepared to respond. If not, you are likely to be too late.

Most of your time as a paramedic will be spent on preparing yourself to do the job properly—not providing emergency care. If you can accept this reality, and if you are willing to undertake the responsibility of preparing for this dynamic occupation, then you are ready to proceed with your education. Remember: The best paramedics are those who make a commitment to excellence.

YOU MAKE THE CALL

The First Response Ambulance Service receives a call for a patient experiencing chest pain and difficulty breathing. You, as a paramedic, and your EMT partner are immediately dispatched to the scene. While en route, the dispatcher tells you that the patient is a 55-year-old male who has had a sudden onset of chest pain shoveling snow in his driveway and has audible labored breathing. The dispatcher also informs you that the patient has a history of heart disease and routinely takes multiple medications.

Approximately 7 minutes later, your ambulance arrives on scene. You observe that your patient, Mr. Yates, is sitting on his porch clutching his chest. His wife and son are sitting beside him. As soon as you and your partner get out of the unit, the son runs to you and starts yelling, "Hurry!" and "Just get him to the hospital!"

While you are performing a primary assessment of the patient, the son continuously exclaims, "Just load my father and get him to the damn hospital!" In 2 minutes, the primary assessment is complete.

Because of the cold weather, you decide to move the patient into the unit. Once inside the ambulance, you quickly complete the history and physical exam and begin to treat the patient. Meanwhile, the patient's wife and son are outside the ambulance yelling at your partner, "Leave immediately, or we'll sue you!" The patient attempts to calm them but is unsuccessful.

After placing the patient on oxygen and connecting him to the monitor, you open the door and ask the family if they are going to ride in the ambulance to the hospital. Mrs. Yates tells you that she will, and she attempts to enter the unit. She is stopped by your partner, who explains that if she is going to ride with the ambulance, she must ride up front in the passenger seat. She immediately and loudly protests. At this point, you ask your partner to sit with the patient. You exit the unit as your partner enters, and you close the unit door. You quickly but calmly explain to Mrs. Yates that First Response Ambulance Service has a policy that requires her to ride in a seat with a seat belt in place, and that the passenger seat is the only seat available. After you explain that during the transport you will keep her updated on her husband's condition, she reluctantly gets into the front seat.

While en route to the hospital, you establish an IV, administer nitroglycerin and aspirin, run numerous ECG strips, and maintain a close watch on the patient's vital signs. Every few minutes you stick your head up front to inform Mrs. Yates about her husband's condition. About 10 minutes from the hospital, you consult with the emergency department, providing them with an estimated time of arrival, the patient's medical history, and the patient's current status.

On arrival, your partner assists you in unloading the patient. After allowing her to talk with her husband, your partner escorts Mrs. Yates to the hospital waiting area. In the emergency department, you provide the hospital staff with a verbal report and assist them in moving the patient to a stretcher. Then you give a copy of the run report to the unit clerk who is responsible for placing it on the patient's chart. You then walk to the waiting area where you find Mrs. Yates and her son. You take a minute to tell them that Mr. Yates is now in the care of Dr. Zimmer, and that he or one of the staff members will be out to speak with them as soon as an assessment is completed.

You and your partner meet outside the hospital and prepare the unit for the next call. The stretcher is made up, and the unit is cleaned and restocked. While driving back to the station, you discuss the difficulty you both had dealing with Mrs. Yates and her son.

1. What were your key responsibilities in the previously detailed scenario?

2. How should you have prepared yourself mentally and physically for this call?

3. Did you and your partner act professionally? If so, explain how.

See Suggested Responses at the back of this book.

REVIEW QUESTIONS

1. During an emergency response, remember that _____ is your number one priority.
   a. patient care
   b. personal safety
   c. documentation
   d. medical direction

2. The force or forces that caused an injury define the:
   a. nature of illness.
   b. chief complaint.
   c. mechanism of injury.
   d. primary illness.

3. _____ trauma patients have very minor injuries and can wait for treatment, or they are dead and no treatment is necessary.
   a. Priority-1
   b. Priority-2
   c. Priority-3
   d. Priority-4

4. _____ trauma center provides the highest level of trauma care.
   a. Level I
   b. Level II
   c. Level III
   d. Level IV

5. Maintaining a complete and accurate written patient care report is essential to:
   a. research efforts.
   b. the flow of patient information.
   c. the quality improvement of EMS systems.
   d. all of the above.

6. Nontraditional careers for paramedics include:
   a. working in the primary care setting.
   b. providing emergency care on off-shore rigs.
   c. taking on the occupational-safety role in an industrial setting.
   d. all of the above.

7. The term _____ refers to the conduct or qualities that characterize a practitioner in a particular field or occupation.
   a. licensure
   b. registration
   c. professionalism
   d. certification

8. _____ are the rules or standards that govern the conduct of members of a particular group or profession.
   a. Ethics
   b. Morals
   c. Etiquette
   d. Protocols

See Answers to Review Questions at the back of this book.

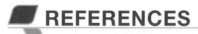

REFERENCES

1. U.S. Department of Transportation/National Highway Traffic Safety Administration. *National EMS Scope of Practice Model*. Washington, DC, 2006.

2. National Registry of Emergency Medical Technicians. 2004 National EMS Practice Analysis. Columbus, OH: National Registry of EMTs, 2005.

3. American College of Surgeons. *Verified Trauma Centers*. [Available at: http://www.facs.org/trauma/verified.html]

4. Feldman, M. J., J. L. Lukins, P. R. Verbeek, et al. "Use of Treat-and-Release Directives for Paramedics at a Mass Gathering." *Prehosp Emerg Care* 9 (2005): 213–217.

5. American College of Emergency Physicians. "Interfacility Transportation of the Critical Care Patient and Its Medical Direction." *Ann Emerg Med* 47 (2006): 305.

6. Harkins, S. "Documentation: Why Is It So Important?" *Emerg Med Serv* 31 (2002): 93–94.

7. Lerner, E. B., A. R. Fernandez, and M. N. Shah. "Do Emergency Medical Services Professionals Think They Should Participate in Disease Prevention?" *Prehosp Emerg Care* 13 (2009): 64–70.

8. Poliafico, F. "The Role of EMS in Public Access Defibrillation." *Emerg Med Serv* 32 (2003): 73.

9. Streger M. R. "Professionalism." *Emerg Med Serv* 32 (2003): 35.

10. Klugman, C. M. "Why EMS Needs Its Own Ethics. What's Good for Other Areas of Healthcare May Not Be Good for You." *Emerg Med Serv* 36 (2007): 114–122.

11. Touchstone, M. "Professional Development. Part 1: Becoming an EMS Leader." *Emerg Med Serv* 38 (2009): 59–60.

12. Bledsoe, B. E. "EMS Needs a Few More Cowboys." *JEMS* 28 (2003): 112–113.

 # FURTHER READING

Bailey, E. D. and T. Sweeney. "Considerations in Establishing Emergency Medical Services Response Time Goals." *Prehosp Emerg Care* 7 (2003): 397–399.

Bledsoe, B. E. "Searching for the Evidence behind EMS." *Emerg Med Serv* 31 (2003): 63–67.

Heightman, A. J. "EMS Workforce. A Comprehensive Listing of Certified EMS Providers by State and How the Workforce Has Changed Since 1993." *JEMS* 5 (2000): 108–112.

Jaslow, D. J., J. Ufberg, and R. Marsh. "Primary Injury Prevention in an Urban EMS System." *J Emerg Med* 25 (2003): 167–170.

National Academy of Sciences, National Research Council. *Accidental Death and Disability: The Neglected Disease of Modern Society*. Washington, DC: U.S. Department of Health, Education, and Welfare, 1966.

Page, J. O. *The Magic of 3 AM*. San Diego, CA: JEMS Publishing, 2002.

Page, J. O. *The Paramedics*. Morristown, NJ: Backdraft Publications, 1979. [No longer available for purchase except as a used book. Entire book can be viewed online at www.JEMS.com/Paramedics.]

Page, J. O. *Simple Advice*. San Diego, CA: JEMS Publishing, 2002.

Persse, D. E., C. B. Key, R. N. Bradley, et al. "Cardiac Arrest Survival as a Function of Ambulance Deployment Strategy in a Large Urban Emergency Medical Services System." *Resusc* 59 (2003): 97–104.

4

Workforce Safety and Wellness

Bryan Bledsoe, DO, FACEP, FAAEM, EMT-P

STANDARD
Preparatory (Workforce Safety and Wellness)

COMPETENCY
Integrates comprehensive knowledge of EMS systems, the safety and well-being of the paramedic, and medical-legal and ethical issues, which is intended to improve the health of EMS personnel, patients, and the community.

OBJECTIVES

Terminal Performance Objective
After reading this chapter you should be able to select behaviors that promote EMS workforce safety and wellness.

Enabling Objectives
To accomplish the terminal performance objective, you should be able to:

1. Define key terms introduced in this chapter.

2. Given a variety of scenarios, recognize potential threats to safety and wellness.

3. Explain the importance of preventing EMS workforce injuries and illnesses.

4. Describe the role and elements of basic physical fitness in EMS workforce safety and wellness.

5. Explain the consequences of addictions and unhealthy habits.

6. Demonstrate work habits that minimize the risk of back injuries.

7. Given a variety of scenarios, select proper Standard Precautions for infection control.

8. Discuss various patient, family, and EMS provider responses to death and dying.

9. Respond professionally and compassionately to patients and family members in situations involving death and dying.

10. Explain the pathophysiology of stress, including stressors, phases of the stress response, signs and symptoms, and consequences of prolonged exposure to stressors.

11. Describe effective stress management strategies.

12. Discuss the effects of shift work on the body and the ability to function effectively.

13. Describe the principles of psychological first aid.

14. Describe the role of disaster mental health services.

15. Given a variety of scenarios, take steps to protect your personal safety, including effective interpersonal relationships and roadway safety precautions.

KEY TERMS

anchor time, p. 71

burnout, p. 71

circadian rhythms, p. 71

cleaning, p. 65

disinfection, p. 66

exposure, p. 66

incubation period, p. 62

infectious disease, p. 62

isometric exercise, p. 58

isotonic exercise, p. 58

pathogens, p. 62

personal protective equipment
 (PPE), p. 62

Standard Precautions, p. 62

sterilization, p. 66

stress, p. 69

stressor, p. 69

CASE STUDY

Howard is a 15-year veteran of a high-volume, inner city EMS service. When he first started his career, Howard thought he knew what he was getting into, but the years have taught him differently.

Right now, Howard is in the spotlight for saving the life of a police officer who was shot in a hostage situation. "That call forced me to reflect on a few important things," he says. "Two years ago, I had a minor heart problem, and it was a good wake-up call. Since then I've been lifting weights and running, so I was able to get to the officer with enough strength to carry him to safety.

"Another thing is that I always use personal protective equipment. I never go to work without steel-toe boots and I never leave the ambulance without a pair of disposable gloves. Can you believe there are still paramedics who knock the concept of infection control? If any one of my partners sticks a needle into the squad bench in my ambulance, they know I'll speak up."

Howard, a mild-mannered, nondescript man, doesn't realize that his young colleagues regard him as a role model. They've seen him handle himself at chaotic scenes as well as when a situation demands sensitivity, patience, and gentleness. "Howard is the man I'd want to tell bad news to my mother," one of his partners says. "He can handle people involved in just about any circumstance—death situations, panicked parents, lonely elderly people, and even hostile drunks. I've never seen anyone treat others with such dignity and respect. He's the best partner anyone could want, especially when we have to manage patients who are thrashing around. But that was not always so, was it, Howard?"

"No, it wasn't," Howard replies. "There was a time when no one wanted to work with me. I was a rebel, and I figured there was only one-way to do things: my way. But an incident that occurred a few years ago changed all that. It's a long story. But the upshot is that when I recovered from the stress, my outlook had been altered. I realized that though I couldn't save the world, I could save myself. That's when I learned how to deal with the effects of a stressful job. I started eating right, lost a bunch of weight, and adopted a new attitude. Anyway, if I can maintain my own well-being, I can do a lot more to help others. Right? Isn't that what we're about?"

INTRODUCTION

The safety and well-being of the workforce is a fundamental aspect of top-notch performance in EMS.[1] As a paramedic, it includes your physical well-being as well as your mental and emotional well-being. If your body is fed well and kept fit, if you use the principles of safe lifting, if you observe safe driving practices, and if you avoid potentially addictive and harmful substances, you stand a chance of having the physical strength and stamina to do the job.

If you seize the information about safe practices and apply them to your life, you will be better able to avoid harm from violent people, roadway hazards, ambulance accidents, and insidious infections. If you let your spirit appreciate the fear and sadness on other faces, you will find ways to combat your prejudices and treat people with dignity and respect. By doing all these things, you will also be able to promote the benefits of well-being to your EMS colleagues.

Death, dying, stress, injury, infection, fear—all threaten your wellness and conspire to interfere with your good intentions. But you can do something about them. Each person has choices about how to live. Every choice has outcomes and consequences. Many patients in nursing homes are living with their choices, paying for lifestyle decisions made decades ago when they were about your age. Is that what you want for yourself?

Most paramedic injuries are caused by lifting and being in and around motor vehicles. Those who train to be physically prepared for their jobs as paramedics stand a better chance of avoiding early forced retirement because of injured backs or knees. Those who train themselves to be mentally alert in the ambulance and at roadway scenes stand a better chance of staying alive and uninjured. Those who can inspire their colleagues to work toward a state of well-being are role models of the highest order.

This chapter introduces the many elements of well-being. If you listen now and enhance your knowledge later, you stand a good chance of enjoying a long and rewarding career of helping others—all because you helped yourself.

PREVENTION OF WORK-RELATED INJURIES

Fortunately, in the twenty-first century there has been a renewed interest in EMS provider safety and injury prevention. Studies have shown that ambulance collisions are a major source of injury for paramedics. Strategies to minimize this have included improving the structural integrity and crashworthiness of emergency vehicles. Also, restraint systems are now available to secure paramedics in the patient compartment while the vehicle is in motion. Since many ambulance accidents occur when emergency lights and sirens are in use, protocols and call screening schemes have been devised to limit the need for these types of responses to patients who actually have a time-critical condition.

The physical act of lifting and moving patients can injure paramedics—especially given the present obesity epidemic in North America. Fortunately, power-lift stretchers are widely available to lift patients once they are on the stretcher. However, in most cases, paramedics must lift patients onto the stretcher and lift the stretcher into the ambulance. Then, once at the hospital, they must lift the stretcher from the ambulance and move it to the ground. Finally, at the bedside, the crew must help move the patient to the hospital bed. Sometimes these lifts and moves are awkward and can result in injury to the provider. Specialized bariatric ambulances with large stretchers, a ramp, and a mechanical winch can help to move the morbidly obese fairly safely. Properly and safely lifting and moving patients is an essential provider skill—regardless of level of training.

Historically, many EMS systems have placed personnel on long shifts, often 24 hours or more, to ensure 24-hour emergency coverage. However, as the volume of EMS calls continues to rise, many paramedics are finding themselves physically and mentally tired long before their shift is over. Also, the lack of sleep has been found to affect the provider's circadian rhythms, causing sleepiness, mental clouding, and lack of energy.[2] These factors can contribute to injury and increase the likelihood of provider injury and illness.[3]

In addition to sleep, nutrition and physical fitness play a role in long-term survival in EMS. While the fire service has long embraced physical fitness, it has only been recently emphasized in EMS. Obese EMS providers caring for and lifting obese patients is a disaster waiting to happen. As EMS providers, it is time we embrace a healthy lifestyle. However, this decision is one that must be made by each individual.

BASIC PHYSICAL FITNESS

Unfortunately, physical fitness has not been a major emphasis in EMS. In a study of back injuries in EMS workers, researchers found that many EMS providers were significantly overweight. This and a lack of general physical fitness were associated with an increase in back injuries.[4] Another study found that physical fitness and satisfaction with current job assignment were modifiable risk factors associated with improvement of back health among EMS personnel.[5]

The benefits of achieving acceptable physical fitness are well known. They include a decreased resting heart rate and blood pressure, increased oxygen-carrying capacity, increased muscle mass and metabolism, and increased resistance to illness and injury. Exercise also slows the progression of osteoporosis, a condition that affects women more often than men. Quality of life is enhanced by physical fitness, too, because of the ability to do more, and there are positive correlations between fitness, personal appearance, and self-image. Other benefits of physical fitness are improved mental outlook and reduced anxiety levels. Finally, a physically fit body enhances a person's ability to maintain sound motor skills throughout life.

Core Elements

Core elements of physical fitness are muscular strength, cardiovascular endurance (aerobic capacity), and flexibility. Like a three-legged stool, if any one of the three is deficient, the whole becomes unstable. Each is equally important.

Be careful about plunging into a well-intended but misguided effort to get in shape. For example, before starting an exercise or stretching regimen, it can be helpful to measure your current state

▶ Dietary Guidelines
  • Enjoy your food but avoid oversize portions
  • Eat more fruits, vegetables, whole grains, and low-fat dairy items
  • Eat less sodium and sugar
▶ Avoid junk foods.

of fitness. There are various methods of assessing the three core elements of fitness. Many EMS agencies have access to facilities where precise assessment methods—with trained personnel—are available. Take advantage of any information available to you.

Muscular strength is achieved with regular exercise that trains muscles to exert force and build endurance. Exercise may be isometric or isotonic. **Isometric exercise** is active exercise performed against stable resistance, where muscles are exercised in a motionless manner. **Isotonic exercise** is active exercise during which muscles are worked through their range of motion. Take time to get in-depth information about the best approach from a trainer or other knowledgeable person.

Weight lifting is an obvious way to achieve muscular strength, and it is excellent all-around training for the body. You can vary the amount of weight lifted, the number of times it is lifted, and the frequency of the demands on the muscle. Whatever type of strength-building exercise is best for you, consider rotating between training the muscles of your upper body and shoulders, muscles of the chest and back, and muscles of the lower body. Do abdominal exercises daily.

Cardiovascular endurance results from exercising at least three days a week vigorously enough to raise your pulse to its target heart rate (Table 4-1). Many people shy away from aerobic exercise, thinking the effort will be too great or the results will take too long. However, there is no need to become a marathon runner to gain aerobic capacity. Try a

brisk walk or ride a stationary bike while watching TV. Make it a daily habit.

Even modest exercise programs, which can be done most days of the week, will improve cardiovascular endurance and muscular strength. Walking briskly from the outer reaches of the employee parking lot, using stairs whenever possible, and playing actively with your children can all "count" toward physical fitness.

Flexibility seems to be the forgotten element of fitness. Without an adequate range of motion, your joints and muscles cannot be used efficiently or safely. A body builder with tight hamstrings may be as much at risk for back injury as anyone else. To achieve (or regain) flexibility, stretch the main muscle groups regularly. Try to stretch daily. Never bounce when stretching; this causes micro tears in muscle and connective tissues. Hold a stretch for at least 60 seconds. A side benefit of good flexibility is prevention or reduction of back pain. Stretching is an excellent TV-time activity. If you are interested, consider studying yoga for improved flexibility.

Nutrition

It is a myth that people in EMS cannot maintain an adequate diet. Even so, the "hit-and-run" nature of emergency care requires planning and awareness of your options. The most difficult part of improving nutrition is altering established bad habits. A change in your behavior requires some commitment and self-discipline, understanding the change process, and patience with what will become long-term self-improvement. Set realistic goals, and understand that backsliding happens. Whatever your goals may be, such as reducing excess weight, gaining weight, or regularly eating more wholesome foods, it is helpful to be able to analyze your progress by using charts or daily intake tallies.

Good nutrition is fundamental to your well-being. The following are dietary guidelines published along with the ChooseMyPlate chart (Figure 4-1 ●) by the U.S. Department of Agriculture.[6]

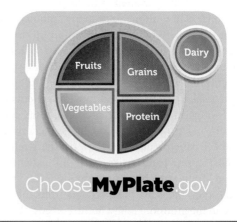

● **Figure 4-1** Dietary guidelines from the U.S. Department of Agriculture are summarized in the ChooseMyPlate chart that uses a dinner-plate-shaped chart to represent appropriate food-group portions. (*USDA Center for Nutrition Policy and Promotion.*)

TABLE 4-1 | Finding Your Target Heart Rate
1. Measure your resting heart rate. (You will use this number later.)
2. Subtract your age from 220. This total is your estimated maximum heart rate.
3. Subtract your resting heart rate from your maximum heart rate, and multiply that figure by 0.7.
4. Add the figure you just calculated to your resting heart rate.
EXAMPLE: In a 44-year-old woman whose resting heart rate is 52, her maximum heart rate would be 176 (220 – 44). Her maximum heart rate minus resting heart rate is 124 (176 – 52). Multiply 124 by 0.7 for a value of 86.8. Resting heart rate plus the calculated figure is 138.8 (52 + 86.8). Rounded up, this person's target heart rate is 140 beats per minute.

Obesity. *Obesity has become a major problem in the United States and other industrialized countries. EMS personnel are not immune to this trend. In fact, EMS personnel are becoming, on the average, progressively more overweight. There are several factors inherent in EMS that can contribute to obesity. First, much of EMS work is sedentary. A great deal of time is spent seated in an ambulance or in a station. Second, physical activity on the job is usually limited to short periods of sometimes intense effort. While these periods of work can be strenuous, they seldom last long enough to provide any significant degree of exercise. Third, the duties of the job often require EMS personnel to "eat on the run," which often means relying on fast food or processed food. These meals provide plenty of "empty calories" and significantly contribute to obesity.*

Obesity can lead to numerous health problems, such as back pain, and can place paramedics at increased risk of sustaining a back injury. Obesity can also lead to cardiovascular disease, diabetes, and other long-term chronic problems. As an EMS professional, you must recognize that, in order to provide the best care for your patient—and to provide a good role model for your patients and the public—you must first care for yourself. This includes watching your weight, finding ways to eat a reasonable diet, and obtaining an adequate amount of exercise. More and more EMS employers are recognizing the obesity epidemic and are developing employee assistance and physical fitness programs designed to minimize the chances of obesity cutting an EMS career short.

10 Tips to a Great Plate

1. *Balance calories.* Find out how many calories YOU need for a day. (Go to www.ChooseMyPlate.gov to find your calorie level.) Physical activity also helps balance calories.

2. *Enjoy your food but eat less.* Take the time to enjoy your food as you eat it. Pay attention to hunger and fullness clues.

3. *Avoid oversized portions.* Use a smaller plate. Portion out foods before you eat. When eating out, choose an appetizer-size portion, share a dish, or take some home for later.

4. *Foods to eat more often.* Eat more fruits and vegetables, whole grains, and fat-free or low-fat dairy products.

5. *Make half your plate fruits and vegetables.* Choose red, orange, and dark green vegetables like tomatoes, sweet potatoes, and broccoli. Add fruit to meals as part of main or side dishes or dessert.

6. *Switch to fat-free or low-fat (1%) milk.* Has the same nutrients as whole milk but fewer calories and less fat.

7. *Make half your grains whole grains.* Eat whole wheat bread instead of white bread. Eat brown rice instead of white rice. Eat oatmeal instead of a sugary cereal.

8. *Foods to eat less often.* Cut back on foods high in solid fats, added sugars, and salt. These include cakes, cookies, ice cream, candies, sweetened drinks, pizza, and fatty meats like ribs, sausages, bacon, and hot dogs. Use these foods as occasional treats, not everyday foods.

9. *Compare sodium in foods.* Use the Nutrition Facts label to choose lower sodium versions of foods like soup, bread, and frozen meals. Select canned foods labeled "low sodium," "reduced sodium," or "no salt added."

10. *Drink water instead of sugary drinks.* Cut calories by drinking water or unsweetened beverages. Soda, energy drinks, and sports drinks are a major source of added sugar and calories.

The standardized Nutrition Facts label provides abundant information about nutritional content. Learn to read it. Be sure to check the serving size to avoid misinterpreting the food's overall nutritional value (Figure 4-2 ●).

Eating on the run can be less detrimental if you plan ahead and carry a small cooler filled with whole-grain sandwiches, cut vegetables, fruit, and other wholesome foods. If you must obtain food during your shift, stop at a local market instead of the fast-food place next door. Buy fresh fruit, yogurt, and sensible deli selections. They are more nutritious and much cheaper than fast foods.

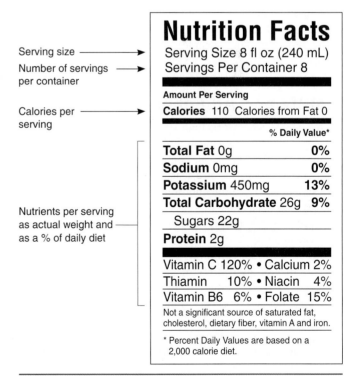

● **Figure 4-2** Example of a standardized food label.

Finally, monitor your fluid intake. Your body needs plenty of fluids to flush food through your system and eliminate toxins. Pay attention to what you are drinking. Fill a "go-cup" with fresh ice water when you stop by the emergency department instead of spending your money on soft drinks. Water is more thirst quenching, cheaper, and much better for you.

Exercising and eating well can help you prevent both cancer and cardiovascular disease. For the typically youthful EMS provider, the likelihood of being hit by either of these diseases may seem remote, but it happens. You can do a lot to prevent these diseases. Minimizing stress through healthy stress management practices, for example, can work wonders. In addition, assess yourself and your family history.

Exercise will improve cardiovascular endurance, help lower blood pressure, and tip the balance of your body composition favorably—all good measures against cardiovascular disease. Know your cholesterol and triglyceride levels and keep them in check. For women who are menopausal, be informed of current research on the risks and benefits of hormone replacement therapy.

Diet can also do much to minimize the chances of getting certain cancers. Certain foods, such as broccoli and high-fiber foods, are thought to help reduce the incidence of cancer; others, such as charcoal-cooked foods, may increase it. The connection between sun exposure and skin cancer is well known. So, take the precaution of using sun blocks, and wear sunglasses and a hat when you can. Watch out for the warning signs of cancer, such as blood in the stools (even in young people, especially men), a changing mole, unexplained weight loss, unexplained chronic fatigue, and lumps.

Be sure to include appropriate periodic risk-assessment screening and self-examination habits in your personal well-being program. That includes tests like mammograms and prostate exams as you gain in years.

Habits and Addictions

Many people who work high-stress jobs overuse and abuse substances such as caffeine and nicotine. These bad habits are rampant in EMS. Each can contribute to long-term diseases such as cancer and cardiovascular disease. Choose a healthier life, and avoid overindulging in these and other harmful substances such as alcohol.

Smoking cessation programs are usually easily accessed in local areas or on the Internet. There are abundant approaches to this common addiction, including medications, behavior modification, nicotine replacement therapy ("patches"), aversion therapy, hypnotism, and "cold turkey." Part of understanding your addiction is knowing whether it is a psychological dependency, sociocultural dependency, or a true physical addiction. Whatever it takes, the message is clear: Get free of addictions, particularly those that threaten your well-being. Substance-abuse programs, nicotine patches, 12-step groups—all exist to help you help yourself. But the first step has to be yours.[7]

Back Safety

EMS is a physically demanding endeavor. Of the host of movements required—scrambling down embankments, climbing ladders or trees, squeezing into narrow spaces, and so on—none will occur more frequently than lifting and carrying equipment and patients. To avoid back injury, you must keep your back fit for the work you do. You also must use proper lifting techniques each time you pick up a load, whether the load is heavy or light.

Back fitness begins with conditioning the muscles that support the spinal column. These are the "guy wires" that stabilize the spine, much the way cables help keep telephone poles upright. Note that the muscles of the abdomen are also crucial to overall spinal-column strength and safe lifting. Never perform old-fashioned sit-ups. They can seriously strain your lumbar spine. Instead, use abdominal crunches, which target only the stomach muscles. Consult an exercise coach or trainer for specifics.

Correct posture will minimize the risk of back injury (Figures 4-3 and 4-4 ●). Good nutrition helps to maintain healthy connective tissue and intervertebral discs. Excess weight contributes to disc deterioration. So does smoking. Thus, proper weight management and smoking cessation are relevant to back health. Finally, adequate rest gives the spine non-weight-bearing time to nourish discs and repair itself.

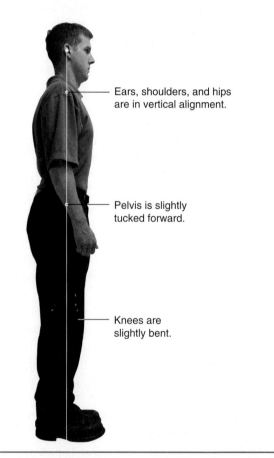

Ears, shoulders, and hips are in vertical alignment.

Pelvis is slightly tucked forward.

Knees are slightly bent.

● **Figure 4-3** Correct standing posture. Note the straight line from ear through shoulder, hip, and knee to arch of foot.

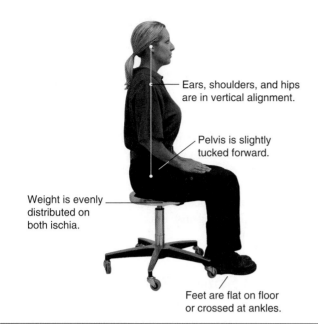

Ears, shoulders, and hips are in vertical alignment.

Pelvis is slightly tucked forward.

Weight is evenly distributed on both ischia.

Feet are flat on floor or crossed at ankles.

● **Figure 4-4** Correct sitting posture.

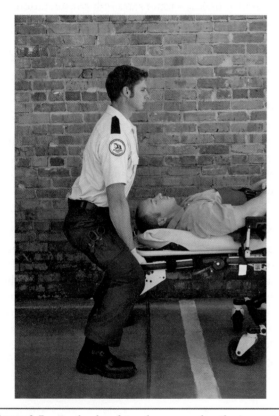

● **Figure 4-5** For back safety, always employ the important principles of lifting.

Proper lifting techniques should ideally be taught by and practiced with a trainer who understands the variety of challenges faced by EMS providers.[8] Important principles of lifting are as follows (Figure 4-5 ●):

● Move a load only if you can safely handle it.

● Ask for help when you need it—for *any* reason.

LEGAL CONSIDERATIONS

● ● ●

Substance Abuse in EMS. *As in the rest of society, substance abuse in EMS is an increasing problem. There is no evidence that substance abuse in EMS is any greater than in other professions. However, the subject has been inadequately studied, and we just don't know. Regardless, there has been an increase in media stories about paramedics stealing and abusing controlled substances such as morphine or fentanyl. Often, clandestine drug use such as this adversely affects patient care. The abuser will often remove the desired drug and replace the drug with water or saline. Another paramedic, unaware of the tampering, may administer the medication to a patient. In this case, the patient will not derive any benefit from the drug and can possibly develop a complication such as infection. Also, if an impaired paramedic is allowed to continue to work, his decision making will ultimately be affected, which can adversely affect patient care.*

Paramedics impaired by substance abuse must be immediately removed from patient care responsibilities while an objective investigation is completed. Substance abuse should be considered a medical condition, a disease, and should be treated as such. This attitude is not intended to excuse illegal behavior such as drug tampering but rather to ensure the paramedic gets the help he needs. States should have a system whereby impaired paramedics can self-report their addiction (or be referred) so that they can obtain the necessary treatment and possibly salvage their careers. These programs, commonly referred to as diversion programs, usually require the impaired provider to enter and complete a substance abuse treatment program. Following completion of the program and other requirements, they may be allowed to return to work under a very strict surveillance program (called an aftercare contract) that includes periodic medical and addiction assessments, randomized observed drug screens, and often participation in 12-step or similar support programs.

Substance abuse is a real problem and must be dealt with swiftly yet compassionately. However, our first consideration should always be the safety of the patient and of coworkers. Diversion programs must be available in each state to preserve the careers of those suffering substance abuse disorders.

● Position the load as close to your body and center of gravity as possible.

● Keep your palms up whenever possible.

● Do not hurry. Take the time you need to establish good footing and balance. Keep a wide base of support with one foot ahead of the other.

● Bend your knees, lower your buttocks, and keep your chin up. If your knees are bad, do not bend them more than 90 degrees.

● "Lock in" the spine with a slight extension curve, and tighten the abdominal muscles to support spinal positioning.

● Always avoid twisting and turning.

● Let the large leg muscles do the work of lifting, not your back.

- Exhale during the lift. Do not hold your breath.

- Given a choice, push. Do not pull.

- Use help when moving patients up and down stairs and into and out of the ambulance.

- Look where you are walking or crawling. If you are walking, take only short steps. Move forward rather than backward whenever possible.

- When rescuers are working together as a team to lift a load, only one person should be in charge of verbal commands.

Heed your own body's signals. You are stronger some days than others. Know when you are physically depleted from exhaustion, lack of food, or minor illness. Use volunteers as helpers wisely, and be sure to ask if their backs are strong enough for the job.

Never reach for an item and twist at the same time. Most back injuries occur because of the cumulative effect of such low-level everyday stresses. Everything you do on behalf of back safety adds up to choices that can mean the difference between a long and rewarding career in EMS, or one shortened by an injury. Be careful!

PERSONAL PROTECTION FROM DISEASE

In recent years the emphasis on infection control has focused on the most devastating diseases, such as HIV/AIDS, hepatitis B, hepatitis C, tuberculosis, and influenza—and rightly so. There is enough risk in EMS without having to worry about dying of a disease you caught while caring for others. Fortunately, there is a lot you can do to minimize your risk of infection. A good first step is to develop a habit of doing the things promoted in this chapter. Eating well, getting adequate rest, and managing stress are among the building blocks of a good defense against infection. In addition, it is a good idea to periodically assess your risk for infection, such as noticing when you are run down or when your hands are dangerously chapped.

Infectious Diseases

Infectious diseases are caused by **pathogens** such as bacteria and viruses, which may be spread from person to person. For example, infection by way of bloodborne pathogens can occur when the blood of an infected person comes in contact with another person's broken skin (cuts, sores, chapped hands) or by way of parenteral contact (stick by a needle or other sharp object). Infection by airborne pathogens can occur when an infected person sneezes or coughs, causing body fluids in the form of tiny droplets to be inhaled or to come in contact with the mucous membranes of another person's eyes, nose, or mouth.

HIV/AIDS, hepatitis B, hepatitis C, and tuberculosis are diseases of great concern because they are life threatening. However, one may be exposed to many different infectious diseases. See Table 4-2 for some common ones, their modes of transmission, and their **incubation periods**.

Even when someone is carrying pathogens for disease, signs of an illness may not be apparent. For this reason, *you must consider the blood and body fluids of every patient you treat as infectious.* Safeguards against infection are mandatory for all medical personnel.

Standard Safety Precautions

Each profession has its occupational hazards and risks. EMS is no different. EMS straddles the disciplines of health care and public safety and the associated risks of both. Anything you do as a paramedic should start with considerations about minimizing risk for you, your patient, your partners, other responders, and the community. Various strategies for this are discussed in detail in this chapter.

Infection Control Measures

Infection control measures are those procedures and practices used by health care personnel to minimize disease transmission and transmission of infectious agents. Infection control is a fundamental tenet of health care and must be practiced proficiently by all EMS personnel.

Standard Precautions

Standard Precautions are strategies that include the major features of what were once called universal precautions (UP)—blood and body fluid precautions designed to reduce the risk of transmission of bloodborne pathogens—and body substance isolation (BSI)—precautions designed to reduce the risk of transmission of pathogens from moist body substances. Standard Precautions apply UP and BSI concepts to all patients receiving care regardless of their diagnosis or presumed infection status. Standard Precautions apply to:

- Blood
- All body fluids, secretions, and excretions except sweat, regardless of whether or not they contain visible blood
- Nonintact skin
- Mucous membranes

Standard Precautions are designed to reduce the risk of transmission of microorganisms from both recognized and unrecognized sources of infection in hospitals.

Standard Precautions dictate that all EMS personnel take the same (standard) precautions with every patient. To achieve this, appropriate **personal protective equipment (PPE)** should

TABLE 4-2 | Common Infectious Diseases

Disease	Mode of Transmission	Incubation Period
AIDS (acquired immune deficiency syndrome)	AIDS- or HIV-infected blood via intravenous drug use, semen and vaginal fluids, blood transfusions, or (rarely) needlesticks. Mothers also may pass HIV to their unborn children.	Several months or years
Hepatitis B, C	Blood, stool, or other body fluids, or contaminated objects.	Weeks or months
Tuberculosis	Respiratory secretions, airborne or on contaminated objects.	2 to 6 weeks
Meningitis, bacterial	Oral and nasal secretions.	2 to 10 days
Pneumonia, bacterial and viral	Oral and nasal droplets and secretions.	Several days
Influenza	Airborne droplets, or direct contact with body fluids.	1 to 3 days
Staphylococcal skin infections	Contact with open wounds or sores or contaminated objects.	Several days
Chicken pox (varicella)	Airborne droplets, or contact with open sores.	11 to 21 days
German measles (rubella)	Airborne droplets. Mothers may pass it to unborn children.	10 to 12 days
Whooping cough (pertussis)	Respiratory secretions or airborne droplets.	6 to 20 days
SARS (severe acute respiratory syndrome)	Airborne droplets and personal contact.	4 to 6 days

be available in every emergency vehicle. The minimum recommended PPE are the following:

- **Protective gloves.** Wear disposable protective gloves before initiating any emergency care. When an emergency involves more than one patient, change gloves between patients. When gloves have been contaminated, remove and dispose of them properly as soon as possible (Figure 4-6 ●).

- **Masks and protective eyewear** (Figure 4-7 ●). These should be worn together whenever blood spatter is likely to occur, such as with arterial bleeding, childbirth, endotracheal intubation and other invasive procedures, oral suctioning, and cleanup of equipment that requires heavy scrubbing or brushing. Both you and your patient should wear masks whenever the potential for airborne transmission of disease exists.

- **HEPA and N-95 masks** (Figure 4-8 ●). Because of the resurgence of tuberculosis (TB), you must protect yourself from infection through the use of a high-efficiency particulate air (HEPA) or N-95 mask. Wear one whenever you care for a patient with confirmed or

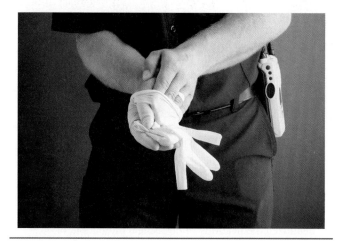

● **Figure 4-6a**   To remove gloves, first hook the gloved fingers of one hand under the cuff of the other glove. Then pull that glove off without letting your gloved fingers come in contact with bare skin.

● **Figure 4-6b**   Then slide the fingers of the ungloved hand under the remaining glove's cuff. Push that glove off, being careful not to touch the glove's exterior with your bare hand.

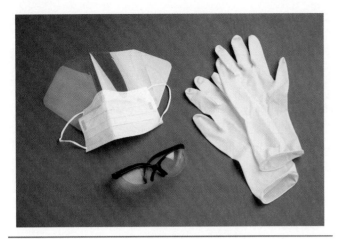

● **Figure 4-7** Proper gloves, eyewear, and mask prevent a patient's blood and body fluids from contacting a break in your skin or spraying into your eyes, nose, and mouth.

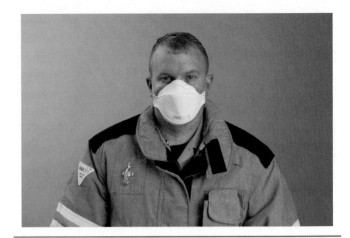

● **Figure 4-8b** An N-95 mask.

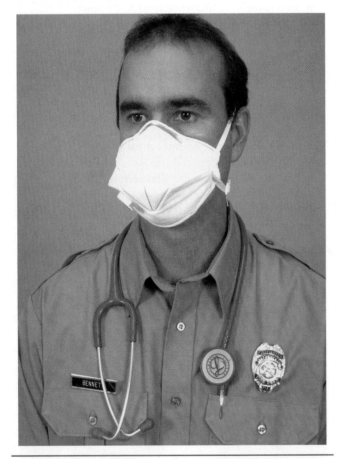

● **Figure 4-8a** A high-efficiency particulate air (HEPA) mask.

suspected TB. This is especially true during procedures that involve the airway, such as the administration of nebulized medications, endotracheal intubation, or suctioning.

● *Gowns.* Disposable gowns protect your clothing from splashes. If large splashes of blood are expected, such as with childbirth, wear an impervious gown.

● *Resuscitation equipment.* Use disposable resuscitation equipment as your primary means of artificial ventilation in emergency care. Such items should be used once, and then disposed of properly.[9]

● *Hand-washing supplies.* Non-water-based hand-washing solutions should be widely available for EMS personnel. These alcohol-based hand sanitizers are available in various forms including gels and prewrapped hand towels. The prewrapped towels can be kept in a pocket for ready use.

The garments and equipment previously described are intended to protect against infection through contact with both potentially contaminated body substances, such as blood, vomit, and urine, and other agents such as airborne droplets. These garments and equipment will assist you in achieving, to the extent possible, the precautions recommended by the Centers for Disease Control and Prevention (CDC).

Infectious diseases also are minimized through the use of appropriate work practices and equipment especially engineered to minimize risk. For example, most invasive equipment is now used on a one-time, disposable basis. Of course, it is important to launder reusable clothing with infection control in mind.

General cleanliness and appropriate personal hygiene will do much to prevent infection. Probably the most important infection control practice is hand washing (Figure 4-9 ●). As soon as possible after every patient contact and decontamination procedure, thoroughly wash your hands. To do so, first remove any rings or jewelry from your hands and arms. Then use soap and water. Lather your hands vigorously front and back for at least 15 seconds up to 2 or 3 inches above the wrist. Be sure to lather and rub between your fingers and in the creases and cracks of your knuckles. Scrub under and around the fingernails with a brush. Rinse your hands well under running water, holding your hands downward so that the water drains off your fingertips. Dry your hands on a clean towel.

Plain soap works perfectly well for hand washing. At those times when soap is not available, you might use an antimicrobial hand-washing solution or an alcohol-based foam or towelette.

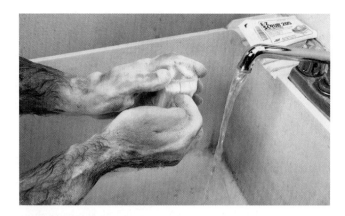

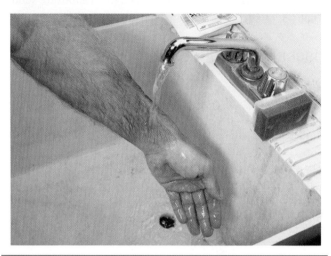

● **Figure 4-9** To wash your hands properly, lather up well and be sure to scrub under your nails. When you rinse off your hands, point them downward so that soap and water run off away from your arms and body.

Vaccinations and Screening Tests

Immunizations against many illnesses are available. Get them. Even "nuisance" illnesses can be avoided if you get vaccinated. Immunizations that are available include those for rubella (German measles), measles, mumps, chicken pox, and other childhood diseases, as well as for tetanus/diphtheria, polio, influenza, hepatitis A, hepatitis B, and Lyme disease. Some, such as tetanus, may require booster shots periodically, so monitor your personal medical history well. Also arrange for routine tuberculosis (TB) screenings and record the results.

Influenza kills thousands of people each year. Some strains of influenza, such as H1N1 (swine flu) or H5N1 (bird flu), can quickly reach pandemic or epidemic states. Health care workers will be among the first to be exposed to novel viruses. Because of this, EMS personnel and other emergency responders are often the first to receive vaccines when a virus becomes a threat. It is important for EMS personnel to follow warnings and recommendations from the World Health Organization (WHO), the Centers for Disease Control and Prevention (CDC), and state and local public health officials.

Decontamination of Equipment

Any personal protective equipment (PPE) designed for a single use should be properly disposed of after use. The same is true of contaminated medical devices designed for a single use. Such materials should be discarded in a red bag marked with a biohazard seal (Figure 4-10a ●). Needles and other sharp objects should be discarded in properly labeled, puncture-proof containers (Figure 4-10b). Once an item is placed in the appropriate container, the container should be disposed of according to local guidelines.

Nondisposable equipment that has been contaminated must be cleaned, disinfected, or sterilized:

● *Cleaning.* Cleaning refers to washing an object with soap and water. After caring for a patient, wash your work areas thoroughly with approved soaps. Throw away single-use cleaning supplies in a proper biohazard container.

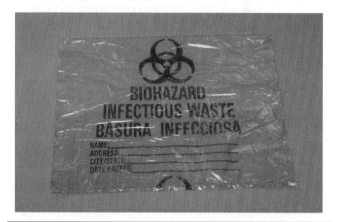

● **Figure 4-10a** Dispose of biohazardous wastes in a bag that is properly marked.

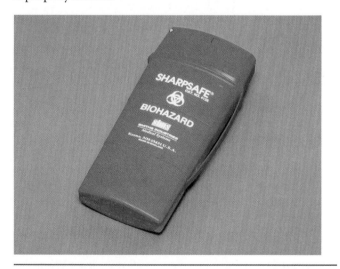

● **Figure 4-10b** Discard needles and other sharp objects in a properly labeled, puncture-proof container.

- *Disinfection.* **Disinfection** means cleaning with a disinfecting agent, which should kill many microorganisms on the surface of an object. Disinfect equipment that had direct contact with the intact skin of a patient, such as backboards and splints. Use a commercial disinfectant or bleach diluted in water (one part bleach to 10 parts water), or follow local guidelines.
- *Sterilization.* **Sterilization** is the use of a chemical or a physical method such as pressurized steam to kill all microorganisms on an object. Items that were inserted into the patient's body (a laryngoscope blade, for example) should be sterilized by heat, steam, or radiation. There are also EPA-approved solutions for sterilization.

If your equipment needs more extensive cleaning, bag it and remove it to an area designated for this purpose. Disposable work gloves worn during cleaning and decontamination should be properly discarded. If your clothing has become contaminated, bag the items and wash them in accordance with local guidelines. After removing contaminated clothing, take a shower before dressing again.

Post-exposure Procedures

By definition, an **exposure** is any occurrence of blood or body fluids coming in contact with nonintact skin or the eyes or other mucous membranes or by parenteral contact (needlestick). In most areas, an EMS provider who has had an exposure should (Figure 4-11 ●):

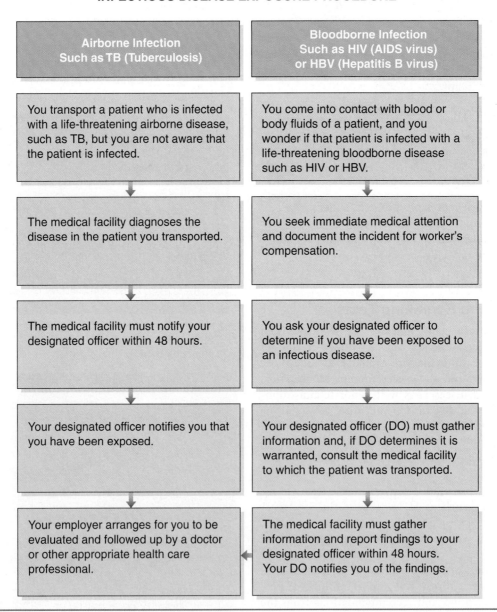

INFECTIOUS DISEASE EXPOSURE PROCEDURE

Airborne Infection Such as TB (Tuberculosis)	Bloodborne Infection Such as HIV (AIDS virus) or HBV (Hepatitis B virus)
You transport a patient who is infected with a life-threatening airborne disease, such as TB, but you are not aware that the patient is infected.	You come into contact with blood or body fluids of a patient, and you wonder if that patient is infected with a life-threatening bloodborne disease such as HIV or HBV.
The medical facility diagnoses the disease in the patient you transported.	You seek immediate medical attention and document the incident for worker's compensation.
The medical facility must notify your designated officer within 48 hours.	You ask your designated officer to determine if you have been exposed to an infectious disease.
Your designated officer notifies you that you have been exposed.	Your designated officer (DO) must gather information and, if DO determines it is warranted, consult the medical facility to which the patient was transported.
Your employer arranges for you to be evaluated and followed up by a doctor or other appropriate health care professional.	The medical facility must gather information and report findings to your designated officer within 48 hours. Your DO notifies you of the findings.

● **Figure 4-11** A federal regulation called the Ryan White Comprehensive AIDS Resources Emergency (CARE) Act outlines procedures to follow after an occupational exposure to human immunodeficiency virus (HIV), hepatitis B, diphtheria, meningitis, plague, hemorrhagic fever, rabies, and tuberculosis.

- Immediately wash the affected area with soap and water.

- Get a medical evaluation.

- Take the proper immunization boosters.

- Notify the agency's infection control liaison.

- Document the circumstances surrounding the exposure, including the actions taken to reduce chances of infection.

In general, the EMS provider should cooperate with the incident investigation and comply with all required reporting responsibilities and time frames.

DEATH AND DYING

Most paramedics agree that of all prehospital situations, those involving death or dying are among the most personally uncomfortable and challenging. There are many reasons for this. Of course, a death is normally a sad event. There is an air of unalterability, of finality. Each person experiences a death in an individual way because of that person's prior experiences of loss, coping skills, religious convictions, and other personal background. Paramedics encounter death much more frequently than most other people do. They often see it as it happens. This can lead to a cumulative sense of overload, which the smart paramedic recognizes and deals with in a healthy manner through appropriate grief work and stress management.

Loss, Grief, and Mourning

For decades, discussing death and dying openly was difficult because of cultural taboos. This began to change when pioneer Elisabeth Kübler-Ross braved the backlash to meet with terminally ill hospital patients to discuss their feelings about death and dying.[10] Before then, it was assumed dying people did not want to talk about the experience. Kübler-Ross learned that there are five predictable stages of grief:

- *Denial, or "not me."* This is an inability or refusal to believe the reality of impending death. It is a defense mechanism, during which the patient puts off dealing with the inevitable end of life.

- *Anger, or "why me?"* The patient's anger is really frustration related to his inability to control the situation. That anger could focus on anyone or anything.

- *Bargaining, or "okay, but first let me. . . ."* In the patient's mind, he tries to make a deal to "buy additional time" to put off or change the expected outcome.

- *Depression, or "okay, but I haven't. . . ."* The patient is sad and despairing, often mourning things not accomplished and dreams that will not come true. The patient withdraws or retreats into a private world, unwilling to communicate with others.

- *Acceptance, or "okay, I'm not afraid."* The patient may come to realize his fate and achieve a reasonable

level of comfort with the anticipated outcome. At this stage, the family may need more support than the patient.

A person experiencing any significant loss usually works through these stages, given enough time. Although there is a tendency to progress from one stage to the next in order, both dying patients and their loved ones experience the stages in their own unique ways. They may jump around among the stages, they may go back and forth, or they may never finish them. It is important for you to remain flexible, so you can decide how best to help, if asked.

Because paramedics encounter death and dying often, there is a mistaken belief that they handle it better. However, paramedics are human, too. Let yourself deal with death and dying when it occurs. Do not shirk the support of friends and family. Do not try to "tough it out." Use every opportunity to process a specific incident in a healthy manner by appropriately grieving losses that have an impact on you.

Grief is a feeling. Mourning is a process. A grieving person feels mostly sadness or distress. A person in mourning is immersed in the process of undergoing, perhaps displaying, and ultimately dissipating the feelings of grief. The sense of loss is predictably most intense immediately after the news is received. Although numerous models for the mourning process exist, a good rule of thumb is that after the loss of a close friend or relative, a period of one year of mourning is normal.

Upon initially hearing the news of a death, a person experiences a paralyzing, totally incapacitating surge of grief that is exactly comparable to the incapacitating pain of an acute blow to an eye or testicle—in that the whole world shrinks down to that acute pain. Typically, the feeling lasts for 5 to 15 minutes. When you deliver the news of a death, remember that a survivor cannot function during this grief spike. After delivering the news, wait until it is past and the survivor is ready and able to receive information and make decisions.

A period of intense feelings that continues for around four to six weeks follows the grief spike. Feelings may include loss, anger, resentment, sadness, and even guilt, depending on the relationship and the circumstances surrounding the death. Gradually, the intensity and immediacy of the loss fade into

CONTENT REVIEW

▶ Stages of Grief

- Denial
- Anger
- Bargaining
- Depression
- Acceptance

CULTURAL CONSIDERATIONS

Responses to Death. *The emotional response to the death of a friend or family member varies significantly among cultures as well as among individuals. Some people will accept the news quietly while others will react with an emotional outburst. Use simple terms and avoid euphemisms. Realize that grieving is a cultural as well as a personal phenomenon, and that it is normal for people to respond to bad news in different ways.*

a phase dominated by a sense of loneliness, which lasts about six months. Finally, a period of recovery usually ensues. The survivor begins to view the loss more objectively and rediscovers an interest in living. Key to the process of mourning is the passage of significant dates and anniversaries, such as birthdays, holidays, and the monthly (then annual) date when the loss occurred.

People cope in various ways with difficult moments such as death. If you are dealing with a child, understand that children's perceptions are different from an adult's. (See Table 4-3 for a summary.) This is true of all the special populations you will encounter, such as the elderly and people with mental disabilities. The elderly, for example, may be particularly concerned about the effects of the loss on other family members, about further loss of their own independence, and about the costs of a funeral and burial. There are a wide variety of responses to death among different peoples and cultures as well. Be flexible, and be ready for anything.

What to Say

As "Do Not Resuscitate" orders and other out-of-hospital death situations increase, EMS personnel are more often placed in the position of telling people that someone has died. It would be nice to have a script for those difficult moments, but the reality is that you have to assess the scene and the people in each situation to determine the safest and most compassionate way to deliver the sad news.

In terms of safety, you never know how people will respond, even if you know them. Most people accept the news quietly. However, some allow their grief to flood out of them in very physical ways, such as throwing things, kicking walls, screaming, or

TABLE 4-3 | Needs and Expectations of Children Regarding Death		
Age Range	**Characteristics**	**Suggestions**
Newborn to age 3	Senses that something has happened in family and notices that there is much activity in the household. Realizes that people are crying and sad. Watch for irritability and changes in eating, sleeping, or other behavioral patterns.	Be sensitive to the child's needs. Try to maintain consistency in routines. Maintain consistency with significant people in child's life.
Ages 3 to 6	Believes death is a temporary state, and may ask continually when the person will return. Believes in magical thinking, and may feel responsible for the death or that it is punishment for own behavior. May be fearful of catching the same illness and die, or may believe that everyone else he loves will die also. Watch for changes in behavior patterns with friends and at school, difficulty sleeping, and changes in eating habits.	Emphasize that the child was not responsible for the death. Reinforce that when people are sad, they cry, and that crying is normal and natural. Encourage the child to talk about and/or draw pictures of his feelings, or to cry.
Ages 6 to 9	May prefer to hide or disguise feelings to avoid looking babyish. Is afraid significant others will die. Seeks out detailed explanations for death, and differences between fatal illness and "just being sick." Has an understanding that death is real, but may believe that those who die are too slow, weak, or stupid. Fantasizes in an effort to make everything the way it was. Denial is the most helpful coping skill.	Talk about the normal feelings of anger, sadness, and guilt. Share your own feelings about death. Do not be afraid to cry in front of the child. This and other expressions of loss help to give the child permission to express his feelings.
Ages 9 to 12	Begins to understand the irreversibility of death. May seek details and specifics of the situation, and may need repeated, explicit explanations. Hard-won sense of independence becomes fragile, and may show concern about the practical matters of his lifestyle. May try to act "adult," but then regress to earlier stage of emotional response. When threatened, expresses anger toward the ill/deceased, himself, or other survivors.	Set aside time to talk about feelings. Encourage sharing of memories to facilitate grief response.
Ages 12 to 18	Demanding developmental processes are an awkward fit with the need to take on different family roles. Retreats to safety of childhood. Feels pressure to act as an adult, while still coping with skills of a child. Suppresses feelings in order to "fit in," leaving teen isolated and vulnerable.	Encourage talking, but respect need for privacy. See if a trusted, reliable friend or adult can provide appropriate support. Locate support group for teens.

running in circles. Before speaking to any survivors, consciously position yourself between them and the door or other escape route. Remember, initially the grief spike has its grip on the survivors. There is little you can do but give them a safe, private place to get through it. Also, for safety, do not deliver the news to a large group. Ask the primary people (no more than four or five) to step aside with you to a private place. Let them tell the others in their own way.

Find out who is who among the survivors. Do not make assumptions. Then address the closest survivor, preferably in a way that shows compassion. That is, avoid standing above the survivor. Instead, sit or squat so that your eyes are at the same level. If the survivor is alone, call for a friend, neighbor, clergy member, or relative. If possible, wait to tell the survivor the news until that person has arrived.

Introduce yourself by name and function. ("My name is Kate. I'm a paramedic with MedicWest EMS.") A careful choice of words is helpful. Although it may seem blunt, use the words "dead" and "died," rather than euphemisms that may be misinterpreted or misunderstood. Use gentle eye contact and, if appropriate, the comforting power of touching an arm or holding a hand. Basic elements of your message should include:

- A loved one has died.
- There is nothing more anyone could have done.

- You and your EMS service are available to assist the survivors if needed. (Sometimes, medical emergencies occur in survivors in the wake of such stressful news.)
- Also give information about local procedures for out-of-hospital death, such as the inspection of the scene by the medical examiner or coroner, and so on.

Do not include statements about God's will or relief from pain or any subjective assumption. You do not know the people well enough to know the details about their relationship or their religious preferences.[11]

When It Is Someone You Know

Many paramedics serve in small communities where calls often involve people they know. Some elements of this are rewarding, and others are heart-wrenching. People may be greatly relieved to see a familiar, trusted face among the ambulance crew. There also is a lot of support for paramedics in small communities, because you are from the community itself and are there to help fellow community members during their most fearful moments. However, being involved when the life of someone you know is threatened—or lost—can have a powerful impact on your own emotions. If it is too much, you must find a way to manage the stress. Often, you must grieve as well. Your well-being demands it.

STRESS AND STRESS MANAGEMENT

Many aspects of EMS are stressful.[12] A time-honored definition of **stress**, according to stress researcher Hans Selye, is "the nonspecific response of the body to any demand."[13] The word *stress* also refers to a hardship or strain, or to a physical or emotional response to such a stimulus. Stress responses are natural reactions that help the organism adapt to a new environment or a sudden change in the usual environment. Stress results from the interaction of events and the capabilities of each individual to adjust to those events. A person's reactions to stressful events are individual and are affected by that person's previous exposure to the stress-causing event, perception of the event, general life experience, and personal coping skills. A stimulus that causes stress is known as a **stressor**.

Stress is both beneficial and detrimental. Stress is usually understood to generate a negative effect, or *distress*, in an individual. There is also "good" stress, which is called *eustress* (for example, seeing a lost loved one for the first time in years). Even eustress, however, generates physiological and psychological signs and symptoms.

Adapting to stress is a dynamic, evolving process. As a person adapts, he uses or develops any or all of the following:

- *Defensive strategies.* While sometimes helpful for the short term, defensive strategies may deny or distort the reality of a stressful situation.
- *Coping.* This is an active process of confronting the stressful situation. By acknowledging the existence

CONTENT REVIEW

► Phases of a Stress Response

• Alarm
• Resistance
• Exhaustion

► Identify your own personal stressors and find out what stress management techniques work for you.

of stressors, the patient is able to gather information about them and then change or adjust as necessary. Coping may or may not serve as the best strategy for the long term.

● *Problem-solving skills.* These skills are regarded as the healthiest approach to everyday concerns. They involve problem analysis, which generates options for action, and determination of a course of action. Mastery—reflected in the ability to recognize multiple options and potential solutions for stressful situations—generally comes only as a result of extensive experience with similar situations.

EMS practice, of course, involves abundant stressors, which provide ample opportunities for the development of problem-solving skills. There are administrative stressors, such as waiting for calls, shift work, loud pagers, and inadequate pay. There are scene-related stressors, such as violent and abusive people, flying debris, vomit, loud noises, and chaos. There are emotional and physical stressors, such as fear, angry bystanders, abusive patients, frustration, exhaustion, hunger or thirst, and lifting heavy objects. Environmental stress may be provided by siren noise, inclement weather, confined workspaces, and the frequent urgent need for rapid scene responses and life-or-death decisions. In addition, the often-difficult world of EMS can strain a paramedic's family relationships and may also lead to conflicts with supervisors and coworkers. Add this to some personality traits commonly found among paramedics, such as a strong need to be liked and often unrealistically high self-expectations, and the combination can lead to disturbing feelings of guilt or anxiety. All these stressors and stress responses take a toll on the paramedic.

To help you manage your own stress, you should learn these things:

● *Your personal stressors.* Each person has an individual list. What is stressful to you may be enjoyable to someone else. What was stressful to you last year may be replaced by new stressors this year.

● *The amount of stress you can take before it becomes a problem.* Stress occurs in a tornado-like continuum. It may start with a few breezes, but it can increase in force until it is whirling out of control. Stopping the "storm" early is key to your well-being. You need to know which stress responses are early indicators for you so you can deal with them at that point.

● *Stress management strategies that work for you.* Again, this is totally individual. Those who seek personal well-being must become well versed about personally appropriate stress-management options.

Adapting to stressors is a dynamic process of receiving, processing, and dissipating stressors and their effects. You bring your life experience, temperament, emotional maturity, spiritual convictions, habits (good and bad), interpersonal skills, ability to be self-aware, gender, and recent activity to each moment of adapting to the world. If a person experiences a pile-on of stressor after stressor without regard for the consequences, the results are likely to be bad. In fact, the U.S. Surgeon General once estimated that stress-related diseases kill 80 percent of people who die of nontraumatic causes. Stress-related disease is avoidable if you make a habit of doing what is necessary to preserve your personal well-being. (Specific stress management techniques will be discussed later.)

Phases of Stress Response

There are three phases of a stress response: *alarm*, *resistance*, and *exhaustion*. At the end there may be a period of rest and recovery.

● *Stage I: Alarm.* The alarm phase is the "fight-or-flight" phenomenon. It occurs when the body physically and rapidly prepares to defend itself against a perceived threat. The pituitary gland begins by releasing adrenocorticotropic (stress) hormones. Hormones continue to flood the body via the autonomic nervous system, coordinated by the hypothalamus. Epinephrine and norepinephrine from the adrenal glands increase heart rate and blood pressure, dilate pupils, increase blood sugar, slow digestion, and relax the bronchial tree. These alarm-stage responses end when the event is recognized as not dangerous.

● *Stage II: Resistance.* This stage starts when the individual begins to cope with the stress. Over time, an individual may become desensitized or adapted to stressors. Physiological parameters, such as pulse and blood pressure, may then return to normal.

● *Stage III: Exhaustion.* Prolonged exposure to the same stressors leads to exhaustion of an individual's ability to resist and adapt. Resistance to all stressors declines. Susceptibility to physical and psychological ailments increases. A period of rest and recovery is necessary for a healthy outcome.

It would be great if we could manage each stressor to the point of recovery before the next one hits, but of course that is not how it works. Typically, people are still dealing with one stress (or the same ongoing one, such as the chronic stress of shift work) when additional stressors pile on, resulting in cumulative stress. If stress accumulates without intervention, the consequences can be serious.

Stress also helps us to function optimally. In fact, heightened stress levels improve our ability to function. You have surely experienced this phenomenon. For example, you are awakened from your sleep to respond to a motor vehicle collision. When you arrive on scene you find several critical patients. Although still sleepy when you are first called to the scene, the stress responses heighten your alertness and your ability to perform the needed skills and procedures (Figure 4-12 ●).

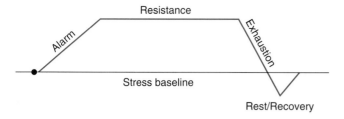

● **Figure 4-12** Phases of stress response. *(Mitchell, Jeff; Bray, Grady, Emergency Services Stress: Guidelines on Preserving the Health and Careers of Emergency Services Personnel, 1st Edition, © 1990. Adapted by permission of Pearson Education, Inc., Upper Saddle River, NJ)*

Shift Work

There will always be shift work in EMS. Because EMS is a 24-hour, 7-days-a-week endeavor, someone has to be functional at all times. But working odd hours is inherently stressful because of disruptions in the biorhythms of the body that are known as circadian rhythms and because of sleep deprivation.

Circadian rhythms are biological cycles that occur at approximately 24-hour intervals. These include hormonal and body temperature fluctuations, appetite and sleepiness cycles, and other bodily processes. When life patterns disrupt the circadian rhythms, such as with extensive travel between time zones, there are biological effects that can be stressful. Sleep deprivation is common among people who work at night. The inherent dangers to paramedics are clear. A recent study estimated that up to 20 percent of fatal crashes resulted from driver fatigue. The hours at which fatigue-related collisions most often occur are between 2:00 A.M. and 6:00 A.M. (early morning) and between 2:00 P.M. and 4:00 P.M. (midafternoon) when our circadian rhythm is at its lowest points. Males ages 18 to 30 are in the high-risk category. They tend to be overconfident about their driving ability and believe they can handle the situation. Women are less likely to be involved in fatigue-related crashes.[14]

If you work at night and have to sleep in the daytime, there are some tips to minimize the stress:

● Sleep in a cool, dark place that mimics the nighttime environment.

● Stick to sleeping at your **anchor time** (times you can rest without interruption), even on days off. Do not try to revert to a daytime lifestyle on days off. For example, if you work 9 P.M. to 5 A.M. and your anchor time is 8 P.M. to 12 noon, then go to bed "early" on days off and on workdays sleep from 8 A.M. to 3 P.M.

● Unwind appropriately after a shift in order to rest well. Do not eat a heavy meal or exercise right before bedtime.

● Post a "day sleeper" sign on your front door, turn off the phone's ringer, and lower the volume of the answering machine.

Signs of Stress

A variety of factors can trigger a stress response. They include the loss of something valuable, injury or the threat of injury, poor health or nutrition, general frustration, and ineffective coping mechanisms.

Remember, each individual is susceptible to different stressors and therefore has a different constellation of signs and symptoms.

However, the signs and symptoms of stress can be beneficial, because they are the body's way of warning that corrective stress management is needed. The warnings typically are mild at first, but left uncorrected they will build in intensity until you are forced to rest. If it means having a heart attack or collapsing, that is what the body will do. So pay attention early.

The signs and symptoms of excessive stress can be physical, emotional, cognitive, or behavioral (Table 4-4). They are unique to each person. Once again, an individual must perform a self-assessment. If you catch a warning sign of excessive stress early and manage it, there is no need to reach the extreme endpoint commonly referred to as **burnout**.

Common Techniques for Managing Stress

There are two main types of defense mechanisms and techniques for managing stress: beneficial and detrimental. Detrimental techniques may provide a temporary sense of relief, but they will not cure the problem. In fact, they make things worse. They include substance abuse (alcohol, nicotine, illegal and prescription drugs), overeating or other compulsive behaviors, chronic complaining, freezing out or cutting off others and the support they could give you, avoidance behaviors, and dishonesty about your actual state of well-being ("I'm just fine!").

It is far better for you to spend your energy on beneficial, or healthy, techniques that dissipate the accumulation of stress and promote actual recovery. When your stress response threatens your ability to handle the moment, try the following:

● *Use controlled breathing.* Focus attention on your breathing. Take in a deep breath through your nose. Then exhale forcefully but steadily through your mouth, so that you can hear the air rush out. Press all the air out of your lungs with your abdomen. Do this two or more times until you feel steadier. This technique helps to reduce your adrenaline levels and slow your heart rate, so you can do your job appropriately.

● *Reframe.* Mentally reframe interfering thoughts, such as "I can't do this" or "I'm scared." Consciously restate your negative thought in a positive way. For example, when you start to think "I can't do this," you might tell yourself, "I will do the best I can and ask another crew member or call medical direction if I need help." When you think, "I'm scared," you might replace that thought with "This is challenging, but I can get through it OK." Be sure to deal with the negative thoughts later, however, or they may continue to interfere with the performance of your duties.

● *Attend to the medical needs of the patient.* Even if you know the people involved, do not let those relationships interfere with your responsibilities as an EMS provider. Later, when it is appropriate to do so, address your stress about the call in some way such as talking it over with family or fellow crew members or seeking spiritual solace or counseling.

TABLE 4-4 | Warning Signs of Excessive Stress

Physical	Cognitive	Emotional	Behavioral
Nausea/vomiting	Confusion	Anticipatory anxiety	Change in activity
Upset stomach	Lowered attention span	Denial	Hyperactivity, hypoactivity
Tremors (lips, hands)	Calculation difficulties	Fearfulness	Withdrawal
Feeling uncoordinated	Memory problems	Panic	Suspiciousness
Diaphoresis (profuse sweating), flushed skin	Poor concentration	Survivor guilt	Change in communications
Chills	Difficulty making decisions	Uncertainty of feelings	Change in interactions with others
Diarrhea	Disruption in logical thinking	Depression	Change in eating habits
Aching muscles and joints	Disorientation, decreased level of awareness	Grief	Increased or decreased food intake
Sleep disturbances	Seeing an event over and over	Hopelessness	Increased smoking
Fatigue		Feeling overwhelmed	Increased smoking
Dry mouth	Distressing dreams	Feeling lost	Increased alcohol intake
Shakes	Blaming someone	Feeling abandoned	Increased intake of other drugs
Headache		Feeling worried	Being overly vigilant to environment
Vision problems		Wishing to hide	
Difficult, rapid breathing		Wishing to die	Excessive humor
Chest tightness or pain, heart palpitations, cardiac rhythm disturbances		Anger	Excessive silence
		Feeling numb	Unusual behavior
		Identifying with victim	Crying spells

For long-term well-being, one of the best stress management techniques is to simply take care of *you*—physically, emotionally, and mentally. Remember that regular exercise does not have to be extreme. Do something that you enjoy and find relaxing. At stressful times, pay especially close attention to your diet. If you smoke, make it a goal to quit.

Create a non-EMS circle of friends, and renew old friendships or activities. Take a vacation or a few days off. Say "no!" to the next offer of an overtime shift. Listen to music, meditate, and learn positive thinking. Try the soothing techniques of guided imagery and progressive relaxation. Some paramedics have even quit EMS for a while. In general, you have many choices. The key principle is to generate positive options for yourself, and keep choosing them until you have recovered.

Specific EMS Stresses

There are three clearly defined types of EMS stresses:

- **Daily stress.** Most EMS stress is unrelated to critical incidents and disasters. Instead, it is related to such things as pay, working conditions, dealing with the public, administrative matters, and other hassles of day-to-day living and working. To help deal with daily stress, all emergency personnel should develop personal stress management strategies such as a personal support system made up of coworkers, family, clergy, and others.

- **Small incidents.** Incidents involving only one or two patients, including incidents that result in injuries or deaths of emergency workers, are best handled by competent mental health personnel in individual or small-group settings. Mental health professionals should be familiar with EMS and be ready to respond when needed. They should then continue to screen affected emergency workers for signs and symptoms of abnormal response to stress. If these are detected, they can refer these workers, as appropriate, to other competent mental health professionals who use accepted treatment methods.

- **Large incidents and disasters.** Most EMS personnel will never encounter a disaster situation. However, all must be ready in case such a catastrophe occurs. The stress of large-scale disasters can be mitigated by a well-coordinated and organized response. Use of the National Incident Management System (NIMS) or Incident Command System (ICS) in large incidents and disasters serves to appropriately direct responding personnel. It also provides for rotating personnel through rehabilitation and surveillance stations. Those who are showing signs of stress or fatigue are removed from duty, at least temporarily. Here, too, there is a role for competent mental health professionals, who should be readily available to provide psychological first aid.

Psychological First Aid

Mental health professionals can provide the information and education needed for rescuers to understand psychological or emotional trauma, what to expect, and where to get help if needed. In addition, competent mental health personnel should be available at all major incidents to provide psychological first aid to rescuers and victims.

The basic principles of psychological first aid as may be practiced by mental health professionals are quite straightforward:

- *Contact and engagement.* Making contact with those in need of assistance; providing practical, instrumental assistance with compassion and care.

- *Safety and comfort.* Taking steps to provide as safe an environment as situations permit; providing as much comfort as circumstances allow.

- *Stabilization.* Attenuating anxiety, providing a calming presence, helping ground and orient the distraught, referring for emergency care where and when clearly indicated.

- *Information gathering (current needs and concerns).* Determining what the pressing needs are *as seen by the person in need;* tailoring assistance efforts to address current needs while anticipating emerging situations.

- *Practical assistance.* Providing practical, instrumental help with identified needs; assisting with problem-solving strategies and access to helping resources.

- *Connection with social supports.* Helping those affected make contact with sources of social support important to them (e.g., friends, family, and community and spiritual resources); integrating their support into problem solving and recovery.

- *Information on coping.* Providing simple, practical, proven tips on managing stress and coping with demands of recovery—timed to match the situations and challenges at hand at any given juncture. Such tips can be useful and well received, especially when delivered in the context of practical assistance and social support.

- *Link to collaborative services.* Since many persons may be unfamiliar with resources available to help with their various needs, providing assistance in navigating the resource network community can be particularly important.

Psychological first aid is not a treatment or packaged proprietary intervention technique. It is an attempt to provide practical palliative care and contact while respecting the wishes of those who may not be ready to deal with the possible onslaught of emotional responses in the early days following an incident. It entails providing comfort and information and meeting people's immediate practical and emotional needs.[15]

Disaster Mental Health Services

The emotional well-being of both rescuers and victims is an important concern in any multiple-casualty incident. In the past, Critical Incident Stress Management (CISM) was recommended for use in emergency services. However, evidence has clearly shown that CISM and Critical Incident Stress Debriefing (CISD) do not appear to mitigate the effects of traumatic stress and, in fact, may interfere with the normal grieving and healing process and should not be used.[16, 17] Instead, mental health practitioners now recommend resiliency-based care. This program includes techniques and activities that promote emotional strength, at the same time decreasing vulnerability to stress, adversity, and challenges.

However, an important role remains for competent mental health professionals in any multiple-casualty incident. Mental health personnel should be available on scene to provide psychological first aid (as already described) to all those affected by an incident—including EMS personnel. At the same time, they can survey rescuers and victims for the development of abnormal stress-related symptoms. In addition, mental health professionals should be available during the two months following a critical incident to screen and assist anyone who may be developing stress-related symptoms. Persons so affected may be referred for additional counseling or mental health care.[18]

GENERAL SAFETY CONSIDERATIONS

The topic of scene safety is vast and requires career-long attention. Considering the many problems that can occur, it is impressive how few injuries there are. Your risks include violent people, environmental hazards, structural collapse, motor vehicles, and infectious disease. Many of these hazards can be minimized with protective equipment, such as helmets, body armor, reflective tape for night visibility, footwear with ankle support, and Standard Precautions against infectious disease. You should use whatever protective equipment you have.

Interpersonal Relations

Safety issues that arise in out-of-hospital care often stem from poor interpersonal relations. Paramedics are public ambassadors of health care. Interpersonal safety begins with effective communication. If you can build a rapport with the strangers you have been sent to serve, you will gain their trust. Suspicious, angry, and upset people are far more likely to be defensive and inflict harm than those who see a reason to trust what you are doing.

Building rapport depends on the ability to put your personal prejudices aside. Everyone has prejudices, but as a representative of an institution far greater than yourself, you must never allow them to interfere with appropriate patient and bystander management. In fact, go beyond curbing prejudice and challenge yourself to treat every person you meet with dignity and respect.

You can begin by taking time to pay attention to the rich array of cultural diversity that exists in our nation and learning to see those differences as valuable and positive. In particular, learn about the different cultural backgrounds of people in your area and how to work with them effectively. For example, although you may like a lot of eye contact, understand that it is regarded as more polite in several cultures to avoid eye contact. Therefore, someone showing you esteem might avoid eye contact with you. This is not wrong; it is just different. Listen well to the stories of other people and see what you can learn. When you learn to accept differences easily, it will become easier for you to work toward win-win situations on the streets.

Roadway Safety

Motor vehicle collisions are the greatest hazard for EMS personnel. The incidence of ambulance and emergency response vehicle collisions is increasing (Figure 4-13 ●). There are several factors that seem to play a role in ambulance crashes. First, ambulances have become larger and more difficult to operate. Most modern ambulances are built on a commercial truck chassis. Many are built on a heavy truck chassis. With this increase in size comes increased braking distances, less responsive steering systems, and slower acceleration (which decreases the ability to avoid certain collisions). Several ambulance types have a high center of gravity or are somewhat unstable. In addition, many times the person designated to drive the ambulance is the person with the least training and the least experience. In many instances, introductory courses for emergency vehicle operations (EVOCs) are not provided or do not have an adequate session to practice driving and emergency techniques.[19]

Roadways are unsafe places. There are good books, classes, and mentors to help you become aware of the various roadway hazards. For all related emergency situations, acquire the necessary training for emergency rescue and for the safe use of emergency rescue equipment. Learn the principles of:

- Safely following an emergency escort vehicle
- Intersection management, when traffic is moving in several directions

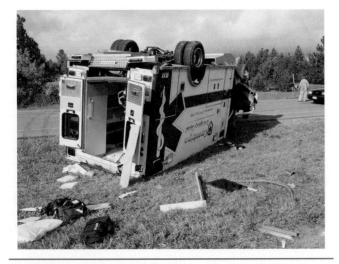

Figure 4-13 Ambulance collisions pose the greatest risk of injury or death for EMS providers. (© *Canandaigua Emergency Squad*)

- Noting hazardous conditions, such as spilled hazardous materials (gasoline, industrial chemicals, and so on), downed power lines, and proximity to moving traffic. Also notice adverse environmental conditions.
- Evaluating the safest parking place when arriving at a roadway incident
- Safely approaching a vehicle in which someone is slumped over the wheel
- Patient compartment safety—in particular, bracing yourself against sudden deceleration or swerving to avoid roadway hazards; and making a habit of hanging on consistently, especially when changing positions. Restraint systems have been developed to help protect EMS personnel while riding in the patient compartment of the ambulance.
- Safely using emergency lights and siren

An ambulance escort can create additional hazards. Inexperienced ambulance operators often follow the escort vehicle too closely and are unable to stop when the escort does. Inexperienced operators also may assume that other drivers know the ambulance is following an escort. In fact, other drivers do not know another emergency vehicle is coming and often pull out in front of the ambulance just after the escort vehicle passes.

Multiple-vehicle responses can be just as dangerous, especially when responding vehicles travel in the same direction close together. When two vehicles approach the same intersection at the same time, not only may they fail to yield, one to the other, but also other drivers may yield for the first vehicle only, not the second one. Extreme caution must be taken when approaching intersections.

Certain equipment is intended to promote your safety on roadways. For example, to be visible to oncoming drivers, who may have dirty, smeared, pitted windshields and may not be sober, wear ANSI/ISEA compliant safety vests. In fact, you also may be issued other protective gear, especially if you are in the fire service. Using respiratory protection, gloves, boots, turnout coat and pants (or coveralls), and other specialty safety equipment is the mark of an aware, professional paramedic. Ask nonmedical personnel to set out flares or cones, if needed. Leave some emergency lights flashing, although you should be careful not to blind oncoming drivers.

To park safely at a roadway incident, make it a habit to scan each individual setting. Notice curves, hilltops, volume, and the speed of surrounding traffic. Ideally, you should park in the front of a crash site on the same side of the street. This facilitates access to the patient compartment and equipment, and it protects you from traffic coming from behind. However, when responding to an incident such as "person slumped behind wheel," maintain the defensive advantage by staying behind the vehicle, and use spotlights to "blind" the person until you know there are no hostile intentions. Walk to the vehicle with cautious alertness until you are sure it is not a trap.

The use of seat belts in the front of an ambulance should be an obvious habit, both for safety and for role modeling. Less obvious is the use of safety restraints in the patient compartment. An improper assumption is that the paramedic is too busy attending to the patient and passengers to wear a seat belt. However, buckling into a seat belt for a safer ride is, in fact, possible during much or most of ambulance transport times. Death and major disability is common when someone is in the patient compartment during a crash. For your well-being, wear a seat belt whenever possible, even "in back."[20]

Because ambulances represent help and hope, it is doubly tragic when a paramedic crew is involved in a motor vehicle crash caused by the misuse of lights and siren. Lights and siren are tools, not toys. They are the paramedic's means for gaining quick access to people in dire need. Those who misuse the mandate to operate them chip away at the public's trust in EMS. Whether using lights and siren or not, the paramedic has a responsibility to drive with due regard for the safety of others. As a professional, you are obligated to study and use safe driving practices at all times.

SUMMARY

The paramedic has the training and responsibility to manage the most complicated health problems posed by out-of-hospital citizens. This makes the paramedic a leader within the prehospital care community. Paramedics who attend to their own well-being are not only helping themselves, but they are also providing a positive role model for other EMS providers and the community at large.

Continuous assessment of personal lifestyle ranges from practices that affect the immediate future to practices that affect the paramedic in old age. They range from wearing personal protective equipment (PPE) and parking safely at a crash site to managing stress daily, eating right, and exercising.

There are numerous elements to the topic of well-being, and the paramedic must strive continually to address each one. Take your knowledge beyond the introduction offered in this chapter. Be a lifelong student of well-being, and you are more likely to have a healthy long life. Your biggest challenge is this: Be well, so that you can help others be well, too.

YOU MAKE THE CALL

It's been a tough year for you on the paramedic squad. Lately, it just seems as if everything that can go wrong does. Arguing (again) with your spouse about paying the mortgage is not helping your irritation one bit. It is 2300 hours. You are tired, and all you ate all day was glazed doughnuts and fast food. Suddenly, the tone alert sounds: "Ambulance 44, respond to the corner of Fero and Bailey on a two-vehicle crash. Number of victims unknown."

You are the second EMS crew to arrive. You prefer the job of triage, and the paramedic who is doing it is too new to know much. Anyway, he has already triaged four patients. As you walk up to the scene, you notice the bumper sticker on one crash vehicle and realize it is your neighbor's daughter's car. You do not see her in the group of patients, and your heart leaps into your throat when you see the DOA covered with a sheet.

You are assigned two patients, one an unconscious teen with a crushed leg and the other an adult with a broken arm.

You take pride in your medical abilities, so handling the immobilization and other medical care is smooth. On the way to the hospital, the teen wakes up and presses you to tell him, "Is Debbie okay? Is she? Please! Tell me, is she all right?" Thus you find out that, indeed, the other person in your neighbor's car was Debbie, their daughter.

After delivering the patients to the hospital, you pop an antacid for your sour stomach and chew out your partner for his bumpy driving.

A couple of days later, you take on yet another overtime shift. Your mortgage payment is due, and besides, you can't face going to the funeral of your neighbor's daughter. You've seen enough death. Who needs another funeral anyway?

1. Are your stress levels inappropriately high? What are the indications?

2. Might it be a good idea for you to go to the funeral? Why or why not?

3. How can you improve stress management in the future?

See Suggested Responses at the back of this book.

REVIEW QUESTIONS

1. Most paramedic injuries are caused by _____ and being in and around motor vehicles.
   a. falls
   b. stress
   c. lifting
   d. violence

2. Which of the following is not a benefit of achieving acceptable physical fitness?
   a. increased muscle mass and metabolism
   b. increased oxygen-carrying capacity
   c. increased resting heart rate and blood pressure
   d. increased resistance to illness and injury

3. According to the U.S. Department of Agriculture dietary guidelines, you should make _____ of your plate fruits and vegetables.
   a. one-fourth
   b. one-third
   c. one-half
   d. two-thirds

4. Which of the following is not an important principle of lifting?
   a. always avoid twisting and turning
   b. keep your palms up whenever possible
   c. move a load only if you can safely handle it
   d. position the load far away from your body and center of gravity

5. A strict form of infection control that is based on the assumption that all blood and other body fluids are infectious, combining aspects of universal precautions and body substance isolation, is termed:
   a. personal protective equipment.
   b. mode of transmission.
   c. incubation period.
   d. standard precautions.

6. _____ is the use of a chemical, or a physical method such as pressurized steam, to kill all microorganisms on an object.
   a. Cleaning
   b. Disinfecting
   c. Sterilizing
   d. Decontaminating

7. How many stages in the grief process are identified by Elisabeth Kübler-Ross?
   a. three
   b. five
   c. seven
   d. eight

8. The first step in the grieving process, as identified by Elisabeth Kübler-Ross, is:
   a. anger.
   b. denial.
   c. depression.
   d. bargaining.

9. This is an active process during which a person confronts the stressful situation.
   a. coping
   b. resistance
   c. defensive strategies
   d. problem-solving skills

10. For safety at a roadway incident it is appropriate to do all of the following except:
    a. ask nonmedical personnel to set out flares or cones.
    b. wear reflective tape and an orange or lime-green vest.
    c. blind a slumped-over passenger with a spotlight as you approach.
    d. park on the opposite side of the street from the crashed vehicle.

See Answers to Review Questions at the back of this book.

REFERENCES

1. Maguire, B. J., K. L. Hunting, G. S. Smith, and N. R. Levick. "Occupational Fatalities in Emergency Medical Services: A Hidden Crisis." *Ann Emerg Med* 40 (2002): 625–632.

2. Boudreaux, E., C. Mandry, and P. J. Brantly. "Emergency Medical Technician Schedule Modification: Impact and Implications on Short- and Long-Term Follow-Up." *Acad Emerg Med* 5 (1998): 128–133.

3. Mitani, S., M. Fujita, and T. Shirakawa. "Circadian Variation on Cardiac Autonomic Nervous System Profile Is Affected in Japanese Men with a Working System of 24-H Shifts." *Int Arch Occup Environ Health* 79 (2006): 27–32.

4. Crill, M. T. and D. Hostler. "Back Strength and Flexibility of EMS Providers in Practicing Prehospital Providers." *J Occup Rehabil* 15 (2005): 105–111.

5. Studnek, J. R. and J. M. Crawford. "Factors Associated with Back Problems among Emergency Medical Technicians." *Am J Ind Med* 50 (2007): 464–469.

6. United States Department of Agriculture (USDA). *ChooseMyPlate.* [Available at: http://www.choosemyplate.gov. For "10 Tips to a Great Plate," go to http://www.choosemyplate.gov/downloads/TenTips/DGTipsheet1ChooseMyPlate.pdf].

7. Bledsoe, B. E., T. Dick, J. O. Page, and M. Taigman. "The Missing Drugs." *JEMS* 29 (2004): 30–36.

8. Friese, G. and K. Owsley. "Backbreaking Work: What You Need to Know about Lifting and Back Safety in EMS." *EMS Mag* 37 (2008): 63–72.

9. Centers for Disease Control and Prevention. *Standard Precautions.* [Available at: http://www.cdc.gov/ncidod/dhqp/pdf/guidelines/Isolation2007.pdf].

10. Kübler-Ross, E. *On Death and Dying.* (Originally published 1969.) Scribner Classics reprint edition. New York: Simon & Schuster, 1997.

11. Olsen, J. C., M. L. Buenefe, and W. D. Falco. "Death in the Emergency Department." *Ann Emerg Med* 31 (1998): 758–765.

12. Boudreauz, E., C. Mandry, and P. J. Brantley. "Stress, Job Satisfaction, Coping, and Psychological Distress among Emergency Medical Technicians." *Prehosp Disaster Med* 12 (1997): 242–249.

13. Selye, H. "A Syndrome Produced by Diverse Nocuous Agents." *Nature* 138 (1936): 32.

14. Cydulka, R. K., C. L. Emerman, B. Shade, and J. Kubincanek. "Stress Levels in EMS Personnel: A Longitudinal Study with Work-Schedule Modification." *Acad Emerg Med* 1 (1994): 240–246.

15. U.S. Department of Veterans Affairs. Psychological First Aid: An Operations Guide. [Available at: http://www.ptsd.va.gov/professional/manuals/psych-first-aid.asp].

16. Bledsoe, B. E. "Critical Incident Stress Management (CISM): Benefit or Rise for Emergency Services." *Prehosp Emerg Care* 72 (2003): 272–329.

17. McNally, R. J., R. A. Bryant, and A. Ehlers. "Does Early Psychological Intervention Promote Recovery from Posttraumatic Stress?" *Psych Sci Pub Int* 4 (2003): 45–79 [Available at http://www.psychological science .org/journals/pspi/index.html].

18. Devilley, G. J., R. Gist, and P. Cotton. "Ready! Fire! Aim! The Status of Psychological Debriefings and Therapeutic Interventions: In the Work Place and After Disasters." *Rev Gen Psych* 10(4) (2006): 318–345.

19. Ray, A. M. and D. F. Kupas. "Comparison of Rural and Urban Ambulance Crashes in Pennsylvania." *Prehosp Emerg Care* 11 (2007): 416–420.

20. Slattery, D. E. and A. Silver. "The Hazards of Providing Emergency Care in Emergency Vehicle: An Opportunity for Reform." *Prehosp Emerg Care* 13 (2009): 388–397.

 FURTHER READING

Becknell, J. *Medic Life.* St. Louis: Mosby Lifeline, 1996.

Dernocoeur, K. B. *Streetsense: Communication, Safety, and Control.* 3rd ed. Redmond, WA: Laing Research Services, 1996.

5

EMS Research

Bryan Bledsoe, DO, FACEP, FAAEM, EMT-P
Michael O'Keefe, MS, NREMT-P

STANDARD
Preparatory (Research)

COMPETENCY
Integrates comprehensive knowledge of EMS systems, the safety and well-being of the paramedic, and medical-legal and ethical issues, which is intended to improve the health of EMS personnel, patients, and the community.

OBJECTIVES

Terminal Performance Objective
After reading this chapter you should be able to critically evaluate published reports of EMS research.

Enabling Objectives
To accomplish the terminal performance objective, you should be able to:

1. Define key terms introduced in this chapter.

2. Explain the relationship between EMS research and EMS practice.

3. Distinguish between the conclusions that can be drawn from research and those that can be drawn from more casual observations of phenomena.

4. Describe each of the steps of the scientific method.

5. Compare and contrast different types of research, including quantitative, qualitative, prospective, and retrospective approaches.

6. Give examples of various experimental designs.

7. Describe different types of studies and their general levels of validity.

8. Given a published research article, discuss its validity.

9. Given a research proposal, identify the ethical considerations for human subjects that must be considered.

10. Discuss the proper use of various descriptive and inferential statistics in a research study.

11. Describe the purpose and intended content of each section of a research paper.

12. Describe how to perform a literature search.

13. Given a variety of research papers, debate the merits of the study with your peers and instructors.

14. Describe the role of published research reports in changing EMS practice.

15. Discuss the roles and responsibilities of EMS providers who participate in research studies.

KEY TERMS

abstract, p. 90

analysis of variance
(ANOVA), p. 90

bench research, p. 85

bias, p. 83

case report, p. 85

case series, p. 85

chi square test, p. 90

cohort study, p. 85

confidence interval, p. 88

control group, p. 83

convenience sampling, p. 93

cross-sectional study, p. 85

data dredging, p. 94

data mining, p. 94

dependent variable, p. 82

descriptive statistics, p. 87

double blind study, p. 84

experiment, p. 81

experimental group, p. 83

experimental study, p. 83

external validity, p. 86

hypothesis, p. 81

in vitro, p. 85

in vivo, p. 85

independent variable, p. 82

inferential statistics, p. 87

institutional review board
(IRB), p. 87

internal validity, p. 86

iterative process, p. 82

mean, p. 88

measures of central
tendency, p. 88

median, p. 88

meta-analysis, p. 84

mixed research, p. 82

mode, p. 88

morbidity, p. 80

mortality, p. 80

National EMS Research
Agenda, p. 80

nominal data, p. 90

nonrandomized controlled
trial, p. 84

null hypothesis, p. 94

observational study, p. 83

odds ratio, p. 90

open access journals, p. 91

ordinal data, p. 90

outcomes-based
research, p. 80

P value, p. 94

parameter, p. 88

peer review, p. 82

placebo, p. 84

population, p. 88

post hoc, p. 95

principal investigator
(PI), p. 95

prospective study, p. 83

PubMed, p. 81

qualitative research, p. 82

qualitative statistics, p. 90

quality of life, p. 80

quantitative research, p. 82

quantitative statistics, p. 90

quasiexperimental
study, p. 83

random sampling, p. 93

randomized controlled trial
(RCT), p. 84

research, p. 80

retrospective study, p. 83

sampling error, p. 88

science, p. 80

scientific method, p. 81

single blind study, p. 84

standard deviation
(SD or σ), p. 88

statistics, p. 87

systematic sampling, p. 93

t test, p. 90

time sampling, p. 93

treatment group, p. 83

validity, p. 86

variance, p. 88

CASE STUDY

One slow day, two EMS crews were sitting in the station, and the conversation soon drifted back to "the way we used to do it." Robert, the most senior paramedic in the agency, had logged more than 30 years in the field. The younger crew members began to question Robert about the various antiquated practices that once were commonplace in EMS.

Robert said, "Well, one thing we routinely did was to give large doses of sodium bicarbonate to cardiac arrest victims." A young EMT piped in and asked, "Why did it stop?" Robert thought for a minute and said, "Well, it was one of those things that looked good on paper but did not work in the field. The research showed that the outcomes from cardiac arrest were not any better for those who received sodium bicarbonate when compared to those who did not. So the American Heart Association took it out of their recommendations, and we stopped giving it."

Steve, a new EMT, said inquisitively, "What about MAST pants for shock or bleeding control?" Robert leaned back in the chair and said, "Ah, MAST pants. We used them all the time for trauma. I'll swear I've seen them work. But, a research study from Houston found them ineffective, if not harmful, and they went the way of the covered wagon."

Robert went on, "We also used calcium chloride in cardiac arrests. I remember giving 100 milligrams of Decadron to head-injured patients—not sure why they had us do that. I have to admit that EMS has changed, and I think it has changed for the better." "What do you mean?" asked Steve. Robert looked pensive and said, "In those days, we did what we did because it seemed like a good idea at the time. Now, EMS is more based on sound scientific principles developed through quality research. The goal has always been to do what was best for the patient. The problem was that we did not always know what was best for the patient. Many of the things that seemed so intuitive as an EMS practice have been proved through research to be ineffective. While I hate to see old practices go by the wayside, it is for the best, I guess. Research is what will drive EMS into the future, and I'm all for that."

The group sat quietly for a while, and finally the conversation took a different turn when Steve looked at his watch, jumped up, and said, "Hey, the Cowboys are playing. Turn on the TV."

INTRODUCTION

Scientific **research** has played a major role in the evolution of modern EMS. When EMS was developed over 30 years ago, there were no scientific studies or objective evidence to guide development. Instead, various practices from other areas (e.g., hospital medicine, fire departments, the military) were applied to EMS. In many instances these practices were based on expert opinions and rational conjecture. Now, as we have moved into the twenty-first century, many EMS practices have been examined through research methods. To the surprise of many, some EMS practices that were considered intuitive, such as endotracheal intubation and medical anti-shock trousers (MAST) have been found to be less effective than once thought.[1, 2] One of the hallmarks of a profession, when compared to a trade, is the ability to change practices and procedures based on evolving research. Thus, a solid and objective research program is what should and will drive EMS practices in the coming years.

The importance of research to EMS cannot be overstated. To continue to receive the required funding and support, EMS must prove that the care and service it provides truly benefit the patients and the community and are cost-effective. This is primarily demonstrated through **outcomes-based research**. Outcomes-based research can help determine whether a procedure, drug, treatment, or similar strategy actually improves patient outcomes (e.g., **mortality**, **morbidity**, **quality of life**). If you can't prove it makes a difference, then why do you do it?

The **National EMS Research Agenda**, published in 2001 by the National Highway Traffic Safety Administration (NHTSA), provided a guide to future EMS research in the United States.[3] The document drew several conclusions about the need for EMS research and made several recommendations. These included:

- Develop a cadre of EMS researchers and support them early in their careers.
- Facilitate collaboration between EMS researchers and those from other disciplines (e.g., social scientists, economists, epidemiologists, and others).
- Establish a reliable funding stream for EMS research within government.
- Establish an alternate funding source for EMS research outside of government.

- Recognize the need for EMS research.
- View research as necessary for the improvement of patient care.
- Enhance ethical approaches to research.

They concluded that a national investment in EMS research infrastructure is necessary to overcome the obstacles that currently impede EMS research. Funding is needed to train new researchers and to establish their careers.

Increased financial support is necessary to develop effective treatments for the diseases that drive the design of the EMS system, including injury and sudden cardiac arrest. Innovative strategies to make EMS research easier to accomplish in emergency situations must be legitimized and implemented.

Researchers must have access to patient outcome information so that the impact of prehospital and out-of-hospital patient care can be evaluated and improved. Incorporating standard scientific methodology into the evaluation of biomedical and technical advances in prehospital/out-of-hospital care is crucial.

In summary, research is the key to maintaining an appropriate focus on improving the overall health of the community in a competitive and cost-conscious health care market. Most important, research is essential to ensure that the best possible patient care is provided in the prehospital and out-of-hospital setting.

This chapter will provide an overview of research and the scientific method. It will detail some of the research methodologies and provide insight in to how EMS personnel should evaluate research studies. Hopefully, it will encourage you, as a paramedic, to venture into the world of research.

RESEARCH AND THE SCIENTIFIC METHOD

The word **science** literally means "knowledge." However, science is generally defined as "knowledge attained through study or practice." Science is the state or fact of having knowledge that is derived through the scientific method (defined next). Use of the scientific method to study a given issue is known as research. Research is patient, careful, systematic study and investigation

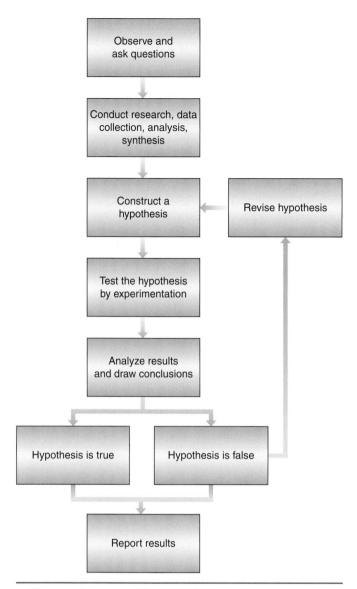

● **Figure 5-1** Steps of the scientific method.

in some field of knowledge, undertaken to discover or establish facts or principles. In EMS, we use research to understand how EMS works and how it does not. However, as you will learn, paramedicine is a part of the discipline of medicine, and medicine is both an art and a science. The knowledge of EMS is science. How we apply that knowledge is art. Excellent paramedics know the science of EMS and use the art of EMS to apply the science.

The fundamental principle behind scientific research is the **scientific method**—a process by which scientists, collectively and over time, endeavor to construct an accurate representation of the world. This representation must be reliable, consistent, and nonarbitrary. The advantage of the scientific method is that it is unprejudiced if properly applied and reproducible.

The scientific method follows these distinct steps (Figure 5-1 ●):

● *Observe and ask questions.* The first step in the scientific method is to observe something in the universe and ask a question. For example, you and your EMS colleagues have observed that calls for psychiatric patients are

more common when the moon is full. So, you decide to determine whether this observation is true. You have made an observation and are now asking a question.

● *Conduct research, data collection, analysis, and synthesis.* The first step in answering your question is to do some background research. Today, this can be easily done through the Internet or through scientific databases such as **PubMed**, which is operated by the U.S. National Library of Medicine.[4] In your study about the effects of a full moon on psychiatric illness, you may find several prior studies and publications on the subject. You can also look at similar perceived phenomena, such as the rate of obstetrical deliveries when the moon is full. When embarking on a study, make it easier on yourself and see if your question or similar questions have already been addressed.

● *Construct a hypothesis.* In your background research you fail to find any study that has looked at whether there is an increase in psychiatric calls when the moon is full, so you decide to move forward with your research. The next step will be to construct a **hypothesis**. Your hypothesis is the specific question your study will answer. It must be something that can be clearly defined and measured. It must be constructed carefully so it will answer your original question. As you move forward with your psychiatric call study, a suitable hypothesis might be, "Psychiatric emergencies are more common when the lunar cycle is in a full moon phase."

● *Test the hypothesis by experimentation.* The next step is to set up an **experiment** to test your hypothesis to determine whether it is true or false. The experiment must be a fair test and must be reproducible (that is, someone else could conduct the same test in the same way). You can conduct a fair test only by changing just one variable in your experiment at a time while keeping all other conditions the same. In your investigation of psychiatric calls, you must clearly define the parameters of the experiment, which may not be as simple as it seems. First, you must define what constitutes a psychiatric call. It could be as easy as stating that a psychiatric call is any call that is marked on a patient run report as psychiatric. Next, you must define a full moon. Different people can look at the moon and have differing opinions about whether it is full. Thus, you might define a full moon as a five-day period that begins two days before the absolute day of the full moon, as stated in a reliable almanac or calendar, and two days after. During this five-day window, the moon will appear full to most people. Finally, you must define the time interval for the study, which might cover, say, three or six months of full-moon periods.

- *Analyze results and draw conclusions.* After you have completed your study, you must collect and analyze the results. This will typically involve some level of statistical analysis. Then, based on your analysis, you can determine whether your hypothesis is true or false. If, in fact, your hypothesis is found false, you can revise or construct a new hypothesis.

- *Revise the hypothesis.* If your hypothesis is found to be correct, you do not need to revise it. However, you might want to revise one parameter and run the experiment again. For example, you decide to change the definition of full moon to the single day of the lunar cycle when the moon is truly full, instead of the five-day definition you were initially using. Interestingly, in your study, you actually find that psychiatric emergencies are slightly less common during full moons, both when defined as a five-day period and when defined as only the day of the true full moon. So now you must revise your hypothesis again to state "Psychiatric emergencies are not more common when the lunar cycle is in the full moon phase." Now your hypothesis is correct according to the data you collected.

- *Report results.* The practice in scientific research, especially medical research, is to share your findings regardless of whether your hypothesis was found to be true or false. In medicine, this primarily occurs through publishing the results in a **peer-review** journal. The publishing of your data opens scientific discussion that will add further insight to your findings and hypothesis.

As you run your experiment or review the results, new information will often become available, causing you to stop and revise some of the steps in your experimental protocol. Stopping, backing up, and repeating a step in the scientific method is common and called an **iterative process**.

TYPES OF RESEARCH

There are various types of research. Typically, research is described as quantitative, qualitative, or mixed. Stated simply, **quantitative research** describes phenomena in numbers while **qualitative research** describes them in words. **Mixed research** is a combination of quantitative and qualitative research and uses both numbers and words to describe the phenomena being studied. These are totally different approaches and each has its strengths and weaknesses (Table 5-1). Most medical research is quantitative.

In addition, research is either retrospective or prospective. Retrospective research examines information that already exists while

TABLE 5-1 | Summary of Research Types

	Quantitative Research	Qualitative Research	Mixed Research
Scientific Method	The researcher tests the hypothesis with data (deductive approach)	The researcher generates a hypothesis after collecting data (inductive approach)	Deductive and inductive
Focus	Narrow topic	Variable topic	Wide topic
Behavior	Studied under controlled conditions	Studied in more than one context	Studied in natural environment
Nature of reality	Objective	Commonsense (pragmatic)	Subjective
Nature of data	Numbers	Numbers and words	Words
Data analysis	Statistical	Statistical and words	Words
Results	Generalizable	May be generalizable	Nongeneralizable
Report	Statistical	Mixed	Narrative

prospective research involves study that starts now and examines what happens from this point forward (or to a predetermined ending date). Occasionally, some studies will have both prospective and retrospective components (e.g., a before and after study).

Quantitative versus Qualitative Research

Quantitative research is objective and specific. It is designed to determine the relationship between one thing (independent variable) and another (dependent or outcome variable) and describe it with numbers (statistics). The **independent variable** is the variable that affects the dependent variable under study. The **dependent variable** (or outcome variable) is the variable being affected or presumed affected by the independent variable. For example, a study that seeks to determine whether faster EMS response times impact patient survival would be considered quantitative research. The EMS response time would be the independent variable while mortality would be the dependent variable.

In addition to experimental quantitative research, as just described, there is nonexperimental and survey-quantitative research. Nonexperimental quantitative research is often used when there are independent variables that cannot be manipulated for one reason or another (e.g., ethical concerns). Nonexperimental research primarily measures what naturally occurs or what has already occurred. Our study of psychiatric patients and the full moon is an example of nonexperimental quantitative research. Survey-quantitative research is a common strategy that is widely used outside medicine and the hard sciences. It is also considered a form of nonexperimental quantitative research. Typically, a survey (either a written questionnaire or an interview) will be performed in the target population. Then, the results will be analyzed and reported. Surveys are commonly used to reflect public opinion and for marketing and social science research.

Qualitative research primarily relies on the collection of qualitative (nonnumeric) data. It primarily seeks the "why" and not the "how" of the phenomena being studied. Qualitative research primarily occurs in a natural setting. For example, many of the studies on stress in EMS have used qualitative methodologies. These studies often evaluate how an individual feels. Qualitative research has an important role in quality assurance. Customer surveys and patient satisfaction programs rely heavily on qualitative methods.

Prospective versus Retrospective Studies

A research project, regardless of whether it has a quantitative or a qualitative design, will be either a **retrospective study** or a **prospective study**. Retrospective studies look at existing data. For example, in our ongoing discussion of the psychiatric patient and full moon study, the design could either be retrospective or prospective. In a retrospective study, all EMS run sheets for a predetermined period of time (e.g., one year) would be carefully reviewed for psychiatric calls. When found, the date of the call and other necessary information would be recorded. In a prospective design, starting on a given day, all psychiatric calls would be flagged and the date recorded. The study would continue until a target date has been reached or a predetermined number of call records have been obtained. Generally speaking, prospective studies have greater validity than retrospective studies. There are several reasons for this. First, prospective studies use a research form or instrument specifically designed for the study. These tend to make the study more objective, accurate, and complete. When looking at historical data, it is often difficult to identify the specific data being sought. Also, there is more chance for the introduction of **bias** in the data gathering for retrospective studies. Despite these problems, there are benefits to retrospective studies. First, the data already exist and are immediately available. Second, retrospective studies are generally less expensive than prospective methodologies.

EXPERIMENTAL DESIGN

Not all studies are created equal. As a rule, the closer a study adheres to the scientific method the more valid the study, and the more valid the study the closer it is to the truth.

There are several types of experimental designs and these have varying degrees of validity. They include experimental studies, quasiexperimental studies, and observational studies. An **experimental study** will have both a **control group** (a group of subjects who do not have manipulation of the independent variable) and a **treatment group**, also called an **experimental group**. Subjects are randomly assigned to one of the groups. The researcher does not assign subjects or affect the assignment of subjects to the groups. The goal of randomization is to ensure that the demographics between the groups are similar. Experimental studies where subjects

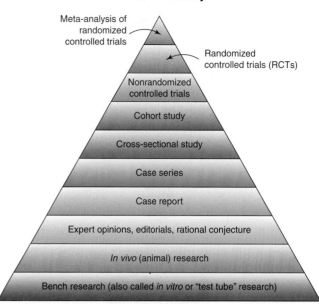

Levels of Validity

● **Figure 5-2** Hierarchy of validity of study types. The most valid type of study is at the top of the pyramid, the least valid at the bottom.

are randomized into either the treatment group or the control group are considered among the most valid of studies.

A similar experimental design is the quasiexperimental study. A **quasiexperimental study** is one in which the scientist does not randomly assign subjects to the study groups. With quasiexperimental studies, there is a greater chance of having groups that are demographically different. Also, there is a greater chance of the introduction of bias (even subconsciously) into the study when subjects are not randomly assigned to the groups. Because of this, quasiexperimental studies are generally considered less valid than experimental studies. However, quasiexperimental studies are quite useful, because in some situations randomization is not possible or is unethical.

An **observational study** is one that does not have a control group. Instead, a single group or multiple groups are studied without comparison to a control. In an observational study, the scientist does not control the variables. Observational studies are considered less valid than experimental or quasiexperimental studies but have an important role in medicine. In many situations it is unethical to withhold treatment from a group simply for the purposes of experimentation. For example, hydroxocobalamin has been found to be a safe antidote for cyanide poisoning, and failing to treat a victim of cyanide poisoning with a safe antidote might result in the victim's death. Because of this, it would be ethically and humanely impossible to study hydroxocobalamin in anything but an observational study. Observational studies are common in medicine.

Specific Study Types

Within the three general categories of scientific research just described (experimental, quasiexperimental, and observational), there are various specific types of study you will encounter in the medical literature. These are presented in a descending order of validity (Figure 5-2 ●).

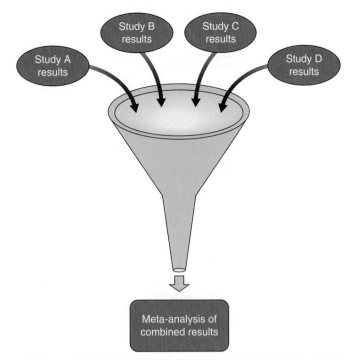

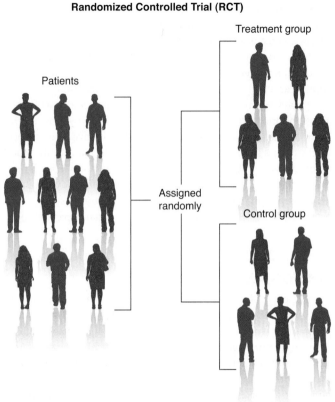

● **Figure 5-3** Meta-analysis is an analysis of the combined results of several prior studies.

● **Figure 5-4** A randomized controlled trial has a treatment group and a control group that is not receiving the treatment being studied. The results of the two groups can be compared.

● *Meta-analysis of randomized controlled trials.* The advent of modern computing has made **meta-analysis** possible. In this study type, researchers locate all available appropriate randomized controlled trials (described next) of a particular area of study. Then, they assimilate the raw data from all these studies into a single database. They subsequently analyze the data and draw conclusions. This is the most valid type of study because it represents a much larger part of the population and often represents a more diverse demographic than each individual study. It is possible to do a meta-analysis of observational studies, but these study types are not common. A meta-analysis is labor intensive and difficult to perform (Figure 5-3 ●).

● *Randomized controlled trials (RCTs).* The **randomized controlled trial (RCT)** closely adheres to the scientific method and is extremely valid. Subjects are randomized into a treatment group (or groups) and a control group (Figure 5-4 ●). The randomization can be achieved in different ways and the researchers cannot have a role in group assignment. One method of avoiding the introduction of bias into an RCT is to "blind" the scientist, the subject, or both. In a **single blind study** the subjects do not know whether they are in the treatment group or the control group. This helps to prevent them from changing behavior during the experiment. In a **double blind study** both the subjects and the experimenters are blinded as to who is in the control group and who is not (Figure 5-5 ●). An example of a double blind study is one that was used to determine whether the administration of morphine

affected subsequent emergency department assessment of patients with possible appendicitis. A pharmacist prepared identical-looking vials, one containing the morphine and the other containing normal saline. When ordered, neither the doctor nor the patients knew if they were getting the drug or the **placebo**. When the experiment was over the data were "unblinded," the analysis completed, and the hypothesis tested.

● *Nonrandomized controlled trials.* **Nonrandomized controlled trials**, also called quasiexperimental studies, as described earlier, have a control group and a treatment group—but assignment to these groups is not randomized (Figure 5-6 ●). This type of study has less validity than an RCT, but it has utility in some circumstances. For example, two battalions of soldiers are going to be tested to determine whether a new IV access device is effective on the battlefield. One battalion serves as the control group and does not receive the new device while the other battalion receives the device. At a given point in time the IV success rate between the groups will be analyzed and compared. The problem in this study design is that there is an increased chance that the two study groups will be different. For example, one battalion is from San Antonio and, incidentally, 25 percent of their soldiers had prior medical training. The other battalion is from Las Vegas and only 12 percent of their group had prior medical training. The prior experience of the San Antonio battalion could affect the results and not give a clear picture of the true effectiveness of the device.

- *Cohort study.* A **cohort study** is an observational study in which subjects who have a certain condition and/or who receive a particular treatment are followed over time and compared with another group who are not affected by the condition under investigation (Figure 5-7 ●). For research purposes, a cohort is any group of individuals who are linked in some way or who have experienced the same significant life event within a given period. A commonly cited example of a cohort study is twin studies. When most twins reach adulthood they typically go their separate ways. Scientists will look at behaviors or characteristics that are different in one twin (e.g., smoking, homosexuality) and compare them to the other twin (who is genetically identical or similar). This can help us to better understand what factors (genetic, social, environmental) are causing the differences.

- *Cross-sectional study.* A **cross-sectional study**, also called a cross-sectional analysis, is an observational study and similar to a cohort study in that various groups are compared without a control. However, unlike a cohort study (which is a longitudinal study that looks at measurements over time), a cross-sectional study looks at a single point in time. For example, a study of EMS providers was completed on a certain date to determine the average number of years of formal education by training level that existed within the group at that time. This would be an example of a cross-sectional study.

- *Case series.* A **case series** is a study that looks at a group of patients (typically a smaller number than found in an RCT) with a similar condition. This is how the AIDS epidemic in San Francisco was first identified. An epidemiologist noted a cluster of patients with similar disease findings (AIDS) and looked at the similarities and differences between these patients in order to isolate a possible cause.

- *Case report.* A **case report** is a structured study of a single patient who is unique or interesting to the medical community in general. These are usually short reports and have limited scientific validity.

- *Expert opinions, editorials, and rational conjecture.* When modern EMS was being planned, there was no identifiable body of knowledge to guide the development of the profession. Instead, physicians and other experts

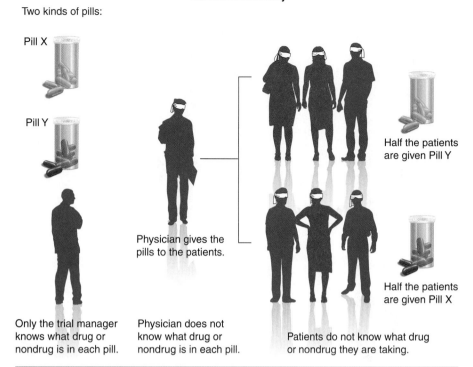

Double Blind Study

Two kinds of pills:

Pill X

Pill Y

Physician gives the pills to the patients.

Only the trial manager knows what drug or nondrug is in each pill.

Physician does not know what drug or nondrug is in each pill.

Half the patients are given Pill Y

Half the patients are given Pill X

Patients do not know what drug or nondrug they are taking.

● **Figure 5-5** In the double blind study illustrated here neither the experimenter nor the subjects know what drug they are taking. (The pills are not identified by drug name but only as "Pill X" and "Pill Y.")

were consulted, and they provided their best opinion about needed practices and procedures. While this strategy is suitable for use before scientific research is available or while scientific research is occurring, it can be problematic when research finally shows that the resulting practices are ineffective or harmful. Many modern EMS practices became established (e.g., spinal immobilization practices, critical incident stress debriefings) because an expert thought them appropriate or effective. However, as additional information has been revealed by the research process, these practices, or specific aspects of these practices, are now considered to be of questionable benefit.

- *Animal research.* Animal research, also called *in vivo* (within the living) research, is important in understanding how certain drugs and procedures affect biological systems. Humans are mammals, and there has certainly been some important information learned from animal research, especially research on other mammals. However, findings in one species do not necessarily apply to other species. Computer modeling is starting to replace some aspects of animal research.

- *Bench research.* **Bench research** is scientific research at its most basic level. This type of research, often called *in vitro* (within the glass) or "test tube" research, is extremely important in learning how the universe functions. Bench research is often the first step in a research strategy that ultimately leads to animal and human research.

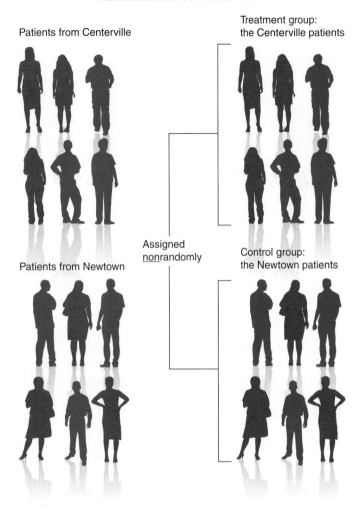

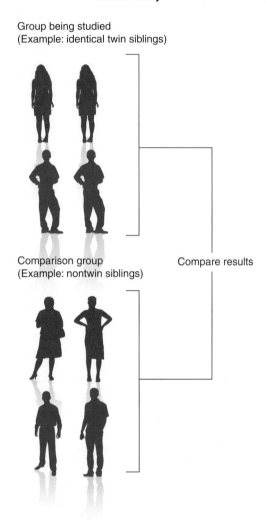

● **Figure 5-6** In a randomized controlled trial, assignments to the treatment group and the control group are made at random. In a nonrandomized study, assignments to the two groups are, as the name indicates, not randomized.

When evaluating the quality of research supporting a clinical practice, reviewers will typically stratify the scientific evidence based on the type and validity of the experimental designs used (Figures 5-8 and 5-9 ●).

Study Validity

Validity is an important part of scientific research. Validity concerns whether or how well the study supports the conclusions—that is, is the interpretation of the results appropriate? We often look at a study as having **external validity** and **internal validity**. External validity assures that the results can be generalized, or possess generalizability (i.e., the results will hold true for other persons at other places and in other times). Internal validity assures that the results can be attributed to the cause (e.g, an increase in psychiatric calls can be attributed to the full moon) and not to other possible causes.

● **Figure 5-7** A cohort is a group of subjects who share a certain characteristic. For example, all may be cancer patients. A cohort study observes and compares the cohort group with a group whose members do not have the cohort characteristic.

LEVELS OF EVIDENCE
Prospective randomized controlled trials
Natural randomized controlled trials
Prospective, nonrandomized controlled trials
Retrospective nonrandomized controlled trials
Case series (no control group)
Animal studies
Extrapolations
Rational conjecture

● **Figure 5-8** The American Heart Association levels of evidence.

LEVELS OF EVIDENCE		
↑	Ia.	Meta-analysis of randomized controlled trials
	Ib.	One randomized controlled trial
	IIa.	Controlled trial without randomization
	IIb.	Other type of quasiexperimental study
	III.	Descriptive studies (e.g., comparative studies, correlation studies, and case-control studies)
	IV.	Expert committee reports or opinions, or clinical experience of respected authorities, or both

• **Figure 5-9** Oxford Center for Evidence-Based Medicine levels of evidence.

ETHICAL CONSIDERATIONS IN HUMAN RESEARCH

While medical research is essential, an overriding concern is the rights of those who serve as subjects in the studies. During the Nazi regime in Germany in the twentieth century, the physician Josef Mengele and others conducted experiments on prisoners, primarily Jews, in German concentration camps. All these studies were performed without the consent of the subjects and often ended in the death of the subject. Some of the experiments had devastating effects, such as when injection of chemicals into the eyes of children to change their eye color resulted in blindness.

After the Nazi experimental atrocities came to light, an international consensus developed that it was necessary to protect the rights of humans who participate in research studies. Following the postwar trials of key Nazis at Nuremburg, Germany, the trial verdict included a set of guidelines to protect human subjects in research. These guidelines, called *The Nuremburg Code of 1947*, were the first code to guide ethical practice in human research.[5]

CONTENT REVIEW

► An overriding concern in medical research is the rights of those who serve as subjects.

The United States has not been free of unethical research, even after the Nuremburg guidelines were promulgated. As a notorious example, between 1928 and 1972 the U.S. Public Health Service and researchers from Tuskegee University in Alabama allowed African American men infected with syphilis to remain untreated in order to study the natural progression of the disease. The men were never told they were infected and little, if any, treatment was provided.[6]

Additional strategies and guidelines regarding protection of human subjects have been developed since the Nuremburg Code. These include the Helsinki Declaration of 1964, developed by the World Medical Association, and amended in 1975, 1983, 1989, 2000, and 2008.[7] The fundamental principles of the Helsinki Declaration are a respect for the individual, the ability of the subject to make an informed decision about participating in the research (initial and ongoing), and assurance by the researcher that the patient's safety will be protected. Partly as a result of the Tuskegee experiment, in 1979 the U.S. Department of Health, Education, and Welfare released the Belmont Report, which was formally entitled *Ethical Principles and Guidelines for the Protection of Human Subjects of Research*.[8] In 1991, 14 other federal agencies joined what is now the Department of Health and Human Services (HHS) in adopting uniform rules for protection of human subjects. The Office for Human Research Protections (OHRP) was also established within HHS.

Institutional Review Boards

To ensure the protection of human subjects in research, institutions that perform these studies must have an **institutional review board (IRB)**. The IRB (sometimes called the ethical review board or independent ethics committee) is a committee that approves, monitors, and reviews human research.[9] The goal of the IRB is to protect human subjects. IRBs have the power to approve or disapprove a study before it begins. They also have the power to require researchers to modify or even terminate a study if they feel the subjects are at risk. Most journals will not consider a study for publication unless it has been formally approved by the IRB.

LEGAL CONSIDERATIONS

The Law and Ethical Medical Research. *The Nuremburg Code did not have the force of law but influenced laws and rules for the same purpose that were subsequently adopted in various countries, including regulations issued by the U.S. Department of Health and Human Services governing federally funded research in the United States.*

Today medical research in the United States is closely regulated. All studies must be approved by an independent review board and subjects must provide informed consent in order to participate. The study is continuously monitored and certain groups (e.g., prisoners) are not allowed to participate. While there is a potential for harm in many studies, overall research is now a much safer endeavor and has provided many of the advancements in modern medical care—including many of those in prehospital care.

AN OVERVIEW OF STATISTICS

Statistics is the mathematics of collecting and analyzing data to draw conclusions and make predictions. It is an essential part of scientific study. There are two general categories of statistics: descriptive statistics and inferential statistics. **Descriptive statistics** are used to describe the basic features of the data obtained in a study. They provide a summary of the sample. Together with simple graphics analysis, they form the basis of virtually every quantitative analysis of data. **Inferential statistics** draw information from the sampled observations of a population and make conclusions about the population. Both kinds of statistics are important in research.[10]

Descriptive Statistics

Descriptive statistics describe the nature of a sample. The most common descriptive statistic you will encounter is the **mean**, or average. It is calculated by adding the values, and then dividing the sum by the number of values involved. This provides the average or typical value of a group of numbers or cases. The mean is especially useful when the data are what statisticians call "normally distributed." This means that if you graphed the data, they would form a shape similar to a bell curve, a symmetrical or nearly symmetrical curve with most data falling in the center of the graph and fewer data falling at the beginning and end. Height of individuals is an example of a normally distributed variable. Most people have a height close to the average, with a few very short and a few very tall people at each end of the graph.

When the data are not normally distributed, the **median** is a better way of finding a typical value. To compute the median, put the values into numerical order and find the middle value. This is the median, also known as the "fiftieth percentile." For example, if you have seven exam scores, to find the median, you put the scores in order and find the fourth highest (or fourth lowest, since it is the same).

Here is an example of how the median can be more useful than the mean in some situations: In many states the number of emergency calls received by EMS agencies is not normally distributed. There are frequently a few very busy services in urban areas, a good number of moderately busy services, and a larger number of services in rural areas that receive a much smaller number of calls. If you were to compute the mean, or average number of calls, it would be skewed by the very busy services, even though there are only a few of them, because they receive such a high number. However, if you computed the median, you would get a smaller number that would better reflect the number of calls received by a typical service.

The mean and the median tell only one part of the story. They are called **measures of central tendency**, because they indicate the center of the group. A different but very important quality to know about a group is how spread out it is, or how dispersed the data are.

There are two closely related measures of dispersion that you are likely to see. The first is called the **variance**. To get it, we take each value and subtract the mean from it. We cannot take the average of these numbers and get anything useful, because the negative numbers will cancel out the positive numbers and we will get zero. To overcome this, we multiply each number by itself (square it) and add up the squared numbers. We then divide this sum by the number of values we started with. (For reasons statisticians can describe, when we are working with samples, we usually divide by one less than the number of values.) This is the variance.

To get the **standard deviation (SD or σ)**, the other common measure of dispersion, we take the square root of the variance. Figure 5-10 ● shows two examples of variance and standard deviation. The standard deviation gives us valuable information about the data. If two groups of data have the same mean, but the second has a standard deviation much larger than the first, the data in the second group are much more spread out than the data in the first group. The SD is also used in many statistical formulas.

Another way we can describe data is to give the **mode**. This is simply the most common value in a set of data. If you graph the data, with the data value on the horizontal axis and the frequency of occurrence on the vertical axis (also known as a frequency distribution), the mode is the value associated with the highest point on the graph.

Inferential Statistics

As noted earlier, the mean, median, variance, standard deviation, and mode are examples of descriptive statistics. They describe the nature of a sample of data taken from a **population**, a group we are interested in.

Descriptive statistics are related to, but quite different from, inferential statistics. Here, instead of describing the sample, we wish to draw inferences about the population the sample came from. In this case, we say we are estimating **parameters** of the population. For example, if the sample is of sufficient size and we make certain assumptions about the population and how the sample was selected, we can estimate the mean value of the population from which we drew our sample. Polling organizations commonly use these techniques in reporting results of their surveys. We must keep in mind, however, the phenomenon of **sampling error**. This is an estimation of the difference between the value obtained from the sample and the value that would be obtained from the entire population, stemming solely from the fact that only a sample of the population was included.

When researchers find that something occurs with a certain frequency, they usually report this proportion as a percentage. For example, survival from cardiac arrest caused by ventricular fibrillation (VF) may be 20 percent in a particular study. But since the study looked at a sample of patients in VF, this proportion is only an estimate and may in reality be higher or lower in the entire group with cardiac arrest. Investigators can calculate how much variability exists in this percentage based on the number of observations, the actual data, and how reliable they wish the estimate to be.

This variability (not the same as the variance) can then be added and subtracted to the original proportion to give what is called a **confidence interval**. For example, suppose the investigators calculated the variability in the previous example with 95 percent confidence and found it was 6 percent. Then we would have a 95 percent confidence interval of 20 percent plus or minus 6 percent. This means that, assuming the hypothesis is true, we can be 95 percent confident that the actual rate of survival under the conditions studied was between 14 percent and 26 percent.

Confidence intervals are very important in interpreting the value of the research results. If the confidence interval for a proportion such as the previous one included zero, then there would be a real possibility that there is no actual difference between the study group outcome and the control group outcome. We would conclude that the results are not statistically significant and that there is insufficient reason to believe there is a difference between the two groups.

Examples of Variance and Standard Deviation

To see how the variance and standard deviation can give valuable information about data, consider this example: Two different EMT-P classes take the same midterm exam. The classes are the same size (seven students each) and have the same mean (or average) score, 85%. If we did not look any further, we might think the two classes performed the same on the exam. By looking at the variance and standard deviation, though, we can see that they are actually quite different.

Class 1

	Score	Mean	Score − Mean	(Score − Mean)^2
	78	85	−7	49
	81	85	−4	16
	82	85	−3	9
	84	85	−1	1
	87	85	2	4
	89	85	4	16
	94	85	9	81
Sum	595		0	176

Recall that to get the variance we must find the mean, then find the differences between the scores and the mean, square these differences, add them up, and divide by one less than the number of scores. The mean is included in the second column to make it easier to calculate the difference between each score and the mean. The variance is then 176/6 = 29.3. The standard deviation is the square root of 29.3, which is 5.4.

Class 2

	Score	Mean	Score − Mean	(Score − Mean)^2
	82	85	−3	9
	83	85	−2	4
	84	85	−1	1
	85	85	0	0
	86	85	1	1
	87	85	2	4
	88	85	3	9
Sum	595		0	28

Again, to get the variance, we sum the squared differences in the last column and divide by one less than the number of scores: 28/6 = 4.7. The standard deviation is the square root of 4.7, or 2.2, less than half the standard deviation of the first class.

This implies that the scores in the first class are much more spread out than the scores in the second class. When we graph the scores, we can see that this is true:

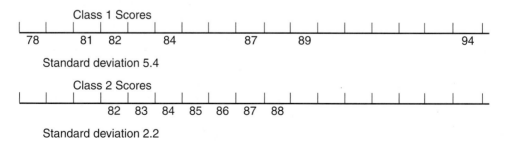

● **Figure 5-10** Examples of variance and standard deviation.

Quantitative and Qualitative Statistics

There are many tests for finding differences between groups. Statisticians frequently classify them into qualitative and quantitative tests. **Qualitative statistics** usually deal with data that are nonnumeric in nature (e.g., female, male) or that are nonnumeric in nature and have been assigned a number indicating ranking or ordering of importance or severity (stage I, II, and III of certain cancers, for example). These are sometimes called **nominal data** and **ordinal data**. Finding the mean of such data may be impossible or absurd since they are categorical in nature. **Quantitative statistics**, however, are numerical in nature, such as temperature measured in degrees on a thermometer or height of an individual measured in centimeters or inches. They are sometimes referred to as continuous data.

Other Types of Data

Commonly used tests you may see in research include **t test**, the **analysis of variance (ANOVA)**, and the **chi square test**. Which test is used depends to a great extent on the kind of data involved and the kinds of differences the investigators are looking for. We will not describe these tests here, but the interested reader can consult some of the sources listed at the end of this chapter.

Another test you may see is the **odds ratio**. This is used in case-control studies and consists of the odds of having a risk factor if the condition is present, divided by the odds of having the risk factor if the condition is not present. Simply put, the odds ratio describes how strong the association is between a risk factor and the condition it is associated with. The larger the risk factor, the stronger is the association. When you see an odds ratio, look for the confidence interval. Since an odds ratio of 1 indicates that there is no risk associated with the risk factor, if the confidence interval includes 1, there is no statistically significant risk.

For example, suppose investigators survey paramedic students regarding how much education they had received before enrolling in their course. They wish to test the hypothesis that having at least a college degree is associated with passing the paramedic certification exam. After the course is over, they perform the proper calculations and determine that the odds ratio is 1.6. This means a student who passes is 1.6 times as likely to have at least a college degree compared to someone who does not pass the exam. The 95 percent confidence interval, though, is 0.8 to 2.4.

This means we are 95 percent confident the true odds ratio lies between 0.8 and 2.4. Since the interval includes 1 (keep in mind an odds ratio of 1 means there is no association), we cannot be 95 percent confident that there really is an association, and so we conclude there is no statistically significant relationship between having at least a college degree and passing the paramedic exam in this group. However, if the 95 percent confidence interval had been 1.2 to 2.0, an interval that does not include 1, we would have concluded with 95 percent confidence that there is a statistically significant relationship and that a person who passes the paramedic exam is between 1.2 and 2.0 times as likely to have at least a college degree.

Many other statistical tests are used for different kinds of studies and different kinds of data. The References section at the end of this chapter lists several sources from which you can learn more about them.

FORMAT OF A RESEARCH PAPER

When authors submit their findings to a journal, they structure their results in a standardized fashion that allows others to quickly understand what the researchers did and what they found (Table 5-2). The first thing to appear after the title and names of the authors is the **abstract**. This is a brief paragraph that summarizes the need for the study, the research methods used, and the results encountered. Many people use the abstract to determine whether or not the paper is one of interest to them and therefore worth reading.

The *introduction* is the first section of the paper itself. This is a brief description of pertinent, previously published papers on the subject of the investigation. It should describe why the study was undertaken and what the purpose of the study was or what hypothesis the authors wanted to test.

Next comes the *methods* section. This describes exactly how the authors conducted the study, including what population they wished to study, how subjects were selected (and excluded), and what intervention was performed, if any. There should be enough information for interested readers to repeat the experiment should they so desire. The authors should also describe how they determined the sample size, how much statistical power there was to detect a difference, which statistical tests they used to analyze the data, and what level of significance they chose for their statistical tests.

The *results* come next. Here the researchers provide their data (or a summary of the data), frequently with tables, charts, and graphs to help make sense of the information they gathered. This section presents the data, but does not elaborate on them.

The *discussion* section is where the authors interpret their findings and describe their significance. There is usually a description of how this new information fits into the field of study and whether it supports or refutes previous research. There should also be a discussion of the limitations of the study, frequently followed by a call for further research to answer the questions raised by the study.

The *summary,* or conclusion, is a very brief (no more than a few sentences) recap of the main findings of the study.

TABLE 5-2	Research Paper Format for Some Emergency Medicine Journals		
Prehospital Emergency Care	**Annals of Emergency Medicine**	**Academic Emergency Medicine**
Abstract	Abstract	Abstract
Introduction	Introduction	Introduction
Methods	Methods	Methods
Results	Results	Results
Discussion	Limitations	Discussion
Conclusions	Discussion	Limitations
References	References	Conclusions
		References

HOW A RESEARCH PAPER IS PUBLISHED

Once the authors of a study have drafted their paper, they submit it to a scientific journal for publication. Each journal has its own rules, but all peer-reviewed journals follow the same general procedure. After receiving the paper, the editor sends it to one or more members of a review board, people who have significant expertise either in the field covered by the journal or in a related area, such as statistics or research methodology. Generally speaking, the reviewers are blinded as to the names of the authors and the institution with which they are affiliated. This serves to ensure objectivity and minimize bias. The reviewers read the paper and evaluate it for its adherence to standards of research methods, its pertinence to the field, and the potential value it has for practitioners. The reviewers send their comments to the editor, who then decides whether to publish it, send it back for revisions, or reject it. A copy editor may review the paper correcting grammar, spelling, and syntax. Many papers submitted by researchers are not published, and some journals have reputations for being very selective.

A note here about the term "abstract": In the preceding section, we mentioned that the first part of a research paper is a brief summary paragraph called the abstract. The term *abstract* more commonly describes a brief form of a longer scientific research paper that is often published before the full research paper. The abstract may be presented at national peer meetings, and responses to the abstract may form the basis for adjustments to the full research paper that is subsequently published. Abstracts are also published and cited in peer-review journals.

The peer-review process has recently begun to receive greater attention than it has in the past. This has been the result, ironically, of several studies looking at the quality of published papers. A surprisingly large number of papers, when evaluated objectively for adherence to principles of research methodology, have been shown to be deficient. This has led at least one journal, *Annals of Emergency Medicine,* to review and revamp its review procedures.[11] Reviewers now get training in what to look for and how to evaluate papers, and closer attention will be paid to how statistics are used. This may be the beginning of a trend that should improve the quality of the research that is conducted and published.

ACCESSING THE SCIENTIFIC LITERATURE

Medical school and university libraries have multiple floors containing stacks and stacks of scientific journals. In the past, accessing the scientific literature was a labor-intensive endeavor. Now, in the Internet age, a great deal of the scientific literature is readily available. For many years, journal publishers have archived their publications online. These can be downloaded as Portable Document Files (PDF) or directly. Most journals require a subscription or library affiliation to access. Some are free and referred to as **open access journals** without financial, legal, or technical barriers. If you don't have access to a medical

or university library, many community college and hospital libraries can access the papers for you.

In addition, the National Libraries of Medicine have long provided an accessible database of the medical and scientific literature called PubMed. It is free and allows users to enter various search terms to find the material needed (Figure 5-11 ●). Then, a page will open that lists all the references that are related to your search term (Figure 5-12 ●). You can further refine your search by choosing all articles or review articles. When you find a reference that meets the needs of your research, you can click on the citation and the information about the article and the abstract for the article will open (Figure 5-13 ●). You can then determine whether this is an article worthy of retrieving and reading. Since searching PubMed is a somewhat complex and specialized task, you may want to have a librarian help you with your search to ensure that you get exactly the information you are looking for. If you do not have access to a library, the National Libraries of Medicine operates a document retrieval service known as Lonsome Doc. It can be accessed through the web.

WHAT TO LOOK FOR WHEN REVIEWING A STUDY

Questions to ask when reviewing a study include the following (Table 5-3):

● *Was the research peer reviewed?* This is no guarantee of quality, but it at least indicates that experts have reviewed the study and found it to have some merit. Keep in mind that some journals will deliberately publish papers they know to be of lower quality than usual in order to stir up debate about an important subject.

● *Was there a clear hypothesis or study purpose?* The paper should have a clear description of exactly what the investigators were evaluating and what their study hypothesis was. When a hypothesis is not clearly spelled out, it is very easy for the investigators to draw unjustified conclusions.

● *Was the study approved by an institutional review board (IRB), and was it conducted ethically?* An IRB is a group of people, usually at a hospital or university, who review study proposals to ensure that patients are protected when they participate in research as study subjects. Virtually all medical journals require IRB approval for research involving human subjects.

● *Was the study type appropriate?* Not every investigation lends itself to the format of the randomized controlled clinical trial. It may be necessary, for ethical or financial reasons, to use another format. Evaluate whether the questions the investigators asked were well suited to the type of study they conducted.

● *What population were the researchers studying?* Is the population similar to the one you see in your community and work?

● *What inclusion and exclusion criteria did the researchers use?* If the investigators excluded the patients most likely to have a condition or patients very similar to the ones you see, the study may have very little to tell you.

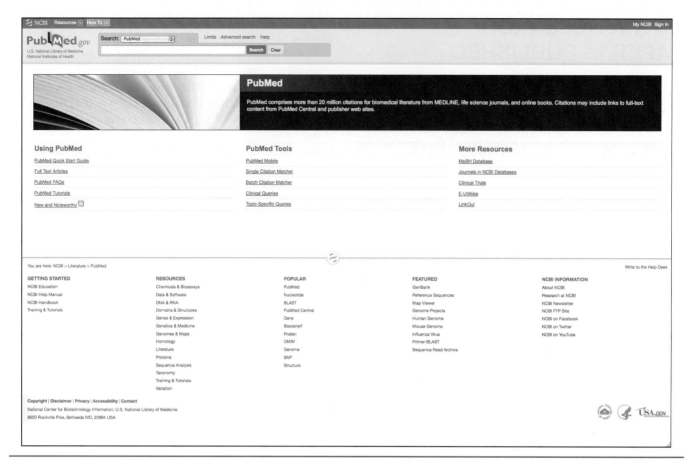

● **Figure 5-11**　Opening screen of the PubMed database search engine.

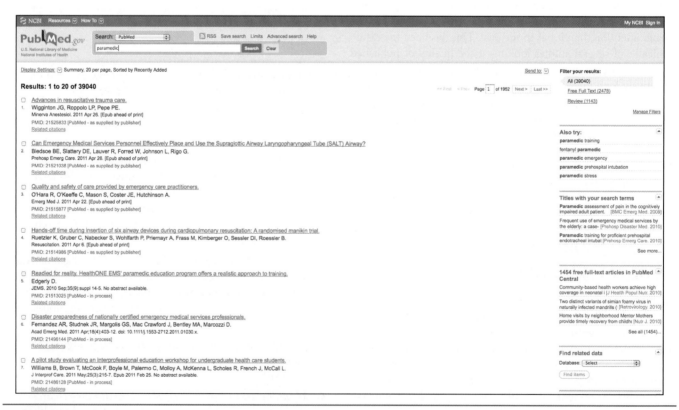

● **Figure 5-12**　Secondary scene of the PubMed database search engine after entering search term "paramedic."

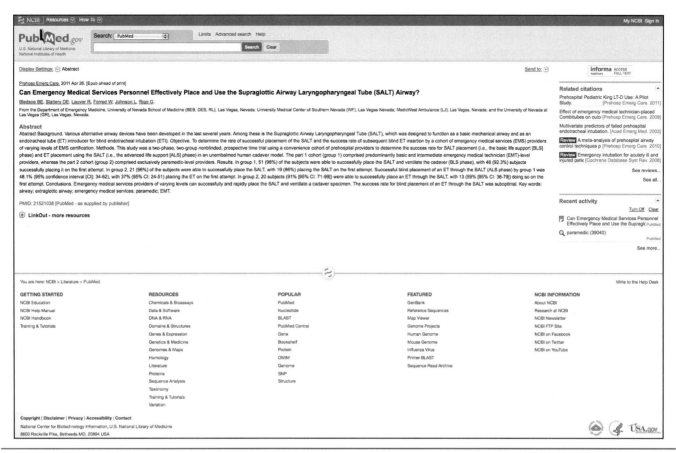

● **Figure 5-13** Individual citation screen of the PubMed database.

TABLE 5-3 | Questions to Ask When Reviewing a Study

- Was the research peer reviewed?
- Was there a clear hypothesis or study purpose?
- Was the study approved by an institutional review board (IRB), and was it conducted ethically?
- Was the study type appropriate?
- What population were the researchers studying?
- What inclusion and exclusion criteria did the researchers use?
- How did the investigators draw their sample?
- How many groups were patients divided into, and were patients assigned to control and study groups properly?
- Were the control and study groups the proper size?
- Were the effects of confounding variables taken into account?
- What kind of data did the investigators collect, and did they analyze the data with the proper statistical tests?
- Were the results reported properly?
- How likely is it that the study results would occur by chance alone?
- Are the author's conclusions logical and based on the data?

- *How did the investigators draw their sample?* Did they use true **random sampling? systematic sampling? time sampling? convenience sampling?**

- *How many groups were patients divided into, and were patients assigned to control and study groups properly?* The effects of bias and confounding must be taken into account for the study to yield worthwhile results. In particular, ask yourself:
  ○ For case-control and cohort studies, were selection bias and recall bias taken into account?
  ○ For randomized controlled studies, were randomization and blind assignment maintained?

- *Were the control and study groups the proper size?* Did the investigators describe the sample size necessary to produce sufficient power to avoid a Type II error (a false negative)? What was the power of the study? (Was the study adequately performed to accurately test the hypothesis in question?)

- *Were the effects of confounding variables (other things that may have affected the study outcome) taken into account?* Did the investigators describe potential confounders and how they prevented them from interfering with the study?

- *What kind of data did the investigators collect, and did they analyze the data with the proper statistical tests?* There are many tests available and more than one may be appropriate for the conditions at hand. You may need to consult a statistician or researcher to determine whether or not the investigators used the right tests on the data. Did the investigators clearly determine before data collection took place which tests they were going to use or was there **data mining**? When the data fail to provide statistically significant results, it is very tempting to perform more tests until one shows significant results. This kind of retrospective testing is called data snooping or **data dredging**. If one continues to perform statistical tests, eventually one will be significant just by chance alone. This inappropriate use of statistics is to be avoided.

- *Were the results reported properly?* When a paper includes a proportion or an odds ratio, is there also a 95 percent confidence interval?

- *How likely is it that the study results would occur by chance alone?* Remember that a *P* value reflects only the odds of seeing the results of a particular piece of research if the study hypothesis is true. A small *P* value may be very impressive, but it does not prove the study hypothesis. Keep in mind also the difference between association and causation. For example, it would be easy to show that the number of drownings increase with sales of ice cream. An inattentive reader might conclude that the sale of more ice cream causes more drownings to occur. In reality, this is an example of association, not causation. Ice cream sales go up when the weather gets warmer, which is also when more people go swimming and drown. This is also an example of confounding.

- *Are the author's conclusions logical and based on the data?* Occasionally a journal publishes a paper that goes against everything you know. It can then be difficult to determine whether you need to change your approach to a particular problem or consider the paper an aberration. After all, by chance alone, some studies will show statistically significant results that are the result of chance or coincidence. Sometimes, the prudent course is to see if anyone else can replicate the experiment before changing your practice. This is a good example of how you should be very cautious in changing your practice based on just one study. If the conclusion is a real one and not spurious, someone else should be able to come up with it, too.

And one more consideration that is very important in EMS research:

- *How "good" was the EMS system in which the study was done?* This factor can have a profound effect on the validity of a study. As an extreme example, how valid would the results of a study of the impact of AED use be if the time from arrest to first responder arrival were 15 minutes? In this scenario, there would likely be no survivors, no matter what intervention was used!

APPLYING STUDY RESULTS TO YOUR PRACTICE

Once you have evaluated a study, you are in a better position to determine whether or not it should change your practice. Before you do so, though, you need to consider several factors. Rarely do clinicians make significant changes on the basis of just one study. Since no study can definitively prove a hypothesis, the reader must look at other studies and his own experience in order to construct an informed opinion. If every other study published on a particular topic comes to very different conclusions than the study at hand, the reader has to wonder whether the study was poorly designed, subject to bias of some sort, affected by unknown confounding variables, or just the result of chance. One must evaluate the field and its knowledge base in order to make an informed decision about how to interpret a piece of research.

The clinical significance is another important piece of the puzzle to consider. A *P* value with lots of zeroes (e.g., $P < 0.0001$) may be very impressive, but not very pertinent. Distinguish between the statistical significance and the clinical significance of the study. Was the difference found in the study large enough to make a real difference to patients?

When investigators conduct their experiments, they have the luxury of selecting patients who meet their criteria and excluding patients who do not. In the real world, things are not quite so tidy. Before we can apply the results of a piece of research to a particular patient, we must be sure the patient is similar enough to the study group to benefit from the intervention.

Finally, EMS providers do not function in a vacuum. Before implementing any significant changes in your practice, speak to the management of your organization and especially to your medical director. You are responsible not only to your patients, but also to your bosses and your medical director. Including them in decision making of this nature is essential and will pay off in better patient care overall.

PARTICIPATING IN RESEARCH

Many EMS systems are not content to watch other people advance their field. They have decided to conduct research themselves. They have found that, by executing well-designed studies, they can not only improve care in their coverage areas, but also improve prehospital care throughout the nation, sharpen the skills of their providers, and rekindle their providers' interest by doing something new and potentially groundbreaking.

Before you participate in such a study, there are certain things you should do and find out (Table 5-4). Usually, the first step is to ask a question. This should involve something of practical importance. Determining the value of a particular intervention (end-tidal CO_2 monitoring, for example) is clearly going to have more impact on EMS than finding out whether ambulances carry 24 four-by-four gauze pads or 48 four-by-four gauze pads.

Once you have focused on the issue and determined exactly what you wish to discover, you can go to the next step. This is where you generate your hypothesis, a statement of exactly what you are going to test. The **null hypothesis** is usually a statement that there is no difference between the groups you are sampling from. The research hypothesis or alternate hypothesis is a statement that there is a difference between the groups. This is often, though not always, what you would like to show.

Once you know what you are evaluating, you need to decide what you want to measure and how you will do it. You also need

TABLE 5-4 | What to Do When You Participate in a Study

- Determine the question.
- Prepare your hypotheses (null hypothesis and research hypothesis).
- Decide what you wish to measure and how you will do it.
- Define the population you are studying.
- Identify the limitations of your study.
- Get the approval of the proper authorities.
- Determine how you will get informed consent from study subjects.
- Gather data, perhaps after conducting pilot trials.
- Analyze the data.
- Determine what you will do with your results (publish, present at a conference, follow up with more studies).

Source: *American College of Cardiology and the American Heart Association, Manual for ACC/AHA Guideline Writing Committees.*

to define the population you will be studying, that is, the group you draw your subjects from and to which you plan to generalize your results.

Closely associated with this step is determining the limitations of your study. This might include limited ability to generalize your results because of the patient-selection methods you used even though you had little or no choice in the methods available to you. Similarly, the population you draw from might be significantly different from other populations.

For example, if you wished to test for improved survival in hypotensive trauma patients, some of whom received a large volume of IV fluids as treatment and some of whom did not, you would need to describe your EMS and trauma care system very carefully. You might have a primarily urban population with predominantly penetrating trauma, short transport times to Level 1 trauma centers, and experienced paramedics. Your results would have limited applicability to a rural population with predominantly blunt trauma, long transport times to small community hospitals, and less experienced emergency medical responders and EMTs.

The best studies limit themselves to a single question or hypothesis. This is desirable because it allows you to focus better on the question at hand. The downside is that you may not find out everything you wanted to. This is usually considered an acceptable trade-off. No single study can answer every question.

The next step in conducting a study is usually to get approval from an institutional review board (IRB). This allows you to get an outside evaluation of your study methodology and reduces considerably the chance you will be accused of conducting an unethical study. One of the items the IRB will undoubtedly be interested in is the issue of informed consent (consent given by the patient based on full disclosure of information regarding the nature, risks, and benefits of the procedure or study).

Several reports in the media over the last few years have described unethical studies in which subjects were not given the opportunity to give or refuse consent because they were not informed of the risks and benefits of participating in the study. In some cases, subjects actually died because they did not receive standard treatment available at the time of the study. These stories have prompted an understandable reluctance on the part of many individuals to participate in research. The U.S. government even came out with standards for government-funded research that describe stringent requirements for informed consent. The IRB process will also determine what kind of consent will be required for your study.

A good **principal investigator (PI)**, the person who oversees the study, will be familiar with these requirements and will be able to guide you through them. The PI should also gain the approval of other appropriate agencies, including the medical director and the head of the service involved.

After you have determined how to gain informed consent, you need to gather your data. Sometimes a pilot trial is undertaken first so you can find unforeseen obstacles to data gathering. Seemingly trivial matters can become very important (such as whether or not busy EMS providers are reluctant to fill out any more forms). A good PI will meet with the EMS providers who are administering the study intervention and collecting the data. The PI should make sure they know how long the study is expected to last. This allows them to make plans and perhaps reschedule certain future activities they had anticipated. The providers collecting data need to know the name of the principal investigator and how to contact him. This is usually, though not always, a physician. Many EMS physicians who conduct field research will recruit a field provider to coordinate and assist with data collection.

Other things to tell participants are the inclusion and exclusion criteria for enrolling patients in the study, the effect of the study on patient care in general, and the risks and potential benefits to patients in the study. Once everyone understands these factors, you will be prepared to go ahead with the study.

After you have collected the data and reached your predetermined sample size, it is time to analyze the data. Use the tests you described in your description of the methods for your study. Be very careful about performing additional tests, especially if your results do not show what you hoped or expected. Data snooping is a dangerous activity. If you perform enough statistical tests, you will eventually find one or more that give you "significant" results. Unfortunately, these results may very well be a product of chance rather than your intervention. When multiple statistical tests are planned for the same set of data, statisticians adjust for this with multiple-testing procedures to avoid such false results. Similarly, *post hoc* analysis of subgroups that were not defined before the study can also be dangerous. This can be a good way of generating hypotheses for future studies, but it is not a good basis for drawing conclusions now.

Once you have finished your data analysis, you must decide what to do with your results. If you feel your study addresses a pertinent timely issue, and you think your methods were well thought out and your study was carefully conducted, you should seriously consider submitting your results to a peer-reviewed journal. This is the best way to get such information out to the EMS community.

Alternatively, you may decide to present your findings at a conference. This usually involves summarizing your methods and results either orally or in the form of a poster, or both. This is less time consuming than writing up a paper for publication but can still get the word out about your results and stimulate others to investigate the same phenomenon.

Do not feel that a "negative" study is worthless. If your study shows no difference in outcome between groups that did and did not receive an intervention, you may have reached important conclusions about the value, or lack of value, of an intervention.

A common result of a well-conducted study is more questions. This frequently stimulates the investigator and others to perform further studies. Once you get involved with researching the answers to questions, you may find yourself a little more skeptical about accepted, untested treatments and more interested in finding out what really works.

EVIDENCE-BASED DECISION MAKING

In the past, traditional medical practices have been based on medical knowledge (often learned during initial education), intuition, and judgment. While all of these are quite important, technology and science change. Thus, medical practice and the use of technology should focus on procedures and practices proven effective in improving patient outcomes. EMS is now at the point where evidence-based decision making and practice

TABLE 5-5 | Applying Classification of Recommendations and Level of Evidence

Estimate of Certainty (Precision) of Treatment Effect	Size of Treatment Effect			
	Class I	**Class IIa**	**Class IIb**	**Class III**
	Benefit >>> Risk **Procedure/Treatment SHOULD be performed/ administered**	Benefit >> Risk Additional studies with focused objectives needed **IT IS REASONABLE to perform procedure/ administer treatment**	Benefit ≥ Risk Additional studies with broad objectives needed; Additional registry data would be helpful **IT IS NOT UNREASONABLE to perform procedure/ administer treatment**	Risk ≥ Benefit No additional studies needed **Procedure/Treatment should NOT be performed/ administered SINCE IT IS NOT HELPFUL AND MAY BE HARMFUL**
Level A Multiple (3-5) population risk strata evaluated General consistency of direction and magnitude of effect	o Recommendation that procedure or treatment is useful/effective o Sufficient evidence from multiple randomized trials or meta-analyses	o Recommendation in favor of treatment or procedure being useful/effective o Some conflicting evidence from multiple randomized trials or meta-analyses	o Recommendation's usefulness/efficacy less well established o Greater conflicting evidence from multiple randomized trials or meta-analyses	o Recommendation that procedure or treatment not useful/effective and may be harmful o Sufficient evidence from multiple randomized trials or meta-analyses
Level B Limited (2-3) population risk strata evaluated	o Recommendation that procedure or treatment is useful/effective o Limited evidence from single randomized trial or non-randomized studies	o Recommendation in favor of treatment or procedure being useful/effective o Some conflicting evidence from single randomized trial or non-randomized studies	o Recommendation's usefulness/efficacy less well established o Greater conflicting evidence from single randomized trial or non-randomized studies	o Recommendation that procedure or treatment not useful/effective and may be harmful o Limited evidence from single randomized trial or non-randomized studies
Level C Very limited (1-2) population risk strata evaluated	o Recommendation that procedure or treatment is useful/effective o Only expert opinion, case studies, or standard-of-care	o Recommendation in favor of treatment or procedure being useful/effective o Only diverging expert opinion, case studies, or standard-of-care	o Recommendation's usefulness/efficacy less well established o Only diverging expert opinion, case studies, or standard-of-care	o Recommendation that procedure or treatment not useful/effective and may be harmful o Only expert opinion, case studies, or standard-of-care

Source: *Reprinted with Permission. Circulation.2008;117:e350–e408. © 2008 American Heart Association, Inc.*

is becoming standard. The use of "best practices" and "clinical pathways" that are based on the best available clinical and scientific evidence available ensures that the care provided is safe, efficacious, and cost-effective. The problem that remains, at least in the EMS setting, is that the available research is, at present, scant or of limited quality. Hopefully, as EMS evolves, this will change.

Evidence-based decision making involves first formulating a question about appropriate treatments. Then the medical literature is searched and organized for additional evaluation. Next, the scientific evidence is stratified based on validity and reliability (See Table 5-5 for the classification recommendations of the American College of Cardiology and the American Heart Association.) Then, if the evidence supports a change in the practice, the change is made. However, the process does not end there. Once the practice has been changed, ongoing evaluation must be carried out to determine whether the practice is correctly applied to the proper group of patients. Also, ongoing outcomes study should occur to determine whether the change in practice is improving essential parameters such as mortality, morbidity, and costs.

 ## SUMMARY

The paramedic of the twenty-first century must have more than a passing knowledge of research. Solid, well-conducted scientific research is the key to improving prehospital care. It is also essential to prove that paramedics make a difference in terms of reducing mortality, morbidity, and pain and suffering. A side benefit to demonstrating the effectiveness of EMS will be an increased (and more appropriate) revenue stream. The future of EMS depends on an aggressive research program, and prehospital research depends on knowledgeable and engaged paramedics.

YOU MAKE THE CALL

One day you and your partner are restocking the ambulance and notice that the crew that precedes you seems to be using a lot more naloxone (Narcan) than your crew. At a shift meeting you bring up the fact that some crews are using more naloxone than others. A discussion ensues, and the general consensus is that there are not a great number of narcotic overdoses in the community so the usage of naloxone might be a misapplication of a protocol. Because you and your partner brought up the issue, you have been asked to study the problem.

So, you and your partner decide to develop a research question. However, you feel that you really need to get a handle on the number of overdoses in the community that required naloxone. So you first do a retrospective study looking at all run reports over the last year. One of your fellow employees, who is on light duty following surgery, goes through all run reports for the prior year. He records the number of total runs, the number of times an opiate overdose was encountered, the number of times naloxone was given, the number of total doses of naloxone administered, and the ID number of the paramedic who administered the drug in each case. These data are placed into an Excel computerized database and analyzed.

When you analyze the data, you see that the incidence of narcotic overdoses requiring naloxone was 0.12 percent of all calls—a pretty low incidence. But, you note that two paramedics were responsible for 45 percent of all naloxone administrations during the study period.

You discuss your findings with your clinical manager and medical director. The medical director directs the clinical manager to provide a continuing education seminar on narcotic overdoses and the usage of naloxone to all paramedics in the system—including the part-timers.

For the next three months you and your partner prospectively monitor the daily run reports and see if any of the parameters in your initial study have changed. At three months you find that the incidence of opiate overdoses requiring naloxone remains low at 0.14 percent. The total amount of naloxone administered diminished significantly, and statistical analysis finds that all paramedics in the system have been using the naloxone similarly. The medical director feels the education program worked and thanks you and your partner for your efforts.

1. What is your study's hypothesis?

2. Did you prove or disprove your hypothesis?

3. What was the derived benefit from the study?

See Suggested Responses at the back of this book.

REVIEW QUESTIONS

1. Proving that the care and service provided by EMS to the community is worthy of funding and support is primarily demonstrated through:
   a. scientific research.
   b. outcomes-based research.
   c. the scientific method.
   d. quantitative research.

2. _____ research describes phenomena in numbers.
   a. Qualitative
   b. Quantitative
   c. Mixed
   d. Scientific

3. _____ research describes phenomena in words.
   a. Qualitative
   b. Quantitative
   c. Mixed
   d. Scientific

4. The variable that affects the dependent variable under study is the _____.
   a. individual variable
   b. independent variable
   c. standard variable
   d. quantitative variable

5. A study that primarily looks at existing data is the _____.
   a. retrospective study
   b. prospective study
   c. independent study
   d. scientific study

6. The closer a study adheres to _____, the more valid is the study.
   a. independent variables
   b. dependent variables
   c. the general hypothesis
   d. the scientific method

7. Which of the following is NOT a randomized controlled trial?
   a. convenience study
   b. single blind study
   c. double blind study
   d. All of the above are randomized controlled trials.

See Answers to Review Questions at the back of this book.

REFERENCES

1. Wang, H. E. and D. M. Yealy. "Out-of-Hospital Endotracheal Intubation: Where Are We?" *Ann Emerg Med* 47 (2006): 532–541.

2. Lateef, F. and T. Kelvin. "Military Anti-shock Garment: Historical Relic or a Device with Unrealized Potential?" *J Emerg Trauma Shock* 1 (2008): 63–69.

3. Sayre, M. R., L. J. White, L. H. Brown, S. D. McHenry; National EMS Agenda Writing Team. "National EMS Research Agenda." *Prehosp Emerg Care* 6 (2002): S1–S43.

4. National Libraries of Medicine. PubMed. Available at: http://www.ncbi.nlm.nih.gov/pubmed/.

5. National Institutes of Health. Directives for Human Experimentation. Available at: http://ohsr.od.nih.gov/guidelines/nuremberg.html.

6. White, R. M. "Unraveling the Tuskegee Study of Untreated Syphilis." *Arch Int Med* 160 (2000): 585–598.

7. World Medical Association. WMA Declaration of Helsinki—Ethical Principles for Medical Research Involving Human Subjects. Available at: http://www.wma.net/en/30publications/10policies/b3/index.html.

8. National Institutes of Health. The Belmont Report: Ethical Principles and Guidelines for the Protection of Human Subjects in Research. Available at: http://ohsr.od.nih.gov/guidelines/belmont.html.

9. Mann, H. "Research Ethics Committees and Public Dissemination of Clinical Trial Results." *Lancet* 360 (2002): 406–408.

10. Goodacre, S. "Critical Appraisal in Emergency Medicine 2: Statistics." *Emerg Med J* 394 (2008): 1–6.

11. Waeckerle, J. F. and M. L. Callaham. "Medical Journals and the Science of Peer Reviewing: Raising the "Standard."" *Ann Emerg Med* 28 (1996): 75–77.

FURTHER READING

Brown, L. H., E. L. Criss, and N. H. Prasad. *An Introduction to EMS Research.* Upper Saddle River, NJ: Pearson/Brady, 2002.

Rumsey, D. *Statistics for Dummies.* Hoboken, NJ: Wiley Publishing, 2003.

Wiersma, W. *Research Methods in Education: An Introduction.* 7th ed. Boston, MA: Allyn and Bacon, 2000.

6

Public Health

Bryan Bledsoe, DO, FACEP, FAAEM, EMT-P

STANDARD
Public Health

COMPETENCY
Applies fundamental knowledge of principles of public health and epidemiology, including public health emergencies, health promotion, and illness and injury prevention.

OBJECTIVES

Terminal Performance Objective
After reading this chapter you should be able to apply principles of public health in your role as a paramedic.

Enabling Objectives
To accomplish the terminal performance objective, you should be able to:

1. Define key terms introduced in this chapter.

2. Identify EMS roles that are within the domain of public health.

3. Describe the components that must be in place for EMS and public health to work together.

4. Discuss ways in which public health efforts have improved the quality of life.

5. Recognize the three categories of public health laws.

6. Explain basic concepts of epidemiology.

7. Give examples of how EMS providers can be involved in injury prevention.

8. Describe the roles of EMS organizations and EMS providers in the prevention of EMS provider illness and injury.

9. Identify areas of need for prevention programs in the community.

KEY TERMS

epidemiology, p. 101

injury, p. 102

injury risk, p. 102

injury surveillance program, p. 102

primary prevention, p. 102

public health, p. 100

secondary prevention, p. 102

tertiary prevention, p. 102

years of productive life, p. 102

CASE STUDY

It's a hot July day and Timmy is spending it with John, whose family has an in-ground pool. At approximately 9:00 A.M., John's mom receives a phone call. The two boys, who had been watching cartoons in the living room, run out to the patio, grab the large inflatable alligator raft, and head for the water. Timmy pronounces himself "king of the alligator killers" as he jumps on the raft. John says he is the "true king" and plops himself down on top of Timmy. In the resulting tussle, Timmy rolls off the raft and into the water. He tries but is unable to get a good enough grasp on the edge of the concrete pool. John watches his friend struggle and, terrified, runs to the side of the house to hide. All this takes about 7 minutes.

At approximately 9:10 A.M., John's mom hangs up the phone. As she steps out onto the patio, she sees Timmy's small form floating face down in the pool. She races to the pool, jumps in, and pulls Timmy out. She checks to see if he is breathing, but he is not. She starts for the phone, but stops short. Where is John? It takes her another minute to find him and another 30 seconds to get to the phone to dial 911.

It takes you and your partner 6 minutes to respond. While waiting, John's mother stays with Timmy, turning him on his side to let the water drain from his mouth and lungs and pleads with him softly to "hang in there." When you arrive on scene, you perform a scene size-up and a primary assessment and start CPR. Timmy begins to breathe in about a minute, but he does not regain consciousness. You rush him to the hospital emergency department. There the staff praises your actions and tells you, "You did the best you could."

Almost a year later, Timmy has still not regained consciousness. The costs for Timmy's care so far have reached more than $650,000. It is difficult to predict the total cost. With good medical care, Timmy could live for many years. This unfortunate situation could have been prevented through the use of relatively inexpensive alarms and locks on doors leading to the swimming pool as well as a pool alarm that detects changes in water displacement when an object falls into the pool.

INTRODUCTION

Many EMS providers are first drawn to emergency medical services because of the opportunity to make a dramatic contribution to society and those in need. We respond to countless scenes of crisis and tragedy and feel genuine excitement when the critically ill or injured patient improves after receiving emergency medical care. But beyond the excitement of the moment is a sobering reality. How often do EMS crews respond to incidents that could easily have been prevented? How often have you thought to yourself, "What a shame" or "I wish there was something I could have done" in the wake of senseless circumstances surrounding an accidental injury or illness?

Such thoughts are all too common after an incident. But what if EMS providers, leaders, and administrators asked these questions *before* an incident occurred? How many injuries could be prevented? How many lives could be saved? This chapter focuses on these questions and discusses the interaction between paramedicine and public health.

BASIC PRINCIPLES OF PUBLIC HEALTH

Public health is defined as the science and practice of protecting and improving the health of a community through the use of preventive medicine, health education, control of communicable diseases, application of sanitary measures, and monitoring of environmental hazards. Public health measures have played a significant role in improving the safety and quality of life of humankind. The primary tenet of public health is to identify and prevent injury and illness—that is, to take steps to remedy a situation *before* it results in an injury or an illness. The roles of public health in modern society are diverse and extremely important (Figure 6-1 ●). As EMS has evolved, it has become clear that EMS has some roles and responsibilities that are clearly within the domain of public health (Figure 6-2 ●). In fact, some communities are working to closely link their EMS and public health systems. In order to achieve this, a community must have the following:

- Strong medical oversight of both public health and EMS
- A desire and an effort to educate both emergency care and public health providers about each others' roles
- Recognition of the role of and a commitment to developing and maintaining relationships between leaders of the component groups through regular meetings, teambuilding exercises, and planning
- Bringing community stakeholders (businesses, clinics, universities, and others) into the planning process
- Creating disaster plans that are developed locally, that involve public health and emergency care, and that are repeatedly drilled
- Aggressively pursuing and securing funding

Public Health Functions

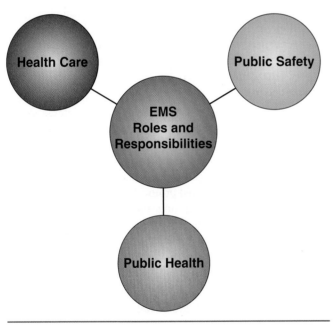

Assessment

Assurance

Policy development

Monitor health

Diagnose & investigate

Inform, educate, empower

Mobilize community partnership

Develop policies

Enforce laws

Link to/provide care

Assure competent workforce

Evaluate

System

Management

Research

● **Figure 6-1** An overview of public health. *(Centers for Disease Control and Prevention)*

● **Figure 6-2** Much of the role of EMS falls within the domain of public health.

Health Care

Public Safety

EMS Roles and Responsibilities

Public Health

ACCOMPLISHMENTS IN PUBLIC HEALTH

Public health has improved both the quality of life and the life span of humankind. These improvements have occurred through research, epidemiology, surveillance, prevention, and

TABLE 6-1 | Public Health Accomplishments (United States)
Public Health Accomplishments (United States)
Vaccination
Motor vehicle safety
Safer workplaces
Control of infectious diseases
Decline in deaths from coronary artery disease and stroke
Safer and healthier foods
Healthier mothers and babies
Family planning
Fluoridation of drinking water
Recognition of tobacco as a health hazard

other strategies. Some of the most important public health accomplishments of the last century are detailed in Table 6-1.

PUBLIC HEALTH LAWS

Public health laws—laws that affect public health practice and strategies—are generally divided into three categories:

● *Illness and prevention.* These laws give public health officials the necessary legal tools to perform their jobs.

● *Police powers for public health agencies.* These laws allow public health entities, when necessary, to act in the general interest of the public. Sometimes these actions are in conflict with individual civil liberties. However, in certain situations such as epidemics and disasters, the needs of the public as a whole generally outweigh the needs of the individual.

● *Epidemiological tools.* These laws give public health agencies the power to use epidemiological tools to analyze legal issues related to public health practice and enforcement.

In 2009, the Public Health Law Research Program (PHLRP) was established at Temple University in Philadelphia. This program, funded by the Robert Wood Johnson Foundation, aids public health entities in promoting effective regulatory and legal solutions to public health problems.[1]

EPIDEMIOLOGY

Epidemiology is the branch of medicine that deals with the incidence and prevalence of disease in large populations. It also works to detect the source and cause of epidemics of infectious disease and other health events. Epidemiology primarily is concerned

CONTENT REVIEW

▶ EMS Roles in Public Health

• Disease prevention
• Disease surveillance
• Disaster management
• Injury prevention

▶ The primary tenet of public health is to identify and *prevent* injury and illness.

with the frequency and pattern of health events that occur in a population.

A number of concepts and terms are used in epidemiology. One such concept is **years of productive life**, a calculation made by subtracting the age at death from 65. (For example, in a liability lawsuit concerning the death of a 45-year-old, a jury might assess damages based on the deceased's loss of 20 years as a wage earner.) Another concept is **injury**, which refers to the intentional or unintentional damage to a person resulting from acute exposure to thermal, mechanical, electrical, or chemical energy or from the absence of such essentials as heat and oxygen. An accident is an *unintentional injury,* but an injury that is purposefully inflicted either on oneself (e.g., suicide) or on another person (e.g., homicide) is an *intentional injury*. Intentional injuries make up about a third of all injury deaths. Other categories of intentional injury include rape, assault, and domestic, elder, and child abuse.

Another concept related to epidemiology is **injury risk**, which is a hazardous or potentially hazardous situation that puts people in danger of sustaining injury. As medical professionals, EMS providers should assess every scene and situation for injury risk and maintain statistics as part of an **injury surveillance program**, which is the ongoing systematic collection, analysis, and interpretation of injury data essential to the planning, implementation, and evaluation of public health practice.

An injury-surveillance program must also include a component for the timely dissemination of data to those who need to know. The final link in the injury-surveillance chain is the application of these data to prevention and control. "Teachable moments" occur shortly after an injury when the patient and observers remain acutely aware of what has happened and may be more receptive to learning about how similar injury or illness could be prevented in the future.

By becoming involved in injury prevention, EMS providers can focus on **primary prevention**, or keeping an injury from ever occurring.[2] Medical care and rehabilitation activities that help to prevent further problems from occurring are referred to, respectively, as **secondary prevention** and **tertiary prevention**.

Epidemiology has six major roles in public health practice:

● *Public health surveillance.* Public health surveillance is the ongoing and systematic collection, analysis, interpretation, and dissemination of health data to aid the public and to aid in health care decision making and action.

● *Field investigation.* Following detection of a health concern through public health surveillance, a field investigation is typically begun. This investigation may be limited to a simple phone call or may involve fieldwork to identify the extent and cause of the health problem in question.

● *Analytic studies.* In most situations, surveillance and field investigations can identify the causes, modes of transmission, and appropriate control and prevention measures for most public health problems. However, when the health problem is more complex (e.g., epidemic), analytic methods are often employed. An example of this was the investigation and detection of AIDS (acquired immunodeficiency syndrome) in 1981. Researchers in both New York and California began to see an unusual form of skin cancer (Kaposi's sarcoma) and an unusual form of pneumonia (*Pneumocystis* pneumonia) among gay men in their communities. This resulted in significant public health efforts to identify the disease and its cause and required the use of analytic methods. In 1983, researchers at the Pasteur Institute in France isolated the human immunodeficiency virus (HIV) that was believed to be the causative agent of what is now called HIV/AIDS. Researchers subsequently backtracked the cases of AIDS that were known at the time and found that a Canadian flight attendant, who was nicknamed "patient zero," was the most likely source for introducing the HIV virus into the general population. By 1985 a test kit for HIV was available and approved by the FDA. In 1987, treatment regimens were developed for HIV. Today, while HIV/AIDS remains a serious infection, the incidence has declined and people with the disease are living almost normal life spans.[3]

● *Evaluation.* Evaluation, from an epidemiological standpoint, is an ongoing process that determines the effectiveness, efficiency, and impact of activities related to public health initiatives. In other words, it is a system to verify that public health policies are doing what they were intended to do and are cost effective.

● *Linkage.* A true public health system requires interaction between various agencies and other entities. As public health policies have been refined, there has been a push to integrate other disciplines such as emergency medical services into public health efforts. Interactions include developing preestablished protocols and agreements, memoranda of understanding, and the sharing of information between organizations. These strategies tie in to the interoperability agreements recommended by the Department of Homeland Security (DHS) and the National Incident Management System (NIMS).

● *Policy development.* In many situations, epidemiologists and other public health professionals have the needed expertise to assist in development of policies, rules, and regulations that positively impact the health and welfare of the population.

EMS Public Health Strategies

Although there are clear differences between EMS practice and public health, at its most fundamental level, EMS is a public health system. Over the last few years, based on the *EMS Agenda for the Future*, there has been a concerted effort to integrate EMS into public health and vice versa.[4]

The numerous roles for EMS in the public health arena include:

- *Health promotion.* EMS personnel can play several important roles in public health. These include such primary prevention strategies as providing health care screenings and vaccinations. With these services, there is an educational component, an opportunity for EMS personnel to inform the public about injury and illness prevention. This can be taken a step further to target high-risk populations in an effort to ensure that they are receiving needed medical care. Many elderly, homeless, and destitute individuals avoid seeking health care because of cost or transportation issues. Many EMS systems, usually in conjunction with social service organizations, periodically assist in helping these high-risk communities.

- *Disease surveillance.* EMS is often the first to encounter an evolving public health emergency such as an epidemic or terroristic activity. By its nature, the EMS system can be an effective monitor of the community. An increase in EMS calls for certain medical conditions or injuries is often an indicator of an evolving larger issue. Several programs provide real-time surveillance. For example, FirstWatch® provides ongoing, live analysis of data to identify patterns and trends as they emerge. This early detection allows actions to be taken quickly, hopefully saving lives and protecting property. When a threat is detected, FirstWatch® automatically sends alerts to authorized, appropriate personnel via email, pager, SMS (short message service) text messaging, or fax. Alerts can contain summary reports, charts, graphs, maps, and other important or mission-critical information (Figure 6-3 ●).

- *Disaster management.* The EMS system is at the core of disaster response. As disasters play out, the mission changes from rescue to recovery. While EMS personnel are well prepared for rescue and emergency medical care endeavors, they are less prepared for recovery efforts. From a medical standpoint, recovery efforts include prevention of disease and further injury and definitive care of injuries that may have been stabilized during the initial hours and days after the onset of the disaster. EMS personnel may be called on to assist in recovery and need the knowledge and skills required to achieve these tasks.

- *Injury prevention.* Though many people believe that injuries "just happen," evidence shows that injuries often result from interaction with identifiable potential hazards in the environment. Thus, it has been suggested that "MVAs" (motor vehicle accidents) should be called "MVCs" (motor vehicle collisions), since driving drunk or at 80 mph and crashing is no accident. In other words, many injuries may be predictable and, thus, preventable. EMS can play an important role in injury prevention. Common strategies include child safety seat classes, bicycle safety training, drunk driving education programs, smoking prevention, and swimming pool safety programs.[5]

PUBLIC HEALTH AND EMS

Other than the victims or survivors and their families, no one experiences the aftermath of illness and trauma more directly than EMS providers. Every day, paramedics witness the tragic effects of preventable injuries and illnesses. Even armed with the best equipment and technology, they cannot save every life. However, by being first on the scene of emergencies, EMS personnel have become prime candidates to be advocates of injury prevention.

EMS providers perform CPR and other lifesaving procedures as part of an everyday routine. In addition, as partners in public health and safety, members of the EMS community must go beyond their normal daily routine and work cooperatively with members of the public to prevent avoidable illness and injury.[6]

EMS providers are widely distributed in the population, often reflecting the composition of their communities. They are often considered to be champions of the health care consumer and are welcome in schools and other community institutions. Medical personnel are high-profile role models and, as such, can have a significant impact on the reduction of injury rates in this country. In rural areas, EMS providers may be the most medically educated individuals, and are often looked to for advice and direction. Essentially, the more than 600,000 EMS providers in the United States comprise a great arsenal in the war to prevent injury and disease.

Organizational Commitment

EMS organizational commitment is vital to the development of any prevention activities. As a member of the EMS community, you should become familiar with available resources and your responsibilities in preventing illness and injury.

- *Protection of EMS providers.* The leadership of EMS agencies must ensure that policies are in place to promote response, scene, and transport safety. The appropriate Standard Precautions and personal protective equipment (PPE) should be issued to protect against exposure to bloodborne and airborne pathogens as well as environmental hazards. An overall commitment to safety and wellness should be emphasized and supported.

- *Education of EMS providers.* EMS personnel must understand the need for involvement in prevention activities. A "buy-in" from employees at every level is key to the success of any prevention program. EMS managers have the responsibility of instructing them in the fundamentals of primary prevention during initial training and in continuing education courses. Public and private sector specialty groups may be called on for specific EMS education and training. EMS providers should also have the skills and training necessary to defend against violent patients or other hostile attackers. Classes in on-scene survival techniques should be commonplace in every EMS agency.

- *Data collection.* Monitoring and maintaining records of patient illnesses and injuries is essential in determining trends and in developing and measuring the success of prevention programs. Each agency should contribute data to local, regional, state, and national systems that track such information.

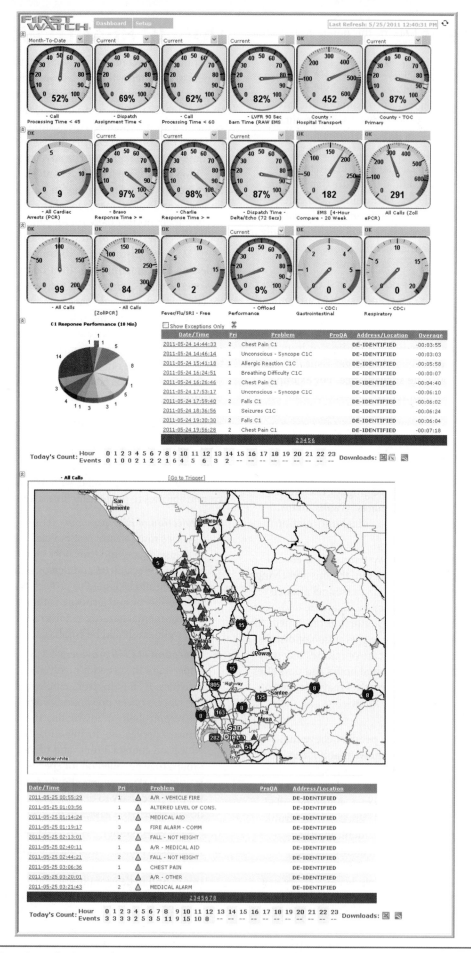

● **Figure 6-3** EMS is often a harbinger for public health events. Early warning systems, such as that provided by FirstWatch®, are now more commonplace. *(www.FirstWatch.net)*

- *Financial support.* An agency's internal budget should reflect support for prevention strategies as a priority. If necessary, support must be sought from outside the organization. Large corporations are often willing to donate funds in exchange for standby coverage at an event or company function. State highway safety offices can offer funding for traffic-related projects, such as those involving child safety seats, seat belts, and drunk driving. Advertising agencies may contribute billboards for safety messages and public service announcements (Figure 6-4 ●). Partnerships with local hospitals can result in advertising safety messages in newsletters and flyers. Community groups such as Mothers against Drunk Driving (MADD) and junior auxiliaries also are great resources for initiating community and school programs.
- *Empowerment of EMS providers.* The ultimate factor in achieving success in a prevention program lies in the hands of the frontline personnel. Managers should identify, encourage, and foster employee interest, support, and involvement. Likewise, such involvement should be recognized and rewarded from top management. In addition, it is also recommended that managers rotate assignment to prevention programs and provide salary for off-duty injury prevention activities.

EMS Provider Commitment

Illness and injury prevention should begin at home and be carried over into the workplace.[7] The priority for EMS providers is to protect themselves from harm. Employers have an obligation to provide a safe working environment. Written guidelines and policies should promote wellness and safety among employees. (See Chapter 4 for more information on the points discussed in the following sections.)

Standard Precautions

Under the guidelines of the Occupational Safety and Health Administration (OSHA), employers and employees share responsibility for ensuring that Standard Precautions are used to assist in preventing contamination from blood and other bodily fluids. Personal protective equipment, such as gloves and eyewear, plays a major role in EMS operations and is one of the provider's basic lines of defense (Figure 6-5 ●).

Physical Fitness

The often hectic and chaotic lifestyle of a paramedic may often interfere with your normal, healthy daily routine. Therefore, you must make an extra effort to consistently incorporate exercise, fitness, and a

health-minded attitude into your life to minimize the risk of injury and to improve your overall quality of life. Encourage your partner, crew members, and other coworkers to do the same. A wellness program that includes a proper diet, cardiovascular fitness, and strength training can increase energy levels, boost immune systems, and help fend off disease and injury.

Note that though lifting and moving techniques and back safety programs have become routine for prehospital staff, back injuries remain a leading cause of disability among EMS workers. Make a solid effort to follow proper lifting techniques in order to prevent bodily injury, strain, and pain.

Stress Management

Members of today's workforce, particularly EMS providers, must learn to control, or at least handle, the stress in their lives. It is often difficult for even the healthiest individual to balance personal, family, and work life. Know your limits and take time out when necessary. Take time to relax. Pick a pastime or hobby that alleviates stress. If work becomes too stressful, speak with a supervisor in order to avoid burnout or future conflicts. Balance your life with exercise, good nutrition, and healthy activities to keep stress in check.

Seeking Professional Care

EMS providers should not be ashamed of needing or asking for professional counseling. Paramedics are called in to assess and treat people during the worst times of their lives. Facing tragedy, disease, death, and despair are part of the daily routine for EMS personnel. Do not forget that paramedics are vulnerable to the same stressors, emotions, illnesses, and injuries as everyone else. If your job or life becomes overwhelming, you may choose to seek counseling from a trained professional.

Many employers will offer employee assistance programs that include counseling, stress management, nutrition, healthy lifestyle inventories, and general wellness. It is often a great

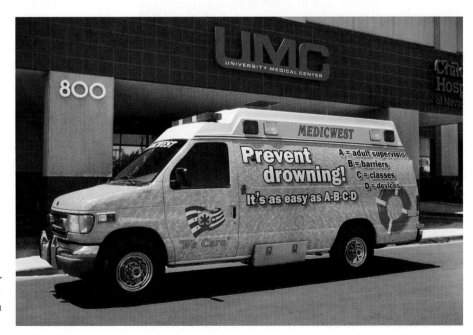

● **Figure 6-4** EMS in the United States needs to be proactive in public education programs. (© Dr. Bryan E. Bledsoe)

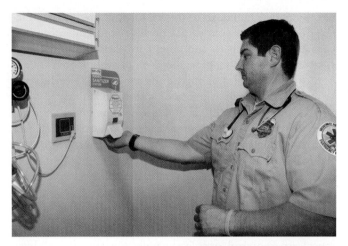

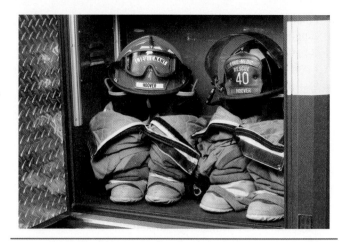

● **Figure 6-6** Every paramedic should have the appropriate safety equipment readily available and in good repair.

addition, you must be able to understand the capabilities and limitations of your emergency vehicle, handle weather and road conditions with precision, and accurately respond to all traffic conditions quickly. Safe emergency operation of EMS vehicles can only be achieved when proper use of warning devices is coupled with sound emergency and defensive driving practices.

Scene Safety

Safety is always your first priority. Once your unit is dispatched to a call, evaluate the dispatch information prior to arrival. Focus your attention on the response and equipment that will be needed (Figure 6-6 ●). Do not approach potentially dangerous scenes until law enforcement has arrived and deemed the scene safe for EMS to enter. On arrival, park the unit in the safest and most convenient place to load the patient as well as to leave the scene. Consider traffic, road conditions, and all other possible hazards. Directing traffic is primarily the responsibility of local law enforcement agencies. The safest method for traffic control at serious vehicle collisions is to stop all traffic and reroute it to different roads. This is for the safety of patients, bystanders, and rescue personnel.

Note that if you are called to an area with potential health hazards, such as an industrial park or a chemical plant or an area with high crime rates, approach the scene with caution. Be sure to protect yourself appropriately. If you do not have adequate protection or are not specifically trained to control the specific hazards, never enter a hazardous scene. Call in specialized teams, such as a hazardous materials crew, if necessary. Law enforcement agencies should be contacted for any violent, potentially violent, or dangerous scene, including those involving domestic abuse or other crimes.

If the scene is safe to enter, be sure to wear reflective clothing to provide added protection on the scene. With Standard Precautions in place, approach patients with your own safety in mind. Determine the mechanisms of injury (forces that caused injury) or the nature of illness. Treat the patient according to protocol.

After patient care is addressed and a transport decision is made, make sure your unit is secure before departure. Have

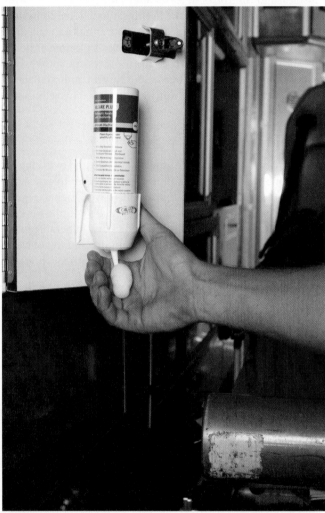

● **Figure 6-5** Disease prevention starts with health care workers. (Top Photo: © *Dr. Bryan E. Bledsoe*)

benefit for employees to take advantage of these opportunities to help themselves through a crisis or stressful time.

Driving Safety

Safe driving is an essential part of EMS response. As an emergency vehicle operator, be familiar with traffic laws and obey them. Never drink and drive. Always fasten your seat belt. In your partner check the outside of the unit to make certain that all doors are secured. The patient should be secured on an ambulance stretcher with at least three straps, as well as shoulder straps if available. If a family member is allowed to accompany the patient, that person should be placed in the passenger seat in the front compartment with vehicle restraints in place. All crew members, including those caring for the patient, should be adequately restrained while the ambulance is in motion.

PREVENTION IN THE COMMUNITY

As a component of health care, EMS has a responsibility to not only prevent injury and illness among EMS workers but also to promote prevention among the members of the public. EMS providers can be an appropriate and effective means of prevention in several situations.

Areas of Need

Infants and Children

Each year, nearly 290,000 infants are born weighing less than 5.5 pounds (2,500 grams), often as a result of inadequate prenatal care. Low birth weight is a key indicator of poor health at the time of birth. Babies born too small or too soon are far more likely to die in the first year of life. Annually, over 4,000 die of low birth weight and prematurity. Among those who survive, an estimated 2 to 5 percent have a disability, and one quarter of the smallest survivors (born weighing less than 1,500 grams) have serious disabilities such as mental retardation, cerebral palsy, seizure disorders, or blindness.[8]

One of every three deaths among children in the United States results from an injury. The number of injuries, of course, far exceeds the number of deaths. The most common causes of fatal injuries in children include motor vehicle collisions, pedestrian or bicycle injuries, burns, falls, and firearms. Injuries generally can be classified into intentional events (such as shootings and assaults), unintentional events (such as motor vehicle collisions), and alleged unintentional events (such as suspicious injury patterns that suggest possible abuse).

In motor vehicle collisions, young children are easily thrown on impact. Because a young child's head is large in proportion to the body, unrestrained children tend to fly head first into the windshield or out of the car when a collision occurs. The back seat is the best seat for children 12 years old or younger. In this location, the properly restrained child is least likely to sustain injuries in a crash. Car safety seats, booster seats (for older children), and seat belts can prevent most severe injuries to passengers of all ages if they are used correctly. Air bags are designed to save people's lives when used with seat belts, and they can protect drivers and passengers who are correctly buckled.

Cars backing up in driveways or parking lots commonly injure infants and toddlers. Children between the ages of 5 and 9 who are struck by cars typically have darted out in front of traffic. Children riding bicycles can be injured when they collide with cars or other fixed objects or when they are thrown from the bicycle. The most serious bicycle-related injuries are head injuries, which can cause death or permanent brain damage. Bicycle safety programs, which promote helmet use and safe riding, can help attenuate this problem.

CONTENT REVIEW

▶ Areas Where EMS Can Be Active in Prevention

- Infants and children
- Motor vehicle collisions
- Geriatric patients
- Work and recreation hazards
- Medications
- Early discharge

Falls are the most frequent cause of injury to children younger than 6 years old. About 200 children die from falls each year. Fire and burn injuries occur in the highest numbers in the very young. Most are caused by scalding from a hot liquid such as when children grab pot handles and spill the contents.

In this modern age of media and the Internet, children and young adults are bombarded with an incredible amount of information and are often faced with some of the same stressors as adults. Sometimes those stressors become overwhelming.

One of the most troubling recent trends is the increased number of violent acts among young people, occurring in the form of self-destructive behavior, gang violence, and assaults. In addition, firearm injury is becoming more common as a result of the accessibility of handguns to children. An increasing number of injuries and deaths occur when children and adolescents take guns to school. The number of firearm deaths has doubled since 1953. About 15 percent of all firearm-related deaths are unintentional, often resulting from improper handling and lack of safety mechanisms.

Motor Vehicle Collisions

For years, the EMS industry and law enforcement have referred to collisions among trucks and automobiles as motor vehicle accidents (MVAs). However, that term does not accurately reflect the circumstances of the incident. The term motor vehicle collision (MVC) more accurately reflects the fact that few collisions are accidents: Something caused the crash to occur. Such crashes are responsible for over half of all deaths from unintentional injuries. Alcohol use is a factor in about half of all motor vehicle fatalities.

Geriatric Patients

Falls account for the largest number of preventable injuries for persons over 75 years of age. As a result of slower reflexes, failing eyesight and hearing, and arthritis, the elderly are at increased risk of injury from falls. Falls frequently result in fractures, since the bones become weaker and more brittle with age. Because the aging brain begins to shrink and stretch the vessels connected to the inner skull, falls in which the head strikes the floor or another object are more likely to cause dangerous bleeding inside the cranium than in a younger person.

Most geriatric patients are coherent, although some may suffer from some degree of dementia. Alzheimer's disease is merely one example of the conditions that can affect the elderly. The associated confusion can contribute to dangerous behaviors such as wandering away from home or into a roadway, which places these patients at greater risk of injury.

► Prevention Strategies
for EMS Personnel

- Preserve response team safety
- Recognize scene hazards
- Document findings
- Conduct on-scene education
- Know your community resources
- Assess community needs

Work and Recreation Hazards

In the workplace, back injuries account for 22 percent of all disabling injuries. Injuries to the eyes, hands, and fingers are responsible for another 22 percent. Even the quietest office setting can be hazardous. Never underestimate the potential dangers in an area that appears to be safe. Many areas and aspects of the work environment are potentially dangerous, including copy machines, electrical cords, faulty wiring, and shoddy building construction, among others.

Sports injuries are commonly seen in persons of all ages as a result of the increased popularity and participation in outdoor recreational activities. Football, soccer, and baseball as well as running, hiking, and biking are among popular sports that can result in fractures, dislocations, sprains, and strains.

Medications

When an illness or injury occurs and treatment is sought, medications are often part of the treatment regimen. These medications are occasionally taken improperly (too much or not enough or in dangerous combinations), or they are taken by others, sometimes causing serious medical problems. Medications of any kind should be taken only by those for whom they are prescribed. They should be stored according to label directions. They should also be continued until the prescription is completed. Following the physician's, the pharmacist's, and the label directions is imperative.

Early Discharge

Managed-care organizations such as HMOs and insurance companies often mandate shorter hospital stays and early discharges from the hospital, urgent care centers, and other outpatient facilities. Such policies often result in more patients being at home sooner with illnesses that are less completely treated. These patients may call on 911 for supportive care and intervention.

Implementation of Prevention Strategies

The following is a list of prevention strategies that you should be able to implement:

- *Preserve the safety of the response team.* Always remember that your first priority is your safety and the safety of your fellow crew members. (If you and other crew members are ill or injured, you cannot help others.) The next priorities are the patient and, finally, bystanders. Do what you can and what is within your training to maintain a safe and secure working area. If there is a chance of risk or further danger on scene, act quickly and appropriately to correct

the situation. Do not hesitate to contact backup units and law enforcement personnel, if necessary.

- *Recognize scene hazards.* To prevent illness or injury to EMS personnel and further illness or injury to patients, size up the scene for potential risks or dangers before entering. Be aware of your surroundings. Is there anyone or anything that could cause harm to you, your crew, or the patient? Does the mechanism that injured the patient still pose a threat to the rescuers? Are there any hazardous materials in the area? Has any crime been committed? Are there structural risks? Are there temperature extremes for which you are unprepared? If the scene is not safe and there is an immediate and imminent danger, retreat immediately and call for the appropriate assistance.

- *Document findings.* Document your patient-care findings at the end of every call. Note that EMS patient forms often can be designed to include specific data on injury prevention in order to benefit researchers and implement future prevention programs. Such a form should include scene conditions at the time of EMS arrival, which may play a major role in determining intentional and unintentional injuries, and the mechanism of injury, which is the best determinant of patient care on scene. It should also include a place where you can describe any risks that were overcome. If protective devices were used (or not used) during the emergency, these should be documented, too (Figure 6-7 ●).

- *Engage in on-scene education.* Taking advantage of a teachable moment is a chance to decrease future emergency responses. Remember that to communicate effectively you must gain your listeners' trust. Remain objective, nonjudgmental, and nonthreatening. Inform them of how they can prevent the recurrence of a similar emergency and, if needed, instruct them on the use of protective devices.

- *Know your community resources.* Treating the medical needs of a patient is often not enough. You must also seek to identify and meet the psychosocial needs of your patient. At times, you may find it appropriate to consider your patient a "customer." Determine what his needs are and how you may assist him. Your patient may require a referral to an outside agency such as a prenatal clinic; a social service organization that offers food, shelter, clothing, mental health resources or counseling; or other services. Your system may also allow for referral or transportation to a clinic, urgent care, or alternative form of health care. Be aware of the presence of both licensed and unlicensed child care centers in your area. Encourage parents to provide

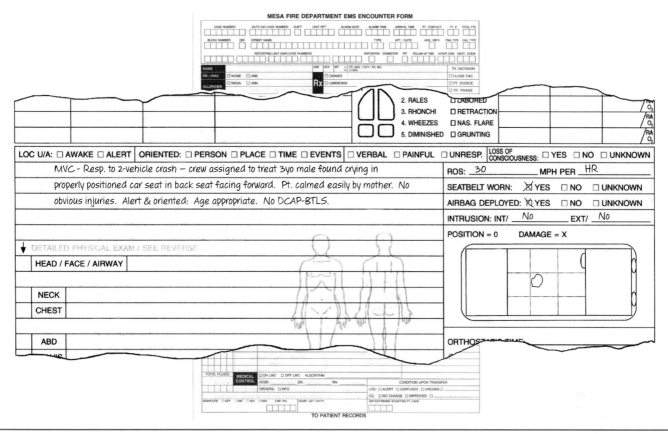

MESA FIRE DEPARTMENT EMS ENCOUNTER FORM

		2. RALES	☐ LABORED
		3. RHONCHI	☐ RETRACTION
		4. WHEEZES	☐ NAS. FLARE
		5. DIMINISHED	☐ GRUNTING

LOC U/A: ☐ AWAKE ☐ ALERT | ORIENTED: ☐ PERSON ☐ PLACE ☐ TIME ☐ EVENTS ☐ VERBAL ☐ PAINFUL ☐ UNRESP. | LOSS OF CONSCIOUSNESS: ☐ YES ☐ NO ☐ UNKNOWN

MVC - Resp. to 2-vehicle crash — crew assigned to treat 3yo male found crying in
properly positioned car seat in back seat facing forward. Pt. calmed easily by mother. No
obvious injuries. Alert & oriented: Age appropriate. No DCAP-BTLS.

ROS: _30_ MPH PER _HR_
SEATBELT WORN: ☒ YES ☐ NO ☐ UNKNOWN
AIRBAG DEPLOYED: ☒ YES ☐ NO ☐ UNKNOWN
INTRUSION: INT/ _No_ EXT/ _No_
POSITION = 0   DAMAGE = X

↓ DETAILED PHYSICAL EXAM / SEE REVERSE

HEAD / FACE / AIRWAY

NECK

CHEST

ABD

ORTHOS...

● **Figure 6-7** Example of documentation of primary and secondary injury prevention.

preexisting consent for treatment and transport in case of illness or injury at a child care facility. Be sure to follow local protocols and report suspected abuse situations to the appropriate child protective agency. Consider developing a social service resource guide for your organization to determine solutions and ideas for these and other situations.

● *Conduct a community needs assessment.* Each community should determine its own specific approaches to prevention. Conducting a formal needs assessment will assist in identifying priorities. Consider the following that your community may already have or may need to develop:

○ Childhood and flu immunizations[9]
○ Prenatal and well-baby clinics
○ Elder-care clinics
○ Defensive driving classes
○ Workplace safety courses
○ Health clinics (cosponsored by local hospitals or health care organizations)
○ Prevention information on your agency's Internet website

These are just a few of the ideas that may be appropriate for your organization. The population served and its ethnic, cultural, and religious makeup may affect the needs and approaches that are most appropriate. Also consider community members who are learning disabled or physically challenged.

CULTURAL CONSIDERATIONS

Immunizing At-Risk Populations. *Many illnesses can be prevented through immunization of at-risk populations. The Centers for Disease Control and Prevention (CDC) and other organizations frequently update and publish a list of recommended immunizations for children and persons at increased risk of contracting a preventable disease. However, for various reasons, some patients are hesitant to obtain these lifesaving immunizations. This is especially true in communities with a large number of illegal immigrants. People who are in the country illegally often will not seek health care for fear their presence in the country will be revealed to immigration authorities and they will be deported. As a result, this population is at increased risk of developing diseases that could be prevented through proper immunization.*

In several areas, paramedics have been called on to provide immunizations as a community service. In these situations, it has been demonstrated that persons unlikely to go to a standard health clinic for immunizations are more likely to attend an immunization session provided by EMS. Thus, by using the trustworthy image of EMS, paramedics can help target populations for preventative immunizations who might not obtain them by traditional means.

It is important to remember that, for many conditions, the best treatment is prevention.

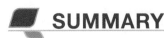

SUMMARY

Each member of EMS shares the responsibility of promoting wellness and preventing illness and injury among coworkers and the community. EMS services have gone beyond the traditional treatment-and-transport-only and followed the steps of the fire service by adding prevention to their repertoire. It is commonplace for EMS services to offer programs to the public such as first aid and CPR classes, infectious disease prevention classes, safe driving classes, child safety seat classes, and even swimming lessons. You should begin to partner with members of your community in new and innovative ways to make everyone more aware of how to prevent avoidable illness and injury. If we can prevent one injury, one disabling disease, or one avoidable death, it will have been more than worth the effort.

YOU MAKE THE CALL

As you walk into work on a sunny, warm Saturday morning, your supervisor greets you at the door. He is beaming with excitement as he tells you, "The boss just approved our budget for EMS Week. And he and I agree that you are just the person to coordinate this year's effort." He continues by insisting that the organization must become "more active" in injury and illness prevention, and EMS Week is the perfect platform to begin such a campaign. You agree to the concept and accept the assignment. The supervisor responds, "Here is the budget overview and the planning kit for this year and last. I would like a preliminary plan from you by the end of today's shift" and wanders back into his office. You briefly scan the packet and proceed to prepare for your shift.

Later, during an hour or so of down time, you and your partner decide to brainstorm ideas on how best to prepare for the event. Your partner mentions that he thinks "this whole idea of us doing prevention is hokey and ridiculous." He continues by saying, "That stuff is for the public health people. I'm a paramedic. I don't have time to be working on prevention." Another paramedic, fresh out of medic school, joins in on the conversation and adds, "Yeah. If we prevented all the injuries and illnesses, we would be out of a job. I don't want that after all I went through to get my certification." You slump slightly into your chair as you begin to discover how difficult this task might become.

1. How will you counter the arguments the two paramedics made?

2. Why is prevention an important responsibility of being a paramedic?

3. List ten ideas for an illness and injury prevention program that may be appropriate in your area.

See Suggested Responses at the back of this book.

REVIEW QUESTIONS

1. The study of the factors that influence the frequency, distribution, and causes of injury, disease, and other health-related events in a population is called:
   a. logistics.
   b. census gathering.
   c. epidemiology.
   d. pathophysiology.

2. Intentional injuries make up about _____ of all injury deaths.
   a. 1/4
   b. 1/3
   c. 2/3
   d. 1/2

3. Rehabilitation after an injury or illness that helps to prevent further problems from occurring is referred to as:
   a. primary prevention.
   b. tertiary prevention.
   c. secondary prevention.
   d. teachable moments.

4. Under the guidelines of _____, employers and employees share responsibility for Standard Precautions.
   a. DOT
   b. FEMA
   c. OSHA
   d. HIPAA

5. It should be noted that, though lifting and moving techniques and back safety programs have become routine for prehospital staff, _____ injuries remain a leading cause of disability among EMS workers.

a. fall

b. back

c. head

d. chest

6. _____ account for the largest number of preventable injuries for persons over 75 years of age.

a. Burns

b. Falls

c. MVCs

d. Head injuries

See Answers to Review Questions at the back of this book.

REFERENCES

1. Public Health Law Research Program. *Public Health Law Research*. Available at: http://www.publichealthlawresearch.org/about-us.

2. Jaslow, D., J. Ufberg, and R. Marsh. "Primary Injury Prevention in an Urban EMS System." *J Emerg Med* 25 (2003): 167–170.

3. Shilts, R. *And the Band Played On: Politics, People, and the AIDS Epidemic.* New York, NY: Stonewall Inn Editions/. Martins Press, 2000.

4. National Highway Traffic Safety Administration. *Emergency Medical Services: Agenda for the Future*. Available at: http://www.nhtsa.dot.gov/people/injury/ems/agenda/.

5. Yancey, A. H., 2nd, R. Martinez, and A. L. Kellermann. "Injury Prevention and Emergency Medical Services: The 'Accidents Aren't' Program." *Prehosp Emerg Care* 6 (2002): 204–209.

6. Weiss, S. J., R. Chong, M. Ong, A. A. Ernst, and M. Balash. "Emergency Medical Services Screening of Elderly Falls in the Home." *Prehosp Emerg Care* 7 (2003): 79–84.

7. Maguire, B. J., K. L. Hunting, G. S. Smith, and N. R. Levick. "Occupational Fatalities in Emergency Medical Services: A Hidden Crisis." *Ann Emerg Med* 40 (2002): 625–632.

8. Streger, M. "Keeping Kids Safe: Injury Prevention Programs in EMS." *Emerg Med Serv* 36 (2002): 24.

9. Mosesso, V. N., Jr, C. R. Packer, J. McMahon, T. E. Auble, and P. M. Paris. "Influenza Immunizations Provided by EMS Agencies: The MEDICVAX Project." *Prehosp Emerg Care* 7 (2003): 74–78.

FURTHER READING

Angle, J. S. *Occupational Safety and Health in the Emergency Services,* 2nd ed. Florence, KY: Delmar/Cengage Learning, 2004.

Sachs, G. M. *The Fire and EMS Department Safety Officer.* Upper Saddle River, NJ: Pearson/Prentice Hall, 2001.

chapter

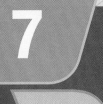

7

Medical/Legal Aspects of Prehospital Care

Bryan Bledsoe, DO, FACEP, FAAEM, EMT-P
Wes Ogilvie, MPA, JD, LP

STANDARD
Preparatory (Medical/Legal and Ethics)

COMPETENCY
Integrates comprehensive knowledge of EMS systems, the safety and well-being of the paramedic, and medical/legal and ethical issues, which is intended to improve the health of EMS personnel, patients, and the community.

OBJECTIVES

Terminal Performance Objective
After reading this chapter you should be able to recognize and appropriately respond to medical/legal issues in the practice of paramedicine.

Enabling Objectives
To accomplish the terminal performance objective, you should be able to:

1. Define key terms introduced in this chapter.

2. Describe the legal, ethical, and moral obligations of the paramedic.

3. Describe the four primary sources of law.

4. Differentiate between civil law and criminal law.

5. Explain the concept of tort law as it applies to paramedic practice.

6. Outline the events that occur in a civil lawsuit.

7. Describe the application of the following legal concepts to paramedic practice:
   a. scope of practice
   b. licensure and certification
   c. motor vehicle laws
   d. mandatory reporting requirements
   e. legal protections for the paramedic
   f. employment laws

8. Given a scenario, determine whether or not the elements necessary for a claim of negligence are present.

9. Describe the paramedic's protections against a claim of negligence.

10. Describe the special liability situations related to:
    a. medical direction
    b. borrowed servant doctrine
    c. civil rights
    d. off-duty practice
    e. airway issues
    f. restraint issues

11. Take measures to protect patients' confidentiality and privacy and comply with HIPAA.

12. Avoid written or spoken statements that could lead to a claim of defamation.

13. Given a variety of scenarios, select the type of patient consent that applies.

14. Given a variety of scenarios, manage withdrawal of consent and refusal of consent situations.

15. Given a variety of scenarios, manage problem patients.

16. Maintain professional boundaries.

17. Avoid situations that could lead to claims of abandonment, assault, battery, false imprisonment, and excessive force.

18. Given a variety of scenarios, manage situations involving advance directives (including Do Not Resuscitate orders), organ donation, and decisions to withhold or terminate resuscitation.

19. Take appropriate actions to avoid destroying evidence at potential crime scenes.

20. Explain the elements of excellent documentation.

KEY TERMS

abandonment, p. 126
actual damages, p. 119
administrative law, p. 115
advance directive, p. 127
assault, p. 126
battery, p. 126
breach of duty, p. 118
civil law, p. 115
civil rights, p. 120
common law, p. 115
competent, p. 122
confidentiality, p. 121
consent, p. 122
constitutional law, p. 115
criminal law, p. 115
defamation, p. 121
Do Not Resuscitate (DNR)
  order, p. 129
duty to act, p. 118

emancipated minor, p. 123
employment laws, p. 131
excited delirium syndrome
  (ExDS), p. 120
expressed consent, p. 122
false imprisonment, p. 126
Good Samaritan laws, p. 117
Health Insurance Portability
  and Accountability
  Act (HIPAA), p. 121
immunity, p. 117
implied consent, p. 122
informed consent, p. 122
intentional tort, p. 117
invasion of privacy, p. 122
involuntary consent, p. 122
legislative law, p. 115
liability, p. 114
libel, p. 121

living will, p. 128
malfeasance, p. 118
minor, p. 123
misfeasance, p. 118
negligence, p. 117
negligence *per se*, p. 118
nonfeasance, p. 118
positional asphyxia, p. 120
professional boundaries, p. 124
proximate cause, p. 119
reasonable force, p. 126
res ipsa loquitur, p. 118
restraint asphyxia, p. 120
scope of practice, p. 116
slander, p. 122
standard of care, p. 118
tort law, p. 115

CASE STUDY

A police officer has pulled a 27-year-old female driver off to the side of the road at the intersection of Quincy Place and Route 122. Because of the dangerous driving he witnessed and the driver's erratic behavior, unsteady gait, and slurred speech, the officer suspects that the driver is intoxicated. To be safe, the officer requests immediate EMS backup.

EMS 117 paramedics arrive on scene in 2 minutes and find a young woman arguing with the police officer. As the paramedics are assessing scene safety, they see the patient turn and lunge at the officer. The officer subdues the patient, who thrashes around briefly before losing consciousness.

At the officer's signal, the paramedics run in to do their jobs. They perform a primary assessment, quickly determining that the patient's airway is clear and breathing and circulation are adequate. They do not detect any immediate life threats, and they begin to review possible causes of the altered mental status. To rule out hypoglycemia, they perform a rapid glucose determination using a glucometer. Then, while one paramedic conducts a physical exam of the patient, the other notes that her blood sugar is 22 mg/dL. Per approved standing orders, an IV is established and 50 mL of 50 percent dextrose is administered. The patient quickly responds, becomes fully oriented, and thanks the paramedics for their help. She then mentions that she has been ill for a few days and has not been eating well.

The paramedics urge the patient to go to the hospital for additional evaluation. She declines, stating that she has recently scheduled a physician's appointment and that she is late for a meeting. The paramedics advise the patient of the risks of refusing care. Nevertheless, she continues to refuse assistance. The paramedics assure themselves that the patient is fully conscious, oriented, and capable of refusing consent. They instruct the patient to go immediately to the mini-mart across the street to get something to eat, and she agrees. They then aseptically discontinue the IV and have the patient sign a "release-from-liability" form, which is witnessed by the police officer. They return their equipment to the ambulance, and notify the dispatcher that they are back in service.

INTRODUCTION

To practice competent prehospital care today, paramedics must become familiar with the legal issues they are likely to encounter in the field. As a paramedic, you must be prepared to make the best medical decisions and the most appropriate legal decisions. This chapter addresses general legal principles in addition to specific laws and legal concepts that affect the paramedic's daily practice.

Note that since laws vary from state to state, and protocols can vary from county to county, the information contained in this chapter cannot be used as a substitute for competent legal advice. Just like the practice of medicine, the practice of law involves some art, some science, and is always heavily dependent on the unique facts present in each situation. If you are faced with a specific legal question, you must rely on the advice of your attorney.

LEGAL DUTIES AND ETHICAL RESPONSIBILITIES

As a paramedic, you have specific legal duties to your patient, crew, medical director, and the public (Figure 7-1 ●). These duties are based on generally accepted standards and are often set by statutes and regulations. The failure of a paramedic to perform his or her job appropriately can result in civil or criminal liability. Your best protection from **liability** (legal responsibility) is to perform a systematic patient assessment, provide the appropriate medical care, and maintain accurate and complete documentation of all incidents.

A paramedic also is responsible for meeting the ethical standards expected of a professional emergency medical care provider. (See Chapter 8 for a detailed discussion of ethics.) Ethical standards are not laws. They are principles that identify

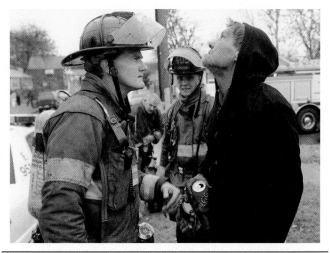

● **Figure 7-1** Each EMS response has the potential of involving paramedics in the legal system. (© *Glen E. Ellman*)

desirable conduct by members of a particular group. Your ethical responsibilities include the following:

- Promptly respond to both the physical and emotional needs of every patient.
- Treat all patients and their families with courtesy and respect.
- Maintain mastery of your skills and medical knowledge.
- Participate in continuing education programs, seminars, and refresher training.
- Critically review your performance, and constantly seek improvement.
- Report honestly and with respect for patient confidentiality.
- Work cooperatively with and respect other emergency professionals.

In addition to the legal and ethical duties, the paramedic will encounter moral issues on a day-to-day basis. Morality, unlike legal obligations, is the principle of right and wrong as governed by individual conscience. Remember, always strive to meet the highest legal, ethical, and moral standards when providing patient care.[1]

The Legal System

Sources of Law

In the United States, there are four primary sources of law: constitutional law, common law, legislative (or statutory) law, and administrative (or regulatory) law.

Constitutional law is based on the Constitution of the United States. The U.S. Constitution sets forth our basic governmental structures, which include the executive branch (the president), legislative branch (Congress), and judicial branch (the Supreme Court). Constitutional law also protects people against governmental abuse. For example, the Fourth Amendment to the Constitution protects people from unreasonable searches and seizures by the government.[2]

Common law which also is referred to as "case law" or "judge-made law," originated with the English legal system and was adopted by Americans in the 1700s. It was derived from society's acceptance of customs and norms over time. Common law changes and grows over the years as established principles are tested and adapted to meet new situations. It is a fundamental principle of our legal system that precedents set by the courts should be followed by other courts. This means that cases with similar facts should be decided in the same way.

For example, the U.S. Supreme Court issued a decision in the case of *Miranda v. Arizona* in 1966. The Court said that a person who is taken into police custody must be informed prior to interrogation that (1) he has the right to remain silent, (2) anything he says can be used against him in court, (3) he has the right to the presence of an attorney, and (4) if he cannot afford an attorney, one will be appointed to him if he so desires. In 2000, the Supreme Court upheld the rules set forth in *Miranda*, affirming that a confession will not be admissable at trial if it is found that the defendant was not advised of his rights before making his statement.[3]

Legislative law (or statutory law) does not come from court decisions. It is created by lawmaking or legislative bodies. Statutes are enacted at the federal, state, and local levels by the legislative branches of government. Examples of legislative bodies include the U.S. Congress, state assemblies, city councils, and district boards. Legislative law is written in a very clear and concise manner and takes precedence over common-law decisions.

Administrative law (or regulatory law) is enacted by an administrative or governmental agency at either the federal or state level. Administrative agencies, such as the Occupational Safety and Health Administration (OSHA), will take a statute enacted by a legislative body and will produce rules and regulations necessary to implement it. The agency is given the authority to make regulations based on that statute; enforce rules, regulations, and statutes under its authority; and hold administrative hearings to carry out penalties for any violations of its rules.

Categories of Law

The United States has two general categories of law: civil law and criminal law. **Criminal law** deals with crime and punishment. It is an area of law in which the federal, state, or local government will prosecute an individual on behalf of society for violating laws meant to protect society. Homicide, rape, and burglary are examples of criminal wrongs. Violations of criminal laws are punished by imprisonment, a fine, or a combination of the two.

Civil law deals with noncriminal issues, such as personal injury, contract disputes, and matrimonial issues. In civil litigation, which involves conflicts between two or more parties, the *plaintiff* (person initiating the litigation) will seek to recover damages from the *defendant* (person against whom the complaint is made). **Tort law**, which is a branch of civil law, deals with civil wrongs committed by one individual against another (rather than against society). Tort law claims include negligence, medical malpractice, assault, battery, and slander.

Note that the United States has a *federal court system* and a *state court system*. The federal court system was created by the U.S. Constitution. Generally, only cases that involve a question of federal law or cases in which the parties are citizens of different states will be heard in a federal court. The state court system is the location for most of the cases in which a paramedic may become involved. In *trial courts,* a judge or jury determines the outcome of individual cases. *Appellate courts* hear appeals of decisions by trial courts or other appeals courts. The decisions of appellate courts may set precedents for later cases.

Anatomy of a Civil Lawsuit

If you have ever been served with legal papers, you know that being sued or even being called to testify at a trial can be very unsettling. A basic understanding of the legal system can help. The following is a brief description of the components of a civil lawsuit:

- *Incident.* For example, a person is driving on a road and fails to see a stop sign. When he passes through the intersection, he hits another car and that driver sustains several injuries.

- *Investigation.* The injured driver's attorney makes a preliminary inquiry into the facts and circumstances surrounding the incident to determine if the case has merit.

- *Filing of the complaint.* The injured driver (now called the "plaintiff") commences the lawsuit by filing a complaint with the court. In some states, the complaint may also be called a petition. The complaint contains information such as the names of the parties, the legal basis for the claim, and the damages sought by the plaintiff. A copy of the complaint is served on the defendant.

● *Answering the complaint.* The defendant's attorney then prepares an answer, which addresses each allegation made in the complaint. The answer is then filed with the court, and a copy is given to the plaintiff's attorney.

● *Discovery.* Before any lawsuit appears in front of a judge or jury, both parties to an action participate in pretrial discovery. This is the stage of the lawsuit when all relevant information about the incident is shared so that parties can prepare trial strategies. Discovery may include:

○ *An examination before trial,* which is also called a "deposition," that allows a witness to answer questions under oath with a court stenographer present.

○ *An interrogatory,* used by either side, is a set of written questions that requires written responses.

○ *Requests for document production* entitle each side to request relevant documents, including the patient care report, records of the receiving hospital, any subsequent medical records, police records, and other records necessary to help prove or defend the lawsuit.

● *Trial.* A trial will be commenced at the appropriate level of trial court. (Some states have different trial courts depending on the type of case and/or amount of money involved.) At the trial, each side will be given the opportunity to present all relevant evidence and testimony from witnesses.

● *Decision.* After deliberations, the judge or jury determines the guilt or liability of the defendant and then decides the amount of damages to award the plaintiff, if any.

● *Appeal.* After the jury's decision is entered by the court, either party may be entitled to an appeal. Generally, grounds for an appeal are limited to errors of law made by the court. Appeals are typically heard by an appellate court.

● *Settlement.* This can occur at any stage of the lawsuit. Generally, the defendant will offer the plaintiff an amount of money that is less than the amount for which he is being sued. The plaintiff may then agree to accept the reduced amount on the condition, for example, that he will no longer pursue the case.

Laws Affecting EMS and the Paramedic

Most of the laws that affect EMS and paramedics are state laws. Although these laws vary from state to state, they share common principles.

Scope of Practice

The range of duties and skills paramedics are allowed and expected to perform is called the **scope of practice**. Usually, the scope of practice is set by state law or regulation and by local medical direction. Often, a state will have a general "medical practice act" that governs the practice of medicine and all health care professionals. These acts prescribe how and to what extent a physician may delegate authority to a paramedic. As you learned in Chapter 3, paramedics may function only under the direct supervision of a licensed physician through a delegation of authority. Generally, paramedics should follow orders given by on-line and off-line medical direction. However, you should not blindly follow orders that you know are medically inappropriate.

Circumstances in which an order from medical direction may be legitimately refused include when you are ordered to provide a treatment that is beyond the scope of your training or inconsistent with established protocols or procedures and when you are ordered to administer a treatment that you reasonably believe would be harmful to the patient. If you are confronted with a situation where an ordered treatment might possibly harm your patient, you should take appropriate action. First, raise the concern with the physician. If the physician still insists, you should refuse to follow the order and document the incident thoroughly on the patient care report.

In addition, every EMS system should have a policy in place to guide paramedics in dealing with intervener physicians (on-scene physicians who are professionally unrelated to the patient and who are attempting to assist with patient care). Generally, such a policy requires that certain conditions be met before the paramedic should allow the intervener physician to assume control of patient care. That is, the physician must be properly identified to the paramedic, licensed to practice medicine in the state, willing to accept the responsibility of continuing medical care until the patient reaches the hospital, and willing to document the intervention as required by the local EMS system.

Licensure and Certification

Other laws that directly affect the paramedic's ability to practice relate to certification and licensure requirements. *Certification* refers to the recognition granted to an individual who has met predetermined qualifications to participate in a certain activity. It is usually given by a certifying agency (not necessarily a government agency) or professional association. For example, after completing an approved paramedic program in New York State, a student who passes an approved written and practical examination will become a certified New York State paramedic.

Licensure is a process used to regulate occupations. Generally, a governmental agency, such as a state medical board, grants permission to an individual who meets established qualifications to engage in a particular profession or occupation. Certification or licensure, or perhaps both, may be required by your state or local authorities for you to practice as a paramedic.

Most states have laws that govern paramedic practice and set forth the requirements for certification, licensure, recertification, and relicensure. It is your responsibility to understand fully the EMS laws and regulations in your state.

Motor Vehicle Laws

As with other EMS-related laws, motor vehicle laws vary from state to state. Generally, there are special motor vehicle laws that govern the operation of emergency vehicles and the equipment they carry. These laws apply to areas such as vehicle maintenance and use of the siren and emergency lights. It is important that you become familiar with the laws of your state. Keep up-to-date with local regulations, too.

Reporting Requirements

Each state enacts different laws designed to protect the public. For example, most states have laws that require a health care worker to report to local authorities any suspected spousal abuse, child abuse and neglect, or abuse of the elderly. In many states, violent crimes, such as sexual assault, gunshot wounds, and stab wounds, must be reported to law enforcement. Emergencies that threaten public health, such as animal bites and communicable diseases, also must be reported to the proper authorities. The content of such reports and to whom they must be made is set by law, regulation, or policy. Become familiar with the circumstances under which you are required to make a report. If you fail to make a required report, you may be criminally and civilly liable for your inaction. In addition, such inaction may place your licensure or certification in jeopardy.

Legal Protection for the Paramedic

In addition to the laws that protect patients, legislative bodies have enacted laws to protect paramedics. For example, some jurisdictions have enacted laws that criminally punish a person who commits assault or battery against a paramedic while he is providing medical care. Others have laws prohibiting the obstruction of paramedic activity.[4]

Immunity, or exemption from legal liability, is another form of protection. Governmental immunity is a judicial doctrine that prohibits a person from bringing a lawsuit against a government without its consent. This type of liability protection, even if allowed under law, generally serves to protect only the government agency, not the individual paramedic, although the specific protections vary from state to state. Therefore, you should not rely on governmental immunity to protect you from claims of negligence. Additionally, governmental immunity would not typically protect a paramedic working for a nongovernment employer. It should be noted that, even with immunity, a plaintiff may still file a lawsuit, which will typically require the paramedic to hire an attorney to defend the claim.

Virtually every state has **Good Samaritan laws**, which provide immunity to people who assist at the scene of a medical emergency. Though these laws vary from state to state, generally, they protect a person from liability if that person acts in good faith, is not negligent (most states will cover acts of simple negligence but not ones of gross negligence), acts within his scope of practice, and does not accept payment for services. The Good Samaritan laws of many states have been expanded to protect both paid and volunteer prehospital personnel.[5]

As a paramedic, you should also become familiar with local laws and regulations governing the use of physical restraints for dangerous or violent patients. There also may be regulations governing entry into restricted areas such as military installations, nuclear power plants, and sites with hazardous materials. Since the laws affecting paramedic practice vary from state to state, your agency should obtain the advice of an attorney in order to minimize potential exposure to liability.

Other laws are designed to protect the paramedic in the event of exposure to bloodborne or airborne pathogens. For example, the Ryan White Comprehensive AIDS Resources Emergency Act (Ryan White CARE Act) requires hospitals and EMS agencies to create a notification system to provide information and assist the paramedic when an exposure occurs. This law allows the paramedic who has been exposed to certain diseases (such as hepatitis B, AIDS, and tuberculosis) access to medical records to determine if the patient has tested positive for, or is exhibiting signs and symptoms of, an infectious disease. The Ryan White CARE Act is a federal law, but many states have enacted similar or even more comprehensive laws to protect paramedics who may have been exposed to infectious diseases. It is important for each agency to appoint an infection control officer and for this individual to implement protocols and an appropriate infection control plan.

LEGAL ACCOUNTABILITY OF THE PARAMEDIC

As a paramedic, you are required to provide a level of care to your patients that is consistent with your education and training and equal to that of any other competent paramedic with equivalent training. You also are expected to perform your duties in a reasonable and prudent manner, as any other paramedic would in a similar situation. Any deviation from this standard might open you to allegations of negligence and liability for any resulting damages.

Most civil claims against EMS providers center around claims for negligence, but some are based on intentional torts. An **intentional tort** is a civil wrong committed by one person against another based on a willful act. Most forms of immunity do not provide protection when the claim is based on an intentional tort.

Negligence and Medical Liability

Negligence is defined as a deviation from accepted standards of care recognized by law for the protection of others against the unreasonable risk of harm. It can result in legal accountability

CONTENT REVIEW

▶ The Four Elements
of Negligence

• Duty to act
• Breach of that duty
• Actual damages
• Proximate cause

and liability. In the health care professions, negligence is synonymous with malpractice (Table 7-1).

Components of a Negligence Claim

In a negligence claim against a paramedic, the plaintiff must establish and prove four particular elements in order to prevail: a duty to act, a breach of that duty, actual damages to the patient or other individual, and proximate cause (causation of damages).

First, the plaintiff must establish that the paramedic had a **duty to act**. That is, he must prove that the paramedic had a formal contractual or informal legal obligation to provide care. Note that the act of voluntarily assuming care of a patient may imply that there was a duty to act, which creates a continuing duty to act. For example, in some states if an off-duty paramedic witnesses a person choking, he may be under no legal duty to act. However, if that paramedic initiates care, then he has a duty to continue care. The rationale behind this rule is if bystanders see that a victim is being helped, they may walk away. If the paramedic rendering assistance walks away after initiating treatment, but not completing it, the patient may actually be left in a worse condition than if the paramedic never tried to help.

Duties that are expected of the paramedic include:

● Duty to respond to the scene and render care to ill or injured patients

● Duty to obey federal, state, and local laws and regulations

● Duty to operate the emergency vehicle reasonably and prudently

● Duty to provide care and transportation to the expected standard of care

● Duty to provide care and transportation consistent with the paramedic's scope of practice and local medical protocols

● Duty to continue care and transportation through to appropriate conclusions

Second, the plaintiff must prove there was a **breach of duty** by the paramedic. A paramedic always must exercise the degree of care, skill, and judgment that would be expected under like circumstances by a similarly trained, reasonable paramedic in the same community. The **standard of care** specific to the paramedic's practice is generally established by court testimony and referenced to published codes, standards, criteria, and guidelines applicable to the situation. In a civil lawsuit, the trier of fact (most often the jury) decides what the standard of care is. A breach of duty may occur by **malfeasance**, **misfeasance**, or **nonfeasance**:

● *Malfeasance,* or the performance of a wrongful or unlawful act by the paramedic. For example, a paramedic commits malfeasance if he assaults a patient.

● *Misfeasance,* or the performance of a legal act in a manner that is harmful or injurious. For example, a paramedic commits misfeasance when he inadvertently intubates a patient's esophagus, fails to confirm tube placement, and leaves the tube in place.

● *Nonfeasance,* or the failure to perform a required act or duty. For example, it would be an act of nonfeasance to fail to properly secure a patient to the stretcher and in the ambulance prior to transport.

In some cases, negligence may be so obvious that it does not require extensive proof. Unlike criminal cases, which require proof "beyond a reasonable doubt," civil cases require only a proof of guilt by a "preponderance of evidence." In most cases, the burden of proving negligence rests on the plaintiff. As a result, when it is difficult to do so, a plaintiff may sometimes invoke the doctrine of *res ipsa loquitur,* which is Latin for "the thing speaks for itself."

To support a claim of *res ipsa loquitur,* the complainant must prove that the damages would not have occurred in the absence of somebody's negligence, the instruments causing the damages were under the defendant's control at all times, and the patient did nothing to contribute to his own injury. After the doctrine of *res ipsa loquitur* is invoked in court, the burden of proof shifts from the plaintiff to the defendant.

For example, a classic situation in which *res ipsa loquitur* might be used occurs when a patient has an appendectomy and wakes to find that a surgical instrument has been left inside his abdomen. To prove negligence in this case, the plaintiff's attorney would show that the damage would not have occurred without the physician's negligence, that the surgical instrument was under the physician's control at all relevant times, and that the patient did not contribute to the injury. Many cases involving incorrect intubations or airway management have a *res ipsa loquitur* claim. Many cases in which *res ipsa loquitur* would be successful are settled out-of-court.

Another situation in which little proof is required occurs when the paramedic violates a statute and injury to a plaintiff results. Some laws state that if a statute is violated and an injury results, a person will be guilty of **negligence** *per se*, or automatic

TABLE 7-1	EMS Liability Claims	
Summary of 275 EMS Liability Claims from a Large National EMS Insurer for a Two-Year Period	
Cause	**Percentage**
Patient Handling	45%
Emergency Vehicle Movement or Collision	31%
Medical Management	11%
EMS Response or Transport	8%
Lack or Failure of Equipment	4%
Other Causes	9%

negligence. For example, if a paramedic, who is driving in non-emergency mode, fails to stop at a red light and hits a pedestrian, the paramedic's negligence is obvious. He violated vehicle and traffic statutes that prohibit a vehicle from running a red light, and he is therefore guilty of *negligence per se.*

After a duty to act and a breach of that duty have been proven, **actual damages** is the third required element of proof in a negligence claim. That is, the plaintiff must prove that he was actually harmed in a way that can be compensated by the award of damages. This is an essential component. A lawsuit cannot be won if the paramedic's action caused no ill effects. The plaintiff must prove that he suffered compensable physical, psychological, or financial damage such as medical expenses, lost wages, lost future earnings, conscious pain and suffering, or wrongful death.

In addition, the plaintiff may seek punitive (punishing) damages. These are awarded only when a defendant commits an act of gross negligence or willful and wanton misconduct. An act of ordinary negligence, such as accidentally allowing an IV to infiltrate, will not support an award of punitive damages. If punitive damages are awarded to the plaintiff, most insurance policies will not cover them. Therefore, the paramedic may become personally liable for any punitive damages awarded to the plaintiff.

Finally, to prove negligence, the plaintiff must show that the paramedic's action or inaction was the **proximate cause** of the damages; that is, the action or inaction of the paramedic immediately caused or worsened the damage suffered by the plaintiff. For example, a cardiac patient who breaks his arm during an ambulance collision while en route to the hospital will likely be able to prove that his injuries resulted from the incident; that is, the collision was the proximate cause of his injuries. However, a patient with a sprained wrist who happens to suffer a stroke while in the ambulance would have difficulty proving the ambulance ride was the proximate cause of the stroke.

Proximate cause may also be thought of in terms of "foreseeability." To show the existence of proximate cause, the plaintiff needs to prove that the damage to the patient was reasonably foreseeable by the paramedic. This is usually established by expert testimony. For example, imagine that a paramedic negligently crashes into a telephone pole with the ambulance. As a result, two people are injured—the patient who was in the back of the ambulance and, two blocks away, a baby who was dropped by his mother when the loud crash startled her. It should be easy for the patient to prove proximate cause, because it was reasonably foreseeable that an ambulance crash could hurt passengers. However,

if the woman who dropped her baby sued the paramedic, she probably would not be able to establish proximate cause. Although the crash was the reason her baby was injured, it was not a foreseeable injury resulting from the ambulance crash.

Defenses to Charges of Negligence

If you are accused of negligence, you may be able to avoid liability if you can establish a defense to the plaintiff's claim. The following is a list of potential defenses to negligence:

- *Good Samaritan laws.* If the paramedic can establish that his or her actions were protected by a Good Samaritan law, liability may be avoided. Note that such laws generally do not protect providers from acts of gross negligence, reckless disregard, or willful or wanton conduct (such as an intentional tort), and they do not prohibit the filing of lawsuits.

- *Governmental immunity.* In many states, these laws do not offer much protection for the individual paramedic accused of negligence. The breadth of governmental immunity established varies from state to state. You may want to become familiar with the governmental immunity law in the state where you practice.

- *Statute of limitations.* This is a law that sets the maximum time period during which certain actions can be brought in court. After the time limit is reached, no legal action can be brought regardless of whether or not a negligent act occurred. Statutes of limitations vary from state to state, so carefully review the laws in your state. Note that they may vary for different negligent acts and for cases involving children.

- *Contributory or comparative negligence.* Some state laws will reduce or eliminate a plaintiff's award of damages if the plaintiff is found to have caused or worsened his own injury. For example, imagine that a patient involved in a car crash complained of neck pain but refused to let the paramedics properly immobilize his spine. The paramedics explained the risks of refusing treatment, but the patient signed a "release-from-liability" form anyway. Later, the patient learns that he has permanent spinal-cord damage and sues the paramedics for negligence. Many courts will find that the paramedics were not negligent because, by refusing necessary treatment, the patient contributed to the exacerbation of his own injury.

To protect yourself against claims of negligence, you should receive appropriate education, training, and continuing education; receive appropriate medical direction, both on-line and off-line; always prepare accurate, thorough documentation; have a professional attitude and demeanor at all times; always act in good faith; and use your own common sense. In addition, it is essential for all paramedics to be covered by medical liability insurance. Although many employers and agencies carry coverage, it is a good idea to obtain your own because your agency's coverage may be inadequate. In addition, several studies have shown that health care providers who have a positive, pleasant attitude are less likely to be the subjects of complaints or lawsuits.

LEGAL CONSIDERATIONS

High Risks for Lawsuits. *Most lawsuits filed against EMS personnel allege negligence or a failure to act. Many involve allegations of misplaced endotracheal tubes, problems related to patient restraint, or medication errors and omissions. Be aware of high-risk areas in EMS practice, make sure that you closely adhere to your system's treatment protocols, and document your care in detail.*

Special Liability Concerns

Medical Direction

If a paramedic makes a mistake in the field and is sued by the injured patient, it is possible that the patient will also sue the paramedic's medical director and the on-line physician. The on-line physician may be liable to a patient for giving the paramedic medically incorrect orders or advice, for the refusal to authorize the administration of a medically necessary medication, or for directing an ambulance to take a patient to an inappropriate medical facility.

A paramedic's medical director may be liable to the patient for the negligent supervision of the paramedic. In order for the patient to be successful in this type of claim, he would have to prove that the physician breached a duty to supervise the paramedic and that breach was the proximate cause of the patient's injuries. Examples include the medical director's failure to establish medication protocols or standing orders consistent with the current standards of medical practice for the paramedic to use in the field; the medical director observed and then failed to correct a paramedic's poor intubation technique; or the medical director received complaints of inappropriate care by a paramedic and then failed to effectively investigate and resolve the problem.[6]

Borrowed Servant Doctrine

As a paramedic, you may find yourself in the position of supervising other emergency care providers, such as EMTs or AEMTs. When doing so, it will be your responsibility to make sure they perform their duties in a professional and medically appropriate manner. Depending on the degree of supervision and the amount of control you have, you may be liable for any negligent act they commit. This is called the "borrowed servant" doctrine. For it to apply, the paramedic accused of negligence must have taken the employees of another employer under his control and exercised supervisory powers over them.

Civil Rights

In addition to suing you for negligence, a patient may be able to sue you under certain circumstances for violating his **civil rights** if you fail to render care for a discriminatory reason. As a paramedic, you may not withhold medical care for reasons such as race, creed, color, gender, national origin, or, in some cases, ability to pay. Also, all patients should be provided with appropriate care regardless of their status, condition, or disease (including AIDS/HIV, tuberculosis, and other communicable diseases).

Off-Duty Paramedics

Liability may also arise in a situation in which an off-duty paramedic renders assistance at the scene of an illness or injury.[7] Generally, any person who provides basic emergency first aid to another person would be protected from liability under a Good Samaritan law. Again, it should be noted that few states have established a legal duty for a paramedic to provide care in an off-duty capacity, regardless of the paramedic's personal moral or ethical beliefs. However, when the off-duty paramedic provides advanced life support, a problem may arise. In many states and in many EMS systems, paramedics cannot practice advanced skills unless they are practicing within an EMS system. To perform paramedic skills and procedures that require delegation from a physician while off-duty may constitute the crime of practicing medicine without a license. Learn the law in your jurisdiction as well as your EMS system's definition of what constitutes being "on duty."

Airway Issues

Issues related to airway management have always been problematic.[8] Failure to secure an airway or failure to recognize that an airway has been improperly placed can result in devastating or fatal injuries for the patient. There have been numerous lawsuits and settlements related to airway management, especially failure to recognize that an endotracheal tube has been improperly placed. The topic of intubation has been further complicated by several studies that question the overall benefit of prehospital endotracheal intubation.

Paramedics must know that intubation is a high-risk procedure and ensure that it is performed properly, that placement is verified by objective measures (e.g., capnography), and that the procedure is properly documented.

Restraint Issues

Almost inevitably, as a paramedic, you will eventually encounter a patient who must be physically or chemically restrained because the patient's behavior is a direct threat to his own health and safety and/or that of others. The cause may be a medical condition, a psychiatric condition, substance abuse, or any combination of these.

Over recent decades, several phenomena have been identified that place restraint patients at risk. **Excited delirium syndrome (ExDS)** is most commonly seen in conjunction with abuse of stimulant drugs. It typically presents as a triad of delirium, psychomotor agitation, and physiological excitation. It has been estimated that approximately 8 to 14 percent of people with ExDS die. An associated phenomenon is called **restraint asphyxia** or **positional asphyxia**. This type of asphyxia may occur alone or in the presence of ExDS. During the process of being restrained, for the reasons just cited or for other reasons, some patients may sustain injury or death. Some studies indicate that restraint maneuvers may impair respiratory excursion. Other studies indicate that the cause is multifactorial. Positional asphyxia often occurs in patients who have used CNS depressants (e.g., alcohol, opiates) and results from the patient being in a physical position that interferes with his airway or with ventilation.[9]

There has been an increase in negligence suits against EMS and law enforcement personnel related to deaths and injuries that occur during restraint. Paramedics must understand and practice safe restraint techniques. The use of medications, especially in ExDS, can help to minimize problems. Paramedics must undertsand that medical restraint is a high-risk issue and ensure that it is performed safely (for all involved, both patient and rescuers), the restrained patient is carefully monitored, and that the circumstances of the call are documented in exquisite detail. (See the section Reasonable Force later in this chapter as well as Volume 4, Chapter 11 for additional information on patient restraint.)

PARAMEDIC-PATIENT RELATIONSHIPS

The relationship you establish with your patient is a very important one. Not only must you provide the best medical care, but you also have legal and ethical duties to protect the patient's privacy and treat him with honesty, respect, and compassion.

Confidentiality

All records related to the emergency care rendered to a patient must be kept strictly confidential. Keeping patient **confidentiality** means that any medical or personal information about a patient—including medical history, assessment findings, and treatment—will not be released to a third party without the express permission of the patient or legal guardian. However, there are specific circumstances under which a patient's confidential information may be released:

- *Patient consents to the release of his records.* A patient may request a copy of his medical records for any reason. If the patient is a child, consent for release of medical records must be obtained from the child's parent or other legal guardian. The request should be accepted only if it is in writing, specifically authorizes the agency to release the records, and contains the patient's signature (or other authorized signature). If the request so directs, it is permissible to forward the records to the patient's physician, insurance company, attorney, or any other party the patient specifies. Be sure your agency retains a copy of the consent document.

- *Other medical care providers have a need to know.* For example, it is not a breach of patient confidentiality to discuss the patient's condition with on-line medical direction or to give a patient report to an emergency department nurse on arrival at the hospital. This is permitted because it allows medical care appropriate for the patient to be continued. It is not acceptable, however, to discuss confidential patient information with medical providers who have no responsibility for the patient's care.

- *EMS is required by law to release a patient's medical records.* Records may be requested by a court order that is signed by a judge, or they may be requested by *subpoena* (a command to appear at a certain time and place to give testimony). When an agency receives a court order or subpoena, it is good practice to consult with an attorney to make sure the order is valid and for assistance with compliance. Failure to comply with a court order or subpoena may result in severe penalties.

- *There are third-party billing requirements.* For EMS agencies that bill patients for services, it is generally necessary to release certain confidential information to receive reimbursement from private insurance companies, Medicaid, or Medicare. If possible, the agency should obtain patient authorization for this purpose.

The law provides penalties for the breach of confidentiality. The improper release of information may result in a lawsuit against the paramedic for defamation (libel or slander), breach of confidentiality, or invasion of privacy. If found guilty, the paramedic may be made responsible for paying monetary damages to the patient.

Health Insurance Portability and Accountability Act

The **Health Insurance Portability and Accountability Act of 1996 (HIPAA)** changed the methods EMS providers use to file for insurance and Medicare payments. It also adds important new layers of privacy protection for EMS patients. The privacy protections provide, among other things, that all EMS employees be trained in HIPAA compliance. Furthermore, EMS providers must develop administrative, electronic, and physical barriers to unauthorized disclosure of patients' protected health information. Disclosures of information—except for purposes of treatment, obtaining payment for services, health care operations, and disclosures mandated or permitted by law—must be preauthorized in writing. HIPAA requires providers to post notices in prominent places advising patients of their privacy rights and provides both civil and serious criminal penalties for violations of privacy.[10]

Patients are given the right to inspect and copy their health records, restrict use and disclosure of their individually identifiable health information, amend their health records, require a provider to communicate with them confidentially, and account for disclosures of their protected health information except for treatment, payment, health care operations, and legally required reporting purposes. The requirements of HIPAA are detailed and every EMS provider must become familiar with them.

Defamation

Defamation occurs when a person makes an intentional false communication that injures another person's reputation or good name. A patient may sue a paramedic for defamation if the paramedic communicates an untrue statement about a patient's character or reputation without legal privilege or consent. Defamation can occur in written form or through verbal statements.

Libel is the act of injuring a person's character, name, or reputation by false statements made in writing or through the mass media with malicious intent or reckless disregard for the falsity of those statements. Allegations of libel can be avoided by completing an accurate, professional, and confidential patient care report. Do not use slang and value-loaded words or phrases in your report (for example, do not refer to a patient as "stupid" or use any derogatory race-based terms). Since many states consider the patient care report part of the public record, never write anything on it that could be considered libelous.

Slander is the act of injuring a person's character, name, or reputation by false or malicious statements spoken with malicious intent or reckless disregard for the falsity of those statements. An allegation of slander can be avoided by limiting oral reporting of a patient's condition to appropriate personnel only. Note that many EMS systems record ambulance-hospital radio transmissions. In addition, scanners, which give the public access to EMS transmissions, are common in the United States. Therefore, information transmitted over the radio should be limited to essential matters of patient care. In most cases, the patient's name and insurance status should not be transmitted over the radio.

Invasion of Privacy

A paramedic may be accused of **invasion of privacy** for the release of confidential information, without legal justification, regarding a patient's private life, which might reasonably expose the patient to ridicule, notoriety, or embarrassment. That includes, for example, the release of information regarding HIV status, other sensitive medical information, or even a potentially embarrassing set of circumstances that the patient was found in. The fact that released information is true is not a defense to an action for invasion of privacy.

Consent

By law, you must get a patient's consent before you can provide medical care or transport. **Consent** is the granting of permission to treat. More accurately, it is the granting of permission to touch. It is based on the concept that every adult human being of sound mind has the right to determine what should be done with his own body. Touching a patient without appropriate consent may subject you to charges of assault and battery.[11]

A patient must be **competent** in order to give or withhold consent. A competent adult is one who is lucid and able to make an informed decision about medical care. He understands your questions and recommendations, and he understands the implications of his decisions made about medical care. Although there is no absolute test for determining competency, keep the following factors in mind when making a determination: the patient's mental status, the patient's ability to respond to questions, statements regarding the patient's competency from family or friends, evidence of impairment from drugs or alcohol, or indications of shock or hypoxia.

Informed Consent

Conscious, competent patients have the right to decide what medical care to accept. However, for consent to be legally valid, it must be **informed consent**, or consent given based on full disclosure of information. That is, a patient must understand the nature, risks, and benefits of any procedures to be performed. Therefore, before providing medical care, you must explain the following to the patient in a manner he can understand:

- Nature of the illness or injury
- Nature of the recommended treatments
- Risks, dangers, and benefits of those treatments
- Alternative treatment possibilities, if any, and the related risks, dangers, and benefits of accepting each one
- Dangers of refusing treatment and/or transport

Informed consent must be obtained from every competent adult before treatment may be initiated. Conscious, competent patients may revoke consent at any time during care and transport. In most states, a patient must be 18 years of age or older in order to give or withhold consent. Generally, a child's parent or legal guardian must give informed consent before treatment of the child can begin.

Expressed, Implied, and Involuntary Consent

There are three more types of consent: expressed, implied, and involuntary. **Expressed consent** is the most common. It occurs when a person directly grants permission to treat—verbally, nonverbally, or in writing. Often, the act of a patient requesting an ambulance is considered an expression of a desire to be treated. However, just because the patient consents to a ride to the hospital does not mean he has consented to all types of treatment (such as the initiation of an IV and/or the administration of medications). You must obtain consent for each treatment you plan to provide. Consent from the patient does not always need to be granted verbally. It may be expressed by allowing care to be rendered.

Unconscious patients cannot grant consent. When treating them or any patient who requires emergency intervention but is mentally, physically, or emotionally unable to grant consent, treatment depends on **implied consent** (sometimes called "emergency doctrine"). That is, it is assumed that the patient would want lifesaving treatment if he were able to give informed consent. Implied consent is effective only until the patient no longer requires emergency care or until the patient regains competence.

Occasionally, a court will order patients to undergo treatment, even though they may not want it. This is called **involuntary consent**. It is most commonly encountered with patients who must be held for mental-health evaluation or as directed by law enforcement personnel who have the patient under arrest. It also is used on occasion to force patients to undergo treatment for a disease that threatens the community at large (tuberculosis, for example). Law-enforcement personnel often will accompany patients who are undergoing court-ordered treatment.

Consent issues also can arise when a paramedic is called by law-enforcement officials to treat a sick or injured prisoner or arrestee. The officers may tell you that they have the legal authority to give consent to treatment for the patient simply because the patient is in police custody. However, a competent adult in police custody does not necessarily lose the right to make medical decisions for himself. In fact, many prisoners have successfully sued health care providers for rendering treatment without consent. Generally, forced treatment is limited to emergency treatment necessary to save life or limb or treatment ordered by the court. Be sure that you are familiar with your local protocols and laws on this issue.

CULTURAL CONSIDERATIONS

Religious and Cultural Beliefs. *Religious and cultural beliefs impact a patient's health care decisions. Some, such as Christian Scientists, prefer to use prayer instead of traditional health care and may refuse treatment on religious grounds. Similarly, Jehovah's Witnesses believe that blood transfusions are prohibited by biblical teachings.*

Special Consent Situations

In the case of a **minor** (depending on state law, this is usually a person under the age of 18), consent should be obtained from a parent, legal guardian, or court-appointed custodian. The same is true of a mentally incompetent adult. If a responsible person cannot be located, and if the child or mentally incompetent adult is suffering from an apparent life-threatening injury or illness, treatment may be rendered under the doctrine of implied consent.

Generally, an **emancipated minor** is considered an adult. This is a person under 18 years of age who is married, pregnant, a parent, a member of the armed forces, or financially independent and living away from home. As an adult, an emancipated minor may legally give informed consent. Anyone else under the age of 18 may not grant informed consent.

Withdrawal of Consent

A competent adult may withdraw consent for any treatment at any time. However, refusal must be informed. That is, the patient must understand the risks of not continuing treatment or transport to the hospital in terms he can fully understand. A common example of a patient withdrawing consent occurs after a hypoglycemic patient regains full consciousness with the administration of dextrose. The patient should be encouraged—*but may not be forced*—to go to the emergency department. If he is competent, the patient may refuse transport. In such cases, advanced life support measures, such as IV fluids, which were initiated when the patient was unconscious should be discontinued. The patient also should complete a release-from-liability form (Figure 7-2 ●).

Sometimes patients choose to accept one recommended treatment, but refuse others. For example, a patient involved in a motor vehicle crash may refuse to be fully immobilized but ask to be transported to the hospital. It is very important for you to do everything in your power to be sure he understands why spinal precautions are necessary and what may happen if they are not taken. If a competent adult continues to refuse care, be sure to thoroughly document his reason for refusal and your attempts to convince him to change his mind. Have the patient and a witness sign a release-from-liability form.

Refusal of Service

Not every EMS run results in the transportation of a patient to a hospital. Emergency care should always be offered to a patient, no matter how minor the injury or illness may be. However, often, the patient will refuse. If this occurs, you must:

- Be sure that the patient is legally permitted to refuse care; that is, the patient must be a competent adult.
- Make multiple and sincere attempts to convince the patient to accept care.
- Enlist the help of others, such as the patient's family or friends, to convince the patient to accept care.
- Make certain that the patient is fully informed about the implications of his decision and the potential risks of refusing care.
- Consult with on-line medical direction.
- Have the patient and a disinterested witness, such as a police officer, sign a release-from-liability form.
- Advise the patient that he may call you again for help, if necessary.

REFUSAL OF TREATMENT AND TRANSPORTATION

I, THE UNDERSIGNED, HAVE BEEN ADVISED THAT MEDICAL ASSISTANCE ON MY BEHALF IS NECESSARY AND THAT REFUSAL OF SAID ASSISTANCE AND TRANSPORTATION MAY RESULT IN DEATH, OR IMPERIL MY HEALTH. NEVERTHELESS, I REFUSE TO ACCEPT TREATMENT OR TRANSPORT AND ASSUME ALL RISKS AND CONSEQUENCES OF MY DECISION AND RELEASE GOLD CROSS AMBULANCE COMPANY AND ITS EMPLOYEES FROM ANY LIABILITY ARISING FROM MY REFUSAL.

SIGNATURE OF PATIENT

WITNESSED BY

DATE SIGNED

● **Figure 7-2** Example of a "release-from-liability" form.

- Attempt to get the patient's family or friends to stay with the patient.
- Document the entire situation thoroughly on your patient care report.[12]

Remember, the refusal of care must be informed. That is, the patient must be told of and understand all possible risks of refusal. Decisions not to transport should involve medical direction. It is a good idea to put the patient directly on the phone with the on-line physician. If all efforts fail, be sure to thoroughly document the reasons for refusal and your efforts to change the patient's mind. If an on-line physician was involved, it is a good idea to obtain his signature on your patient care report. (See Figure 7-3 ● for an example of an EMS patient refusal checklist.)

Problem Patients

As a paramedic, you will occasionally encounter a "problem patient," one who is violent, a victim of a drug overdose, an intoxicated adult or minor, or an ill or injured minor with no adult available to provide consent for medical treatment. Such a patient can present you with a medical/legal dilemma. For example, consider the patient who has allegedly taken an overdose of medication. Concerned family members may panic and activate the EMS system. However, on your arrival at the scene, you find the patient alert, oriented, denying that he has taken any medication, and refusing to give consent for treatment or transport.

In a case such as this, attempt to develop trust and some rapport with the patient. If he continues to refuse, and remains alert and oriented, a refusal form should be completed and witnessed by a police officer. If the patient will not sign the form, have a police officer or family member sign it, indicating that the patient verbally refused care. If, however, the situation becomes dangerous, or you have reason to suspect the patient has tried to injure himself, police officers or family members should consider legal measures to force the patient to receive treatment.

The intoxicated person who refuses treatment and transport also poses a problem for the paramedic. Every effort should be made to encourage the patient to accept care and transport to the hospital. If the patient refuses, explain to him in a calm and detailed manner the implications of refusal. However, if you determine that the patient cannot understand the nature of his illness or the consequences of his refusal, then he may not refuse treatment because he is not competent to do so. Involve law enforcement at this point. If the patient is competent to make such a decision, then have him sign a refusal form. Your conversation with the patient and his refusal should be witnessed by a disinterested third party, such as a police officer.

Regardless of the type of problem patient, always document the encounter in detail. Your records should include a

---

PATHO PEARLS

Patients with Mental Disorders. *Several types of mental disorders are frequently encountered with problem patients. In addition to intoxication with alcohol or drugs, many problem patients suffer from personality disorders. These disorders cloud judgment and significantly impact interactions with others.*

---

description of the patient, the results of any physical examination (or reasons for the lack of one), important statements made by the patient and other persons at the scene, and the names and addresses of any witnesses. If you are going to include an important statement from the patient or witnesses in your patient care report, put the exact statement in quotation marks.

Ideally, a police officer should respond to the scene of all problem patients and should either sign the patient care report as a witness or, if the paramedic's safety is at risk, accompany the patient and paramedic to the emergency department.

Boundaries Issues

There are ethical and societal limits to the interactions between paramedics or other health care personnel and the patients they serve. These are called **professional boundaries** and serve to protect both the paramedic and the patient. EMS professionals have certain legal and ethical responsibilities to their patients, themselves, and the EMS system. Crossing professional boundaries can result in breaching these responsibilities. Danger zones for boundary crossing include being tired, being seduced, and being unprepared.

- *Being tired.* Fatigue can lead to problems such as medication errors, poor decision making, vehicle crashes, and more. EMS must be provided 24 hours a day, and long shifts and a heavy workload are common. You owe it to yourself and your patients to see to it that you are well rested and clear headed.

- *Being seduced.* In modern society "being seduced" is generally thought of as being enticed into some sort of sexual liaison. But, by definition, "being seduced" means being led away from one's principles, ethics, faith, or allegiance. Certainly, a sexual relationship between a health care provider and a patient is unethical and must be avoided at all costs. But, there are other temptations that may cause some to stray from honorable and appropriate behavior, such as money, food, items of value, and drugs. The physical and mental demands of EMS work, including the isolation, can sometimes lead to addictive behavior and lapses in judgment.

- *Being unprepared.* The motto of the Boy Scouts is "Be Prepared," and preparation is also a fundamental tenet of EMS. At some point in your EMS career you will encounter a situation that your education and experience has not prepared you for. Unfortunately, when we don't have the time and opportunity to think through a situation, we make errors. For example, several years ago, two paramedics encountered a pregnant woman who was killed in a motor vehicle collision. The death was sudden, and their response time was short. They decided to attempt to save the life of the baby through a postmortem Cesarean section. This was a procedure that their education and experience had not prepared them for, and it was met with sanctions from the state and the local medical director.

Boundary issues can be avoided by adhering to one's personal ethics and integrity and to the ethics expected of the profession.[13] Try to look down the road and see if any of your

EMS PATIENT REFUSAL CHECKLIST

PATIENT'S NAME:_____ AGE:_____

LOCATION OF CALL:_____ DATE:_____

AGENCY INCIDENT #:_____ AGENCY CODE:_____

NAME OF PERSON FILLING OUT FORM:_____

I. ASSESSMENT OF PATIENT (Check appropriate response for each item)

    1.   Oriented to: Person?   ☐ Yes ☐ No

                          Place?   ☐ Yes ☐ No

                          Time?   ☐ Yes ☐ No

                          Situation? ☐ Yes ☐ No

    2.   Altered level of consciousness?   ☐ Yes ☐ No

    3.   Head injury?   ☐ Yes ☐ No

    4.   Alcohol or drug ingestion by exam or history? ☐ Yes ☐ No

II. PATIENT INFORMED (Check appropriate response for each item)

    ☐ Yes ☐ No   Medical treatment/evaluation needed

    ☐ Yes ☐ No   Ambulance transport needed

    ☐ Yes ☐ No   Further harm could result without medical treatment/evaluation

    ☐ Yes ☐ No   Transport by means other than ambulance could be hazardous in light of patient's illness/injury

    ☐ Yes ☐ No   Patient provided with Refusal Information Sheet

    ☐ Yes ☐ No   Patient accepted Refusal Information Sheet

III. DISPOSITION

    ☐ Refused all EMS assistance

    ☐ Refused field treatment, but accepted transport

    ☐ Refused transport, but accepted field treatment

    ☐ Refused transport to recommended facility

    ☐ Patient transported by private vehicle to_____

    ☐ Released in care or custody of self

    ☐ Released in care or custody of relative or friend

        Name:_____ Relationship:_____

    ☐ Released in custody of law enforcement agency

        Agency:_____ Officer:_____

    ☐ Released in custody of other agency

        Agency:_____ Officer:_____

IV. COMMENTS: _____

_____

_____

_____

● **Figure 7-3**   Some EMS systems have checklists for procedures to follow when a patient refuses care and/or transport.

thoughts, actions, or circumstances could cause problems in the future. Generally, signs of potential trouble will be obvious. Keep in mind that loneliness and isolation can lead to boundary crossings. Always maintain a healthy lifestyle and have a life and circle of friends outside EMS. Keep your priorities straight and maintain high standards and ethics. As Ralph Waldo Emerson said, "Character is higher than intellect."

Legal Complications Related to Consent

There are many legal complications related to consent to treatment. If the paramedic does not obtain the proper consent to treat or fails to continue appropriate treatment, he may be liable for damages based on a tort cause of action, such as abandonment, assault, battery, or false imprisonment.

Abandonment

Abandonment is the termination of the paramedic-patient relationship without providing for the appropriate continuation of care while it is still needed and desired by the patient. You cannot initiate patient care and then discontinue it without sufficient reason. You cannot turn the care of a patient over to personnel who have less training than you without creating potential liability for an abandonment action. For example, a paramedic who has initiated advanced life support should not turn the patient over to an EMT or an AEMT for transport.

Abandonment can occur at any point during patient contact, including in the field or in the hospital emergency department. Physically leaving a patient unattended, even for a short time, may also be grounds for a charge of abandonment. If, for example, you leave a patient at a hospital without properly turning over his care to a physician or nurse, you may be liable for abandonment. It is always a good idea to have the nurse or physician to whom you have passed responsibility for patient care sign your patient care report.

Assault and Battery

Failure to obtain appropriate consent before treatment could leave the paramedic open to allegations of assault and battery. **Assault** is defined as unlawfully placing a person in apprehension of immediate bodily harm without his consent. For example, your patient states that he is scared of needles and refuses to let you start an IV. If you then show him an IV catheter and bring it toward his arm as if to start an IV, you may be liable for assault.

Battery is the unlawful touching of another individual without his consent. It would be battery to actually start an IV on a patient who does not consent to such treatment. A paramedic can be sued for assault and battery in both criminal and civil contexts.

False Imprisonment

False imprisonment may be charged by a patient who is transported without consent or who is restrained without proper justification or authority. It is defined as intentional and unjustifiable detention of a person without his consent or other legal authority, and may result in civil or criminal liability. Like assault and battery, a charge of false imprisonment can be avoided by obtaining appropriate consent.

This is a particular problem with psychiatric patients. In most cases, you can avoid allegations of false imprisonment by having a law enforcement officer apprehend the patient and accompany you to the hospital. If no officer is available, you should attempt to consult with medical direction and carefully judge the risks of false imprisonment against the benefits of detaining and treating the patient. You should determine whether medical treatment is immediately necessary and whether the patient poses a threat to himself or to the public when you are making your decision to treat or transport.

Reasonable Force

If it is safe to do so, you may use a reasonable amount of force to control an unruly or violent patient. **Reasonable force** is the minimum amount of force necessary to ensure that the patient does not cause injury to himself, you, or others. Use of excessive force can result in liability for the paramedic. Force used as punishment will be considered assault and battery, for which the patient may be able to recover damages, and the paramedic may face criminal charges.

The use of restraints may be indicated for a combative patient. Restraints must conform to your local protocols. Restraining devices typically used by EMS providers include straps, jackets, and restraining blankets. Paramedics should take special care to prevent positional asphyxia in restrained patients. As discussed under the section Restraint Issues earlier in this chapter, positional asphyxia occurs when a patient's position prevents him from being able to breathe or to breathe adequately. In some EMS systems, paramedics are authorized to use chemical restraints, such as benzodiazepines and antipsychotics, in lieu of or in addition to physical restraints. In most EMS systems, paramedics are not authorized to apply law enforcement restraints such as handcuffs or leg irons. In the event that a paramedic accompanies a patient who is handcuffed, it is imperative that a law enforcement officer also accompany the patient in case the restraints need to be removed.

For the combative patient, an EMS team's goal is to use the least amount of force necessary to safely control the patient while causing him the least amount of discomfort. Whenever the use of force and/or the use of restraints is indicated, involve law enforcement officials (Figure 7-4 ●). For more information on the use of restraints, see Volume 4, Chapter 11.

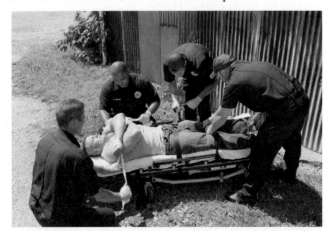

● **Figure 7-4** Patient restraint is a high-risk endeavor. The safety of personnel and the patient should be the highest priority.

Patient Transportation

The transportation of patients to a health care facility is an integral part of the patient-care continuum. During transportation to a health care facility, be sure to maintain the same level of care as was initiated at the scene. This means that if you, as a paramedic, initiate advanced emergency care procedures, you must either ride with the patient to the hospital or ensure that another paramedic will accompany the patient. If you fail to do so, and the patient is harmed as a result, you may be liable for abandonment.

One of the greatest areas of potential liability for paramedics is emergency vehicle operations. It is essential that you become familiar with your state and local laws. The laws that provide exceptions from driving rules and regulations may allow you, for example, to drive at a rate of speed in excess of a posted speed limit, but if you are negligent at any time during the operation of your vehicle, you will not be protected from liability.

Another issue that will arise is patient choice of destination. If you work in a small area with only one hospital, you are not likely to encounter difficulties. However, many paramedics work in areas that have many hospitals and medical centers to choose from. Over the past few years, increasing numbers of lawsuits involving facility selection have been brought by patients. Some have sued paramedics themselves, claiming negligence based on the failure to transport to the nearest or most appropriate hospital.

An additional issue you may need to address involves the patient's insurance company protocols. In some situations, it may be appropriate to respect a patient's choice of facility based on his insurance company's facility-choice protocols. Local restrictions by insurance companies and health care maintenance organizations may determine under what conditions and to what facilities patient transport may be authorized and paid for. While most areas are not yet being confronted with restrictions on service provision, it may be only a matter of time. However, never put patient care in jeopardy by transporting to a less-appropriate facility because of insurance concerns.

In general, facility selection should be based on patient request, patient need, and facility capability. Local written protocols, the paramedic, on-line medical direction, and the patient should all play a role in facility selection. The patient's preference should be honored unless the situation or the patient's condition dictates otherwise. Become familiar with your system's protocols regarding hospital destinations as well as the capabilities of specialty care facilities such as trauma centers or stroke centers.

RESUSCITATION ISSUES

Advances in medical technology have saved and prolonged thousands of lives. However, in some instances, the use of sophisticated medical technology may only prolong pain, suffering, and death. When a person is seriously injured or gravely ill, family members must make difficult decisions regarding the intensity of medical care to be provided, including the use or withdrawal of life-support systems.

Generally, you are under obligation to begin resuscitative efforts when summoned to the scene of a patient who is unresponsive, pulseless, and apneic (not breathing). There are times, however, when you will determine that resuscitation is not indicated. This occurs with patients who have a valid Do Not Resuscitate (DNR) order, with patients who are obviously dead (decapitated, for example), with patients with obvious tissue decomposition or extreme dependent lividity (gravitational pooling of blood in dependent areas of the body), or with a patient who is at a scene that is too hazardous to enter.

As more is learned about resuscitation, it is now becoming common practice, in selected cases, either not to begin resuscitation or to terminate resuscitative efforts in the field. For example, pulseless victims of blunt trauma have virtually no chance of survival. Because of this, many EMS systems now have protocols in place whereby resuscitation of pulseless blunt trauma victims is not attempted. Likewise, resuscitation research has shown that patients who are not resuscitated from standard ALS measures in the prehospital setting will not benefit from transportation to the hospital. In this circumstance too, many EMS systems have established protocols for termination of resuscitation efforts in the field.

Always follow your state laws, local protocols, and medical direction. The role of medical direction should be clearly delineated and included in your agency's protocols. If you are authorized to determine that resuscitative efforts are not indicated, be sure to thoroughly document your decision and the criteria on which it was based.

Advance Directives

To improve communication between patients, their family members, and physicians regarding such matters, the federal government enacted the Patient Self-Determination Act of 1990. This act requires hospitals and physicians to provide patients and their families with sufficient information to make informed decisions about medical treatment and the use of life-support measures, including cardiopulmonary resuscitation (CPR), artificial ventilation, nutrition, hydration, and blood transfusions.

Patients and their families are therefore more likely than ever to have prepared a written statement of the patient's own preference for future medical care, or an **advance directive**. An advance directive is a document created to ensure that certain treatment choices are honored when a patient is unconscious or otherwise unable to express his choice of treatments. Advance directives come in a variety of forms. The most common encountered in the field are living wills, durable powers of attorney for health care, Do Not Resuscitate orders, and organ donor cards.

The types of advance directives recognized in each state are governed by state law and local protocols. Medical direction must establish and implement policies for dealing with advance directives in the field. Those policies should clearly define the obligations of a paramedic who is caring for a patient with an advance directive. They should also provide for reasonable measures of comfort to the patient and emotional support to the patient's family and loved ones. Some states do not allow paramedics to honor living wills in the field but do allow them to honor valid Do Not Resuscitate orders. Be sure you are familiar with your state law and local policies.

Living Will

A **living will** is a legal document that allows a person to specify the kinds of medical treatment he wishes to receive should the need arise (Figure 7-5 ●). For example, many states allow patients to

---

LIVING WILL

I, _____ _____ , make the following Living Will declaration to my family, physicians, hospitals, and other health care providers and any Court or Judge:

After thoughtful consideration and while I am of sound mind, I make this statement as an expression of my settled and firm wishes if the time comes when I can no longer take part in decisions about my own future health.

My Wishes. If at any time I have a terminal condition, and in the opinion of my attending or treating physician there is no reasonable probability that I will recover and the condition can be expected to cause my death within a relatively short time if medical procedures which serve only to prolong the process of dying are not used, or if I am in a persistent vegetative state in which I have no voluntary action or cognitive behavior and cannot communicate or interact purposefully and which is a permanent and irreversible condition of unconsciousness, **I request that I be allowed to die naturally and not be kept alive by artificial means.** I ask that all life-prolonging procedures, including medical assistance to eat and drink when it is highly unlikely that I will regain the capacity to eat and drink without medical assistance, be withheld or withdrawn in such a situation.

Resuscitation. It is my further wish that no cardiopulmonary resuscitation shall thereafter be administered to me if I sustain a cardiac or respiratory arrest. In those circumstances I consent to an order not to resuscitate, and direct that such an order be placed in my medical record.

I direct that these decisions shall be carried into effect even if I am unable to personally reconfirm or communicate them, without seeking judicial approval or authority.

I recognize that there may be instances besides those described above for which life-sustaining treatment should be withheld or withdrawn and this instrument shall not be construed as an exclusive enumeration of these circumstances.

Revocation and Responsibility. This instrument and its instructions may be revoked by me at any time and in any manner. However, no physician, hospital, or other health care provider who withholds or withdraws life-sustaining treatment in reliance upon this Living Will or upon my personally communicated instructions shall have any liability or responsibility to me, my estate, or any other persons for having withheld or withdrawn treatment.

I intend this declaration to be accepted in the circumstances described as an exercise of my legal right to refuse medical treatment even if I am unable to personally reconfirm or communicate that. It is made in the presence of the witnesses who have signed below.

Signed on (date): _____

Signature: _____

Witness: _____

Witness: _____

● **Figure 7-5**   Example of a living will.

include in living wills their wishes concerning dying in a hospital or at home, receiving CPR, and donation of their organs and other body parts. In addition, patients with prolonged illnesses sometimes invoke the right to choose a person who may make health care decisions for them in the event that their mental functions become impaired. They might formalize this decision by way of a special notation in a living will. (They may also do this through execution of a document called a "Durable Power of Attorney for Health Care" or "Health Care Proxy.") Living wills, once signed and witnessed, are effective until they are revoked by the patient.

Be sure you know your local protocols concerning living wills. If any question arises on scene, contact medical direction for instructions.

Do Not Resuscitate Orders

A **Do Not Resuscitate (DNR) order** is a common type of advance directive (Figure 7-6 ●). Usually signed by the patient and his physician, the DNR order is a legal document that indicates to medical personnel which, if any, life-sustaining measures should be taken when the patient's heart and respiratory functions have ceased. DNR orders generally direct EMS personnel to withhold CPR in the event of a cardiac arrest. When you honor a DNR order, do not simply pack up your equipment and leave the scene. You still may have the patient's family and loved ones to attend to. Provide emotional support as appropriate.

PREHOSPITAL DO NOT RESUSCITATE ORDERS

<u>ATTENDING PHYSICIAN</u>

In completing this prehospital DNR form, please check Part A if no intervention by prehospital personnel is indicated. Please check Part A and options from Part B if specific interventions by prehospital personnel are indicated. To give a valid prehospital DNR order, this form must be completed by the patient's attending physician and must be provided to prehospital personnel.

A) _____ **Do Not Resuscitate (DNR):**
No Cardiopulmonary Resuscitation or Advanced Cardiac Life Support to be performed by prehospital personnel

B) _____ **Modified Support:**
Prehospital personnel administer the following checked options:
_____ Oxygen administration
_____ Full airway support: intubation, airways, bag-valve mask
_____ Venipuncture: IV crystalloids and/or blood draw
_____ External cardiac pacing
_____ Cardiopulmonary resuscitation
_____ Cardiac defibrillator
_____ Pneumatic anti-shock garment
_____ Ventilator
_____ ACLS meds
_____ Other interventions/medications (physician specify)

Prehospital personnel are informed that (print patient name)_____
should receive no resuscitation (DNR) or should receive Modified Support as indicated. This directive is medically appropriate and is further documented by a physician's order and a progress note on the patient's permanent medical record. Informed consent from the capacitated patient or the incapacitated patient's legitimate surrogate is documented on the patient's permanent medical record. The DNR order is in full force and effect as of the date indicated below.

_____   _____

Attending Physician's Signature

_____   _____

Print Attending Physician's Name   Print Patient's Name and Location
                                                  (Home Address or Health Care Facility)

_____

Attending Physician's Telephone

_____   _____

Date   Expiration Date (6 Mos from Signature)

● **Figure 7-6**   Example of an EMS Do Not Resuscitate (DNR) order.

DNR orders pose a particular problem in the field. Paramedics are often called to nursing homes or residences where they find a patient in cardiac arrest and in need of resuscitation. As a rule, you are legally obligated to attempt resuscitation. If a physician has written a specific order to avoid it, the paramedics should not have been summoned. Even so, people tend to panic and will call for help. Valid DNR orders should be honored as your protocols allow. Note, however, that if there is any doubt as to the patient's wishes, resuscitation should be initiated.

Occasionally, you may be requested to treat a patient as a "slow code" or "chemical code only." This is not legally permitted. Cardiac resuscitation is an all-or-nothing proposition. Treating a cardiac arrest with only medications would mean abandoning airway management and defibrillation. To do so, even at the request of the family, amounts to negligence and must be avoided.

Potential Organ Donation

Over the past few years, advances in medicines have led to an increased number of organ transplants and a higher survival rate of transplant patients. As organs and tissues are in very high demand and short supply, many EMS systems are now becoming a vital link in the organ procurement and transplant process. Some have developed protocols that specifically address organ viability after a patient's death. These include providing circulatory support through IV fluids and CPR and ventilatory support via endotracheal tube. Whether or not your EMS has protocols in place for potential organ donation, it is important for you to consult with on-line medical direction when you have identified a patient as a potential donor (Figure 7-7 ●).

Death in the Field

Whether you arrive at the scene of a patient who has died prior to your arrival or you make an authorized decision to terminate resuscitative efforts, a death in the field must be appropriately dealt with and thoroughly documented. Paramedics should carefully follow state and local protocols. It is also important for the paramedic to contact on-line medical direction for guidance.

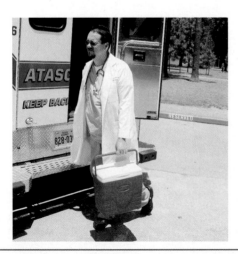

● **Figure 7-7** Transporting organs for transplantation. (© *LifeGift Organ Donation, Houston, TX*)

CRIME AND ACCIDENT SCENES

Since it may be your duty as a paramedic to treat a patient found at a crime scene, you should be aware of crime-scene preservation issues. However, you must not sacrifice patient care to preserve evidence or to become involved in detective work. You can best assist investigating officers by properly treating the patient and by doing your best to avoid destroying any potential evidence. As a paramedic, your responsibilities at a crime scene include the following:

- If you believe a crime may have been committed on scene, immediately contact law enforcement if they are not already involved.
- Protect yourself and the safety of other EMS personnel. This should always be your primary consideration. You will not be held liable for failing to act if a scene is not safe to enter.
- Once a crime scene has been deemed safe, initiate patient contact and medical care.
- Do not move or touch anything at a crime scene unless it is necessary to do so for patient care. Observe and document the original placement of any items moved by your crew. If the patient's clothing has holes made by a gunshot or a stabbing, leave them intact, if possible. If the patient has an obvious mortal wound, such as decapitation, try not to touch the body at all. Do your best to protect any potential evidence.
- If you need to remove items from the scene, such as an impaled weapon or bottle of medication, be sure to document your actions and notify investigating officers.

You should treat the scene of an accident in the same way. Your goals are to ensure your own safety and the safety of your crew and to treat your patients as medically indicated. Use the resources available to you, and be prepared to summon additional personnel and rescue equipment as necessary.

DUTY TO REPORT

As a paramedic, you have an ethical duty to protect those at risk—especially the more vulnerable among us. During the course of your work you may encounter patients who may have been abused or neglected. When abuse or neglect is suspected, you must balance the need to protect patient confidentiality against the need to notify the proper authorities. As a rule, you should always act with the patient's best interest in mind.

Abuse of the elderly, children, and the invalid is all too common. Many states have rules that require EMS personnel to report suspected abuse to the proper authorities. If abuse or neglect is suspected, you should report your concerns to the proper authority in an objective and timely manner. You should not confront the abuser. It is not necessary for you to prove that abuse or neglect occurred before reporting. As a rule, you will be doing the proper thing if you report acting in the patient's best interest. You should learn and review the rules and requirements for reporting abuse and neglect in your state. Oftentimes, the failure to report abuse or neglect is a bigger liability than reporting.

DOCUMENTATION

The importance of developing and maintaining superior documentation skills and habits cannot be overemphasized. As a paramedic, you must recognize that the treatment of your patient does not end until you have properly documented the entire incident from initial response to the transfer of patient care to the hospital emergency department staff.

A complete well-written patient care report is your best protection in a malpractice action. In fact, a well-written report may actually discourage a plaintiff from filing a malpractice case in the first place. In general, a plaintiff's attorney will request copies of all medical records, including the paramedic's report, before filing a lawsuit. If the paramedic's report is sloppy, incomplete, or otherwise not well written, this may encourage the plaintiff to sue, even if the paramedic's conduct was not negligent.

A well-documented patient care report has the following characteristics:

- *It is completed promptly after patient contact.* It should be made in the course of business, not long after the event. Any delay could cause you to forget important observations or treatments. If possible, a copy of the completed report should be left with the emergency department staff before you leave the hospital. This copy will become part of the patient's permanent medical records. Proper documentation is so important that some EMS systems now require paramedics to dictate their reports, which are later transcribed and placed in the patient's permanent records. Some systems use template-driven electronic records (Figure 7-8 ●).

  Note: Never delay patient care to attend to a patient care report.

- *It is thorough.* The report should paint a clear and complete picture of the patient's condition and the care that was provided. Its main purpose is not simply to record patient data, but also to support the diagnosis and treatment that you provided to the patient. All actions, procedures, and administered medications should be documented as well. Remember this saying: "If you didn't write it down, you didn't do it."

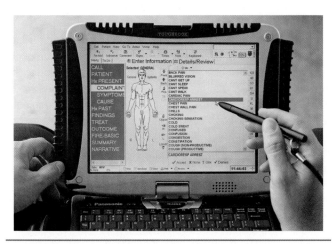

● **Figure 7-8** Template-driven electronic patient records are becoming more common in modern EMS.

- *It is objective.* Avoid the use of emotional and value-loaded words. Not only are they irrelevant to patient care, but they also may be the cause of a libel suit against you.

- *It is accurate.* Be as precise as possible, avoiding the use of abbreviations and jargon that are not commonly understood or are approved within your EMS system. Also try to limit your report to information that you have personally seen or heard. If you need to document something that you do not have personal knowledge of, be sure to indicate the source of your information. Document your observations, not your assumptions, and do not draw a medical conclusion that you are not competent to make. For example, you cannot conclusively diagnose a patient as having pneumonia. You can, however, report your suspicion of pneumonia and document findings that are consistent with this condition.

- *It maintains patient confidentiality.* Your agency should have well-defined policies regarding the release of patient information. Whenever possible, patient consent should be obtained prior to release of information.

The medical record should never be altered. An intentional alteration amounts to an admission of guilt by the paramedic. If a patient care report is found to be incomplete or inaccurate, a written amendment should be attached to the report. The date and time the amendment was written, not the date of the original report, should be noted on the addendum. Also, be sure to send a copy of the addendum to the receiving hospital so that it will become a part of the patient's medical records. For computerized medical records, amendments and corrections are generally automatically flagged and dated as such.

Medical records need to be maintained for a period of time that is prescribed by state law. For example, in New York State patient care reports must be maintained by an EMS agency for a period of six years, or for three years after the patient reaches the age of 18, whichever is longer. Be sure to become familiar with the record retention requirements in your state.

EMPLOYMENT LAWS

Employment laws are laws that address employee/employer relationships. Even volunteer agencies fall under the jurisdiction of many of these laws. Employment law can be complex and you should consult an attorney with expertise in this area of law should a problem arise. There are several employment laws that paramedics should be familiar with.

- *Americans with Disabilities Act. The Americans with Disabilities Act (ADA),* enacted in 1990, prohibits private employers, state and local governments, employment agencies, and labor unions from discriminating against qualified individuals with disabilities in job application procedures, hiring, firing, advancement, compensation, job training, and other terms, conditions, and privileges of employment. The ADA covers employers with 15 or more employees, including state and local governments. It also applies to employment agencies and to labor organizations.

The ADA's nondiscrimination standards also apply to federal employees as well. An employer is required to make a reasonable accommodation to the known disability of a qualified applicant or employee if it would not impose an "undue hardship" on the operation of the employer's business. Reasonable accommodations are adjustments or modifications provided by an employer to enable people with disabilities to enjoy equal employment opportunities. EMS agencies should abide by the ADA.

- *Title VII.* A federal law that prohibits workplace harassment and discrimination, *Title VII* is a part of the *Civil Rights Act of 1964.* It covers all private employers, state and local governments, and educational institutions with more than 15 employees. It prohibits discrimination against employees on the basis of race, color, national origin, religion, and gender. It has been extended to protect against discrimination on the basis of pregnancy, sex stereotyping, and sexual harassment. EMS agencies, regardless of the type, should have well-established policies and procedures to address the requirements of Title VII.

- *Amendments to Title VII.* The Civil Rights Act of 1964 has been amended several times. The *Equal Employment Opportunity Act of 1972* made discrimination in employment illegal. Equal Employment Opportunity programs include affirmative action for employment as well as processing of and remedies for discrimination complaints. All employees, including supervisors, managers, former employees, and applicants for employment, regardless of grade level or position, are covered under this legislation. The *Age Discrimination and Employment Act of 1967 (ADEA)* and the *Age Discrimination Act of 1975* prohibit discrimination on the basis of age and protect individuals who are 40 years of age or older from employment discrimination based on age.

- *Family Medical Leave Act (FMLA).* The *Family and Medical Leave Act of 1993 (FMLA)* allows eligible employees to take off for up to 12 workweeks in any 12-month period for the birth or adoption of a child, to care for a family member, or if the employees themselves have a serious health condition. This act was amended in 2008 to permit a spouse, son, daughter, parent, or next of kin to take up to 26 workweeks of leave to care for a member of the Armed Forces.

- *Fair Labor Standards Act (FLSA).* The *Fair Labor Standards Act of 1938* was enacted following the Great Depression and established certain standards in regard to employment. It has been amended multiple times over the years. FLSA establishes the minimum wage, overtime pay, recordkeeping, and child labor standards. It applies to both full-time and part-time workers in the private sector as well as those employed in federal, state, and local government.

- *Occupational Safety and Health Act (OSHA).* The *Occupational Safety and Health Act (OSHA)* was signed into law in 1970. The purpose of OSHA was to ensure that employers provide employees with an environment that is healthy and safe. The act also established the Occupational Safety and Health Administration to oversee workforce safety and the National Institute for Occupational Safety and Health (NIOSH) to guide occupational health and safety research.

- *The Ryan White Care Act.* The *Ryan White Care Act* was enacted in 1990 and was designed to fund programs to improve the availability of health care for victims of AIDS and their families. The act also mandated that EMS personnel learn whether they have been exposed to life-threatening diseases while providing emergency care. The Ryan White act was set to expire on September 30, 2009, but the Ryan White HIV/AIDS treatment extension act of 2009 extended the benefits for an additional four years.

SUMMARY

The very nature of a paramedic's job requires interaction with law enforcement authorities and frequent involvement in situations that can give rise to litigation. For example, not only will police be called to the same emergencies to which paramedics are called, such as motor vehicle collisions or scenes where violence caused injuries, but paramedics also may become material witnesses to crimes or domestic disputes. It is therefore in your best interest to learn and follow all state laws and local protocols related to your practice as a paramedic.

Also be sure to receive good training and keep current by attending continuing medical education programs and conferences, reading industry journals, and obtaining recertification or relicensure as required by state law.

Remember, a paramedic is not immune from allegations of negligence or malpractice. However, the potential for liability may be limited or avoided by adhering to the following guidelines:

- Always obtain informed consent before initiating treatment and/or transport.
- Practice only those skills and procedures that a reasonable and prudent paramedic would, given the same or similar circumstances.

- Practice only those procedures that you are trained to perform and are directly authorized to perform by a medical-control physician or by approved local standing orders.

- Prepare accurate, legible, and complete medical records that thoroughly document the entire EMS incident, from initial response to the transfer of patient care to hospital emergency department staff.

- Discuss patient information with only those who need to know. Limit writings and oral reports to information essential to patient care.

- Purchase and maintain malpractice insurance, and see that your employer does the same.

- Be nice to your patients and their families.

Always act in good faith and use your common sense. High-quality patient care and high-quality documentation are always your best protection from liability.

YOU MAKE THE CALL

You and the rest of the crew of EMS Unit 116 receive a call to assist an unconscious 5-year-old girl. On arriving at the scene, you are met by the child's babysitter, who states that for the past hour the child had been acting "strangely," after which she fell asleep and would not wake up. The babysitter also tells you that the child had been playing in her bedroom alone all afternoon. You ask the babysitter to call the child's parents immediately. She tells you that they are unreachable but are expected home in approximately 20 minutes.

While your partner searches the child's room, you assess the patient and note the following physical findings: respiratory depression, hypotension, bradycardia, and constricted pupils. Quickly searching, your partner finds an empty bottle of Darvocet under the child's bed. You now suspect a narcotic overdose and determine that the child needs immediate medical intervention and transport to an appropriate medical facility. You prepare to start an IV, when the babysitter tells you that she will not consent to treatment and tells you to wait for the parents to return home. A neighbor arrives on scene and insists that the child's parents would want only the family physician to treat her, and begs you to drive her there.

1. You believe that the child needs emergency care, but the child's parents are unavailable. What should you do?

2. If you decide to treat the child without consent, can you be sued for doing so?

3. What would you do if the parents returned home and refused to grant permission for treatment?
See Suggested Responses at the back of this book.

REVIEW QUESTIONS

1. _____ _____ originated with the English legal system and was adopted by Americans in the 1700s.
   a. Common law   c. Criminal law
   b. Civil law   d. Constitutional law

2. _____ _____ is enacted by an administrative or governmental agency at either the federal or state level.
   a. Civil law   c. Legislative law
   b. Criminal law   d. Administrative law

3. The _____ _____ is the location of most of the cases in which a paramedic may become involved.
   a. appellate court system
   b. state court system
   c. federal court system
   d. supreme court system

4. On-scene licensed physicians who are professionally unrelated to the patient and who are attempting to assist with patient care are called:
   a. intervener physicians.
   b. direct control physicians.
   c. on-line medical control.
   d. indirect control physicians.

5. Legislative statutes that generally protect the person who provides care at no charge at the scene of a medical emergency are called:
   a. medical practice laws.
   b. scope of practice laws.
   c. Good Samaritan laws.
   d. standard of care laws.

6. In a negligence claim against a paramedic, the plaintiff must establish and prove four particular elements in order to prevail. Which of the following is not one of those elements?
   a. proximate cause
   b. duty to act
   c. level of compensation
   d. breach of the duty to act

7. The law provides penalties for the breach of confidentiality. The improper release of information may result in a lawsuit against the paramedic for:
   a. defamation.
   b. invasion of privacy.
   c. breach of confidentiality.
   d. all of the above.

8. This court-ordered type of consent is most commonly encountered with patients who must be held for mental-health evaluation or as directed by law enforcement personnel who have the patient under arrest.
   a. implied   c. involuntary
   b. expressed   d. guardianship

9. _____ is the termination of the paramedic-patient relationship without providing for the appropriate continuation of care while it is still needed and desired by the patient.
   a. Libel   c. Neglect
   b. Slander   d. Abandonment

10. A well-documented patient care report is:
    a. accurate.   c. thorough.
    b. objective.   d. all of the above.

See Answers to Review Questions at the back of this book.

 ## REFERENCES

1. Sine, D. M. and N. Northcutt. "A Qualitative Analysis of the Central Values of Professional Paramedics." *Am J Disaster Med* 3 (2008): 335–343.

2. United States of America. *Constitution of the United States*. Available at: http://www.archives.gov/exhibits/charters/constitution.html.

3. *Miranda v. Arizona,* 384 U.S. 436 (1966).

4. Hoffman, S., R. A. Goodman, and D. D. Stier. "Law, Liability and Public Health Emergencies." *Disaster Med Public Health Prep* 3 (2009): 117–125.

5. Nagorka, F. W. and C. Becker. "Immunity Statutes: How State Laws Protect EMS Providers." *Emerg Med Serv* 36 (2005): 47–52.

6. Hall, S.A. "Potential Liabilities of Medical Directors for Actions of EMTs." *Prehosp Emerg Care* 2 (1998): 76–80.

7. Erich, J. Where Duty Ends: "The Perils and Pitfalls of the Off-Duty Response." *Emerg Med Serv* 33 (2004): 49–52.

8. Wang, H. E. and D. M. Yealy. "Out-of-Hospital Endotracheal Intubation: Where Are We?" *Ann Emerg Med* 47 (2006): 532–541.

9. Chan, T. C., G. M. Vilke, and T. Neuman. "Reexamination of Custody Restraint Position and Positional Asphyxia." *Am J Forensic Med Pathol* 19 (1998): 201–205.

10. Department of Health and Human Services. *Health Information Privacy Act*. Available at: http://www.hhs.gov/ocr/privacy/.

11. Ayres, R. J., Jr. "Legal Considerations in Prehospital Care." *Emerg Med Clin North Am* 11 (1993): 853–867.

12. Graham, D. H. "Documentation of Patient Refusals." *Emerg Med Serv* 30 (2001): 56–60.

13. Maggiore, W. A. "Professional Boundaries: Where They Are & Why We Cross Them." *JEMS* 32(12): 68–76, 2007. (This article is available on-line at http://www.jems.com. Click on JEMS/issues to locate a pdf of this article in Volume 32 Issue 12, December 2007.)

 ## FURTHER READING

The Ambulance Service Guide to HIPAA Compliance. Mechanicsburg, PA: Page, Wolfberg, & Wirth, 2003.

Cohn, B. M. and A. J. Azzara. *Legal Aspects of Emergency Medical Services.* Philadelphia: W. B. Saunders, 1998.

Lee, N. G. *Legal Concepts and Issues in Emergency Care.* Philadelphia: W. B. Saunders, 2001.

Louisell, D. and H. Williams. *Medical Malpractice.* New York: Matthew Bender, 1995.

Page, J. O. "Anatomy of a Lawsuit." *JEMS* 1989: 14.

Schneid, Thomas D. *Fire and Emergency Law Case Book.* Albany, NY: Delmar Publishing, 1997.

Wang, H. E., R. J. Fairbanks, M. N. Shah, and D. M. Yealey. "Tort Claims from Adverse Events in Emergency Medical Services." *Prehospital Emergency Care* 11 (2007): 96–97.

8

Ethics in Paramedicine

Bryan Bledsoe, DO, FACEP, FAAEM, EMT-P

STANDARD
Preparatory (Medical/Legal and Ethics)

COMPETENCY
Integrates comprehensive knowledge of EMS systems, the safety and well-being of the paramedic, and medical/legal and ethical issues, which is intended to improve the health of EMS personnel, patients, and the community.

OBJECTIVES

Terminal Performance Objective
After reading this chapter you should be able to apply the ethical principles of paramedicine to your work as a paramedic.

Enabling Objectives
To accomplish the terminal performance objective, you should be able to:

1. Define key terms introduced in this chapter.
2. Describe the relationship between ethics and morals, laws, and religion.
3. Compare and contrast different approaches to ethical decision making.
4. Identify codes of ethics that serve to guide health care professionals, including EMS providers.
5. Explain the fundamental principles of ethics.
6. Given a variety of scenarios, recognize ethical dilemmas.
7. Given a variety of scenarios involving ethical dilemmas, take actions you can defend on the basis of ethical principles of paramedicine and tests of ethical decisions.

KEY TERMS

autonomy, p. 139	ethics, p. 136	morals, p. 136
beneficence, p. 139	justice, p. 139	nonmaleficence, p. 139

CASE STUDY

Mrs. Weinberg has fractured her hip. Her right lower extremity is obviously shortened and externally rotated. Fortunately, she has no apparent life-threatening injuries. As you and your partner tend to her, you notice that she seems more anxious than other patients you have seen with a similar problem. When your partner goes to the ambulance to retrieve additional pillows, she whispers to you, "I would really prefer if you took care of me."

"Why?" you ask.

She rolls up her sleeve and shows you a tattoo of a number on her left forearm. "This is why," she says. "When I was a little girl back in Germany, I was in a Nazi concentration camp. Your partner reminds me of the men who worked there. They killed my family, and they almost killed me. Could you take care of me on the way to the hospital?"

You do not have much time to think about this question, but you promise to help. Before you leave the scene, you approach your partner discreetly. "Heinz," you say to him, "this patient is a concentration camp survivor. Apparently your blond hair, blue eyes, and German accent remind her of the men who killed her family. Would you mind driving to the hospital on this call? I realize you enrolled in an exchange program to gain experience in patient care here in the United States, but there will be other calls." Heinz has no objection, so he drives to the hospital, and you take care of Mrs. Weinberg in the back of the ambulance.

After the call, the two of you discuss what happened. "Boy," you say, "I've never had a patient make a request like that. I think it was really great of you to accommodate her. Did it make you uncomfortable?" "No," he says, "but it surprised me. The Holocaust was long before my time. It remains an embarrassment for all of us in my country." You agree that the best way to make Mrs. Weinberg comfortable was to switch places. You also agree that the two of you handled a difficult situation gracefully.

Later, when you think about the call a little more, you realize that this situation was truly a first for you. Is it right, you wonder, to accommodate a request like this? Heinz was not going to harm her. Were you assuaging her fears or validating her prejudices? What if the patient had been an elderly man who asked you to switch places with your black partner? Would the patient's ignorance have been enough of a reason to accommodate him? What if the patient had been a neo-Nazi skinhead who insisted on having a white person care for him?

Was the situation just a matter of being courteous, as you first thought? After all, no one was hurt, and it was only a minor inconvenience for you and your partner to switch positions. Or was it actually a matter of ethics? You realize you are not quite sure how to determine the best thing to do under circumstances like these. It is time, you realize, to brush up on your ethics.

INTRODUCTION

Consider the following: A physician administers 15 milligrams of intravenous morphine to a dying patient to alleviate pain and suffering. Another physician administers 15 milligrams of intravenous morphine to a dying patient to end the patient's life. What's the difference? Although the question is seemingly simple, it is actually quite complex. Is there a moral difference between these two actions?

When asked what the most difficult part of the job is, most paramedics do not say "ethics." Nonetheless, in one recent survey almost 15 percent of advanced life support calls in an urban EMS system generated some ethical conflict.[1] In another survey, EMS providers responded that they frequently have ethical problems related to patients refusing care, conflicts regarding hospital destination, and difficulties with advance directives.[2] Other aspects of prehospital care present potential ethical problems. These include patient confidentiality, consent, the obligation to provide care, and research.

Although ethical problems often have a legal aspect, most ethical problems are solved in the field and not in a courtroom. However, there are times when ethical problems spill over into the legal arena and become the subject of legislation or regulations. The federal government, for instance, recently instituted rules to protect patients who are unable to consent to emergency care.

Ethical issues often begin with specific circumstances and lead to broad general rules or principles for behavior. This chapter examines how the most common principles and approaches are applied to common prehospital situations.

OVERVIEW OF ETHICS

Ethics and morals are closely related concepts. **Morals** are generally considered to be social, religious, or personal standards of right and wrong. **Ethics**, also known as moral philosophy, is a branch of philosophy that addresses questions about morality.

Generally speaking, ethics more often refers to the rules or standards that govern the conduct of members of a particular group or profession and how our institutions should function. Both ethics and morals address a question Socrates asked: "How should one live?"

Relationship of Ethics to Law and Religion

Ethics and the law have a great deal in common, but they are distinctly separate disciplines (Figure 8-1 ●). Although ethical discussions have an unfortunate tendency to degenerate into arguments about what is legal and who might be liable, ethics is not the same as law. In general, laws have a much narrower focus than ethics. Laws frequently describe what is wrong in the eyes of society. Ethics goes beyond examining what is wrong. It also looks at what is right, or good, behavior. As a result, the law frequently has little or nothing to say about ethical problems. In fact, laws themselves can be unethical. For example, for many years, laws existed and were enforced that perpetuated racial segregation in the United States. These were ethically wrong and, ultimately, made legally wrong.

Even though ethics and the law are different, ethical discussions can sometimes benefit from techniques developed by the law over the centuries. In particular, the law emphasizes impartiality, consistent procedures, and methods to identify and balance conflicting interests.

Just as ethics differs from the law, it also differs from religion. In a pluralistic society such as ours, ethics must be understood by and applied to people who hold a broad range of religious beliefs, or no religious beliefs at all. Thus, ethics cannot derive from a single religion. It is true, however, that religion can enhance and enrich one's ethical principles and values.

Relationship of Ethical and Legal Issues with Medicine

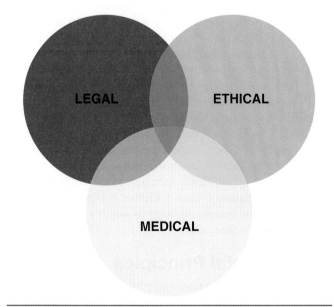

● **Figure 8-1** The relationship of ethical and legal issues and medicine.

Making Ethical Decisions

There are many different approaches one can use to determine how a medical professional should behave under different circumstances. One approach is to say that each person must decide how to behave and whatever decision that person makes is okay. This approach is known as *ethical relativism*. People sometimes say they believe in ethical relativism. However, when questioned, they typically admit they do not find it satisfactory. For example, no reasonable person would say that it was acceptable for the Nazis, especially Nazi physicians, to behave as they did.

A similar approach is to say, "Just do what is right." This sounds fine but in reality it does not answer the question of how a health care professional should act. This occurs because different people have different beliefs about what is "right." Ethics and morality overlap, but professional ethics go beyond what one individual thinks is right or wrong. Even the Golden Rule— "Do unto others as you would have them do unto you"—is not a sufficient guideline. What happens when the person making the decision has desires and values that are radically different from the patient's? It becomes clear that reason and logic must be used and emotion must be excluded as much as possible from the decision-making process.

Another approach is to say that people should just fulfill their duties. This is known as the *deontological method*. A very simple example of this approach is someone who says, "Just follow the Ten Commandments." Unfortunately, although the Ten Commandments provide useful instruction, they do not provide enough guidance for medical professionals who must make difficult ethical decisions in health care situations.

A very different approach is *consequentialism*. Followers of this school of thought believe that actions can be judged as good or bad only after we know the consequences of those actions. Utilitarians, who believe that the purpose of an action should be to bring the greatest happiness to the greatest number of people, are consequentialists. One difficulty with the utilitarians' approach is determining what constitutes happiness. Another challenge arises when the happiness of one person is in conflict with the happiness of another person. Utilitarianism offers a "bankbook" approach to resolving these conflicts, asking the decision maker to weigh relative "amounts" of happiness.

Codes of Ethics

Over the years, a number of organizations have drafted codes of ethics for the members of their organizations. The American Medical Association and the American Osteopathic Association have a code of ethics for physicians. The American College of Emergency Physicians has a code of ethics specifically for emergency physicians.[3] The American Nurses Association and Emergency Nurses Association both have codes for practitioners in their fields. The National Association of EMTs adopted a code of ethics for EMTs in 1978 (see Chapter 3). Most codes of ethics address broad humanitarian concerns and professional etiquette. Few provide solid guidance on the kind of ethical problems commonly faced by practitioners.

Ethical codes often address the following areas:

- Honesty
- Objectivity
- Integrity
- Carefulness
- Openness
- Legality
- Confidentiality
- Responsible publication
- Responsible mentoring
- Respect for colleagues
- Social responsibility
- Nondiscrimination
- Competence
- Respect for intellectual property
- Human subjects protection

Many of the areas listed above have direct application to EMS.[4]

Impact of Ethics on Individual Practice

Only by consistently displaying ethical behavior will paramedics gain and maintain the respect of their colleagues and their patients. It is vital that individual paramedics exemplify the principles and values of their profession. Paramedics must understand and agree to abide by the responsibilities, both implicit and explicit, of their profession. Occasionally, this can be a problem. A paramedic is expected to work, for example, in an uncontrolled environment that is sometimes dangerous. A person who is unwilling to enter a scene until every risk has been totally eliminated is not acting in accordance with the expectations of the profession. Conversely, a paramedic is expected to refrain from entering a hazardous area until the risks have been made manageable. Common sense should help in resolving conflicts such as these.

The Fundamental Questions

The single most important question a paramedic has to answer when faced with an ethical challenge is "What is in the patient's best interest?" Most of the time the answer to this question is obvious: The patient wants reassurance, relief from pain, and prompt, safe transport to a hospital emergency department. But sometimes the answer to this question is not so obvious. For example, what is in the best interest of a terminally ill patient who goes into cardiac arrest? Is it to resuscitate him? Or is it to not start resuscitation in order to prevent further suffering?

Under ideal circumstances, a written statement describing the patient's desires will be available. In many states, such a statement (which meets other specified state and local requirements) is in fact required before a paramedic may elect not to start resuscitation efforts. In less extreme circumstances, the patient may state verbally what he wishes you to do and not do. As long as the patient is competent and the desires are consistent with good practice, the paramedic is obligated to respect the patient's desires.

Traditionally, family members have been an important source of information for physicians in determining the wishes of a patient. This approach, however, is not necessarily appropriate in the field. In the hospital or especially in the years before a hospital admission, physicians are able to spend time with the patient and the patient's family and develop a relationship with them. In the field, paramedics typically do not know the patient or the family. There is usually not enough time for a paramedic to develop the same kind of relationship that physicians do in their practices. Additionally, the family is under a great deal of stress when the paramedic encounters them.

For these reasons and others, a paramedic must be very cautious in accepting a family's description of what a patient desires. The paramedic must also take into consideration the state and local laws regarding patient resuscitation desires and documentation of those desires.

It may sometimes be difficult for a paramedic to agree with a patient's wishes, but it is important that he respect them. Only by demonstrating "good faith" in following a patient's wishes does a paramedic show respect for the patient. A paramedic must also realize that the family may not agree with the patient's desires. This may lead family members to substitute their own desires for the patient's. This is another reason why the paramedic should not necessarily accept a family's description of a patient's desires at face value.

Fundamental Principles

A common approach to resolving problems in bioethics today is to employ four fundamental principles or values. These principles are beneficence, nonmaleficence, autonomy, and justice.

Beneficence is related to a more familiar term, *benevolence*. Both come from Latin and concern doing good. However, *benevolence* means the *desire* to do good (usually the main reason people become paramedics), whereas *beneficence* means actually *doing* good (the paramedic's obligation to the patient).

Maleficence means doing harm, the opposite of *beneficence*. **Nonmaleficence** means *not* doing harm. Few medical interventions are without risk of harm. Under the principle of nonmaleficence, however, the paramedic is obligated to minimize that risk as much as possible. This includes, for example, making the scene safe and protecting the patient from impaired or unqualified health care providers. The Latin phrase, *primum non nocere*, which means "first, do no harm," sums up nonmaleficence very well.

Autonomy refers to a competent adult patient's right to determine what happens to his own body, including treatment for medical illnesses and injuries. The paramedic has an obligation to respect this right of self-determination. Under ordinary conditions, a patient must give consent before the paramedic can begin treatment. There are, of course, exceptions to this, including the patient who is not competent and for whom the doctrine of implied consent applies. But the competent patient must receive accurate information in order to make an informed decision. This implies that the paramedic must be truthful in describing to the patient his condition and the risks and benefits of treatment for it. It also implies respect for the patient's privacy.

Justice refers to the paramedic's obligation to treat all patients fairly. For example, the paramedic should provide necessary emergency care to all patients without regard to sex, race, ability to pay, or cultural background, among other conditions.

Resolving Ethical Conflicts

Even if everyone agreed on the same principles and procedures for resolving ethical difficulties, there would still be disagreements in specific situations. These disagreements can be resolved at different levels. Even the government sometimes takes action when issues become very important to the public. For example, there are now laws to protect the rights of hospitalized patients and members of managed-care organizations. Many states have implemented laws or regulations that allow for the use of advance directives. The federal government has instituted rules to protect the rights of patients in emergency research when they are unable to consent.

The health care community has also responded to the challenge. Long before the federal government instituted rules regarding consent in emergency research, hospitals and universities set up institutional review boards (IRBs). These groups serve to protect the rights of subjects participating in research projects. Hospitals throughout the world have had ethics committees for many years to assist in clarifying patients' desires and in weighing competing interests in ethically challenging situations.

The paramedic, however, cannot depend on these institutions to assist in the field. He needs to have a system for resolving these conflicts, one that will allow him to weigh the various factors, including all relevant facts, principles, and values, that lead to responsible, defensible actions. One such system or method

of resolving ethical issues before or after they arise is illustrated in the following scenario:

> You are the official representative of your service to the regional EMS coordinating agency. At the most recent meeting, the head nurse for the emergency department of the largest hospital in the county mentioned how recent cutbacks in support staff had led to more difficulty retrieving patients' medical records in a timely manner. This has led to a number of difficulties in treating patients. As a result, the emergency department (ED) was considering asking incoming ambulances to give patients' names and dates of birth on the radio. This would give the ED staff additional time to search for the patient's medical records.

After the meeting, you consider the issue's ethical aspects. First, you identify the problem, which in this case is: Is it justifiable to breach patient confidentiality in order to expedite the retrieval of medical records? Second, you list the possible actions that might be taken in this situation. Possibilities include:

- Provide all patients' names and dates of birth on the radio.
- Continue the current policy of identifying patients only by age and sex.
- Provide selected patients' names and dates of birth on the radio.

To reason out an ethical problem, first state the action in a universal form. Then list the implications or consequences of the action. Finally, compare them to relevant values (Figure 8-2 ●). The application of this method to the scenario described would be as follows:

> To state an action in a universal form, describe what should be done, who should do it, and under what conditions. For example, EMS (who) will volunteer names and dates of birth for all patients (what) on the radio (condition).

The immediate implications are that the ED will be able to get records sooner for patients who have records at that hospital. There will be no change for most patients because hospital records are often irrelevant to emergency care. The ED admitting staff may be able to admit patients more quickly. However, patients' names and dates of birth will be broadcast to thousands of people listening with scanners. The long-term consequences are that people with scanners will learn more about patients who go to the hospital via EMS. Because private information may be broadcast, patients may become reluctant to call EMS. Conceivably, there may be more burglaries at homes of patients who use EMS.

Finally, compare those consequences to values that are relevant. A list of values that pertain to this case might include beneficence, nonmaleficence, autonomy, and confidentiality. That

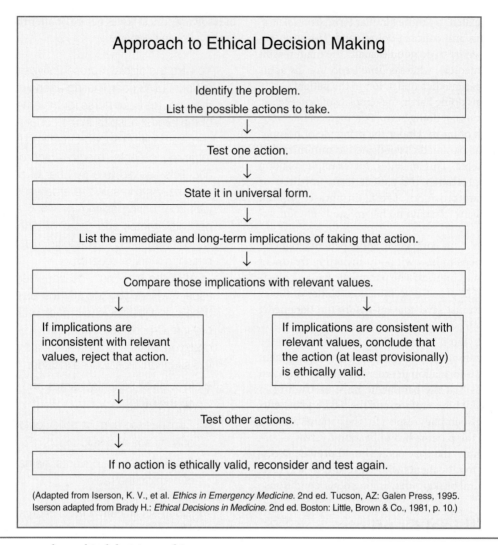

Approach to Ethical Decision Making

Identify the problem.
List the possible actions to take.

↓

Test one action.

↓

State it in universal form.

↓

List the immediate and long-term implications of taking that action.

↓

Compare those implications with relevant values.

↓   ↓

If implications are inconsistent with relevant values, reject that action.

If implications are consistent with relevant values, conclude that the action (at least provisionally) is ethically valid.

↓

Test other actions.

↓

If no action is ethically valid, reconsider and test again.

(Adapted from Iserson, K. V., et al. *Ethics in Emergency Medicine.* 2nd ed. Tucson, AZ: Galen Press, 1995. Iserson adapted from Brady H.: *Ethical Decisions in Medicine.* 2nd ed. Boston: Little, Brown & Co., 1981, p. 10.)

● **Figure 8-2** An approach to ethical decision making.

is, if EMS provided names and dates of birth for all patients on the radio, what would be the benefit to the patient (beneficence)? A few patients might be cared for sooner because their records arrived sooner. Most patients will see no benefit because they have no records at that hospital or time is not a significant issue (such as for a laceration that requires sutures). Furthermore, from a legal standpoint, such a practice would probably violate patient confidentiality laws such as HIPAA.

Autonomy suffers under this arrangement because the patient is not given the opportunity to consent (or decline). The patient's name and date of birth go out over the air without his permission. And, in this case, nonmaleficence and confidentiality are intertwined. There is potential for harm to the patient and to future patients who lose faith in the EMS system's ability to maintain privacy.

So, since the possible consequences of providing all patients' names and dates of birth on the radio are not compatible with the values we consider important and relevant, you must go back and test another action using this same method.

When you evaluate the choice of continuing the current policy of identifying all patients over the radio only by age and sex, you may find the following consequences: People listening to scanners can learn facts about patients EMS is transporting,

but no more than they have in the past; a few patients may get care that is delayed or less than optimal because their hospital records do not arrive quickly enough; and the ED staff are still stressed because they cannot get records in a timely manner. A comparison with relevant values reveals that patient confidentiality and patient confidence in EMS are unchanged, but the patients who might benefit from earlier arrival of their records may be suffering.

Continue to evaluate any other options you listed. In this case, the third and final one is: Provide selected patients' names and dates of birth on the radio. A comparison with relevant values shows that there is some potential benefit for selected patients, a breach of confidentiality for patients who might benefit, and no breach of confidentiality for patients who would not benefit. Therefore, the scenario may conclude as follows:

The third option sounds closer to being acceptable, but you might wonder if there is a way to further limit loss of confidentiality. You revise your rule to read, "EMS broadcasts the initials and dates of birth of selected patients who meet predetermined criteria when there is no other private means of communication available." This strictly limits the loss of confidentiality to patients who may benefit from it and encourages both EMS and the ED to find other less public means of identifying patients. For example, paramedics could broadcast a patient's age, sex, and hospital card number or, if the patient does not have a hospital identification card available and time allows, someone at the scene could telephone the ED to relay the patient's name and date of birth privately.

The method just described is useful when you come upon a new ethical problem and time is not an issue. In situations where time is limited, an abbreviated method can sometimes be used (Figure 8-3 ●). First, ask yourself whether the current problem is similar to other problems for which you have already formulated a rule. Then, if the answer is yes, follow that rule. If the answer is no, determine if you can do something to buy time. Finally, if you can find a reasonable way to postpone dealing with the issue for a while, do so. If you cannot, analyze the best rule you have against three tests suggested by Iserson: the *impartiality test*, the *universalizability test*, and the *interpersonal justifiability test*:

- **Impartiality test**—asks whether you would be willing to undergo this procedure or action if you were in the patient's place. This is really a version of the Golden Rule (do unto others as you would have them do unto you), which helps to reduce the possibility of bias.

- **Universalizability test**—asks whether you would want this action performed in all relevantly similar circumstances, which helps the paramedic to avoid shortsightedness.

- **Interpersonal justifiability test**—asks whether you can defend or justify your actions to others. It helps to ensure that an action is appropriate by asking the paramedic to consider whether other people would think the action reasonable.[5]

CONTENT REVIEW

▶ Quick Ways to Test Ethics
- Impartiality test
- Universalizability test
- Interpersonal justifiability test

When there is little time to consider a new ethical problem, these three questions can help a paramedic navigate murky waters, allowing him to find an acceptable solution in a short time.

ETHICAL ISSUES IN CONTEMPORARY PARAMEDIC PRACTICE

The first part of the chapter built a foundation for ethical decision making by describing and demonstrating methods for dealing with these types of issues. The following discussion is meant to help you apply those principles to several commonly encountered situations. It also describes some of the ethical considerations to take into account in less common situations you may face.

Resuscitation Attempts

Consider the following scenario:

You are leaving the emergency department in your ambulance when an approximately 50-year-old woman jumps out of a window on the third floor of the hospital and lands on the road in front of you. Your partner

---

Quick Approach to New Ethical Problems

Consider the ethical problem.

*Do you already have a rule for dealing with this problem?

*Or, can you reasonably extend a rule to apply to the situation?

If yes to either of the above, follow the rule.

If no to the above,

*Can you buy time to consider a solution without causing significant risk to the patient?

*If you cannot, then apply the impartiality test, the universalizability test, or the interpersonal justifiability test.

(Based on Iserson, K. V., et al. *Ethics in Emergency Medicine.* 2nd ed. Tucson, AZ: Galen Press, 1995.)

● **Figure 8-3** A quick approach to new ethical problems. *(Based on Iserson, K.V., et al. Ethics in Emergency Medicine. 2nd ed. Tucson, AZ: Galen Press, 1995)*

stops the vehicle, and you get your equipment to begin assessment and management of the patient. As you reach her, a breathless aide runs out the door and says, "Don't do anything! She's got a DNR order!" How does this affect the care you administer?

You have virtually no time to think about what to do for this woman, who is bleeding on the street and appears unresponsive. Your instincts say, treat her now and let the hospital sort things out later if she survives.

In this case, your instincts are probably steering you in the right direction for a number of reasons. First, every state that has laws or rules regarding Do Not Resuscitate (DNR) orders requires that you see the order and verify its legitimacy in some manner. In this case, the order is not available for you to see so you are under no legal obligation to withhold care.

Second, if the patient is alive (as she appears to be), even a valid DNR order would not prevent you from assessing the patient and administering basic care, including comfort care.

Third, the principle of nonmaleficence says do no harm. Refraining from helping her might cause irreversible harm, including perhaps death. The principles of beneficence and nonmaleficence both urge you to help the patient. The potential conflict arises when you consider autonomy. The competent patient of legal age has a right to determine what happens to her body. You have some reason to believe she has determined that she does not wish resuscitation efforts if her heart stops but, in this case, the accuracy of this information cannot be verified.

The conclusion of the scenario is as follows:

Considering the lack of verifiable information and the severe time limitations you are facing, you and your partner go ahead and assess the patient. You find that she responds to verbal stimuli by moaning, her airway is open, ventilations are adequate, and she has several lacerations and apparent fractures. Since you are literally in front of the hospital, you limit your interventions to quick immobilization on a spine board with bleeding control and oxygen by mask. You rapidly move her to the ED and turn her over to the team there.

Later you discover that she had originally been admitted for evaluation of new onset seizures. When the doctors told her she might have a brain tumor, she signed a DNR form. Fortunately, no tumor was found and her prognosis is actually quite good. The trauma team finds no life-threatening injuries from her fall and expects her to be able to begin psychiatric treatment before she leaves the hospital. This additional information makes you very glad you decided to go ahead with treatment.

More and more states are passing laws or regulations allowing prehospital personnel to withhold certain treatment when the patient has a DNR order. A valid order consists of a written statement describing interventions a particular patient does not wish to have that is recognized by the authorities of that state.

Before following a DNR order, the paramedic must be aware of several things.

First, the order must meet state and local requirements regarding wording and witnesses (a standardized form is usually available). Also, there may be a time limit on how long a DNR order is valid in certain jurisdictions. A patient with a valid prehospital DNR order may be required to wear or have nearby a particular means of identification, such as a bracelet with a special symbol. There should be a clear description of which interventions are to be withheld and under which circumstances. And finally, every patient is still entitled to reasonable measures intended to make the patient more comfortable (comfort care). Similarly, the family and loved ones are entitled to emotional support from EMS providers. (See Chapter 7 for legal aspects of DNR orders.)

Paramedics spend a great deal of time and energy learning how to assess and treat patients with life-threatening problems. It becomes difficult, then, for a paramedic to watch someone die without doing something to try to stop it. You must nonetheless respect the patient's wishes when a competent patient has clearly communicated what he really wants. DNR orders make this easier because they typically must be signed or approved by a physician, increasing the likelihood that the decision was thoroughly thought through.

When there is no such order, however, it becomes more difficult for the paramedic to determine what the patient's wishes truly are. Family members may be able to describe the patient's desires, but they can have conflicts of interest that make their statements less credible. For example, the patient may have accepted his impending death before his family has. They may want you to attempt resuscitation when that was clearly against the patient's expressed wishes. A less common situation is one in which the patient wishes all resuscitation efforts, but the family does not because they do not wish to prolong their own suffering or they have other less noble motivations.

The general principle for paramedics to follow in cases such as these is: "When in doubt, resuscitate." This usually satisfies the principles of beneficence and nonmaleficence, admittedly perhaps at the expense of autonomy, but one of the biggest advantages to this approach is that, unlike the alternative, it is not irreversible. If you refrain from attempting resuscitation, it is certain that the patient will die. If you attempt resuscitation, there is no guarantee the patient will survive, but the patient can be removed from life-sustaining equipment later if that is deemed appropriate. Another advantage is that there will be more time later to sort out competing interests.

What about not attempting resuscitation when the situation appears futile? This option may appear attractive at first glance. After a little investigation, though, the issue becomes much more complex. How would a reasonable person or society define "futile"? This is an issue that has received a good deal of attention and the conclusion is that, except at the extreme ends of the spectrum, there is no consensus on what constitutes a futile attempt at resuscitation.

In addition, there is the issue of who would actually make the decision that a resuscitation attempt is futile in a particular case. Is it the experienced paramedic who has seen very few lives saved under similar circumstances or the new paramedic who is still excited about the prospect of saving lives every day? How can it be fair to have such wide disparities in such an important decision? Clearly, the concept of futility does not provide a useful guide for whether or not to attempt resuscitation.

Another related topic is what to do when an advance directive is presented to you after you have begun resuscitation. Once you have verified the validity of the order and the identity of the patient, you are obligated ethically (and perhaps legally, depending on your state) to cease resuscitation efforts. This can be a very difficult situation for you emotionally, but you have an obligation to respect the patient's autonomy and stop doing something to him that he did not want. Follow your local protocols regarding procedures for cessation of resuscitation efforts.

Confidentiality

Consider this scenario:

You are called at one o'clock in the morning to a local hotel for a man reported to be unresponsive (but breathing) at the front desk. When you arrive, one of the guests at the hotel meets you at the front door. He tells you that he tried to call the front desk from his room to request a wake-up call but got no answer. When he went to the front desk, he found the clerk slumped over in his chair, apparently unconscious, with what smelled like alcohol on his breath.

When you approach the patient, you see an approximately 25-year-old male who appears to be unresponsive. His skin appears normal, and he is moving air well. He does not respond when you call him by the name on his name plate, which is Howard. He has a strong, regular radial pulse that is within normal limits. You do not smell anything except for a faint minty odor. When you shake his shoulder and call his name again, he moans. Further shaking and shouting eventually bring him to the point where his eyes are open, he is looking around, and he asks, "Who are you?"

You explain to Howard that you were called by a concerned guest who could not wake him up. Howard says he is fine now and does not want to go to a hospital. He is alert and oriented to person, place, and time. He denies any complaints, takes no medications, and has no past medical history. His vital signs are within normal limits. He denies any alcohol intake or use of any other drugs. The physical exam is unremarkable.

By your protocols and standard operating procedures, you have no reason to attempt to force the patient to go to a hospital. You complete the appropriate documentation for a refusal of transport and are leaving the lobby when the guest who called 911 stops you. "Aren't you going to take him to the hospital?" he asks. No, you reply, he does not want to go. "But what if there's a fire in the hotel and he's passed out and unable to help guests evacuate?"

This makes you stop and think, and you begin to weigh the rights of the hotel guests against the rights of your patient.

Your obligation to the patient is to maintain as confidential the information you obtained as a result of your participation in this medical situation. Clearly, the most beneficial thing you can do for his privacy is not to notify anyone about his condition. Additionally, there are questions regarding what you could accurately report. The patient denies alcohol and drug intake, and you could find no objective signs to dispute his claim. He might just be a heavy sleeper. Reporting that he is or may be under the influence of alcohol or drugs might lead to the loss of his job and to legal trouble for you.

However, what if there is an emergency in which the desk clerk's assistance is needed and he is unable to provide it? That is an unlikely, though certainly a conceivable, possibility. However, there is no clear and present danger that would require you to report. In fact, you may, depending on the state you're in, have a legal obligation to maintain confidentiality under circumstances such as these.

There are a number of reasons to respect confidentiality in general. In an emergency, a patient typically has little choice about who is going to come to his aid. He is assuming that he can be honest with these strangers who have come to help him because they will protect his privacy. If that trust was routinely violated without sufficient cause, patients might very well be embarrassed or humiliated. This would undermine the public's trust in EMS and any particular patient's trust in the paramedics and others coming into his home. If word got around that private information was being made public, patients might not be forthcoming in giving their medical histories, potentially leading to disastrous consequences. For example, a man who had recently taken sildenafil (Viagra) for erectile dysfunction might deny taking it before you give him nitroglycerin. This drug interaction is potentially serious, possibly even fatal.

There are nonetheless times when it is appropriate and necessary to breach confidentiality. Every state has laws requiring the reporting of certain health facts such as births, deaths, particular infectious diseases, child neglect and abuse, and elder neglect and abuse. These last requirements have the most applicability to EMS. They are considered justifiable reasons to breach confidentiality because, in the eyes of society, the benefit to someone who is defenseless (protection from harm and perhaps even death) and to the public (a safer environment for children) outweighs the right to privacy of a particular person. A valid court order is also considered a reasonable justification for breaching confidentiality. So is a clear threat by a patient to a specific person, as well as informing other health care professionals who will care for the patient.

Clearly, patient confidentiality is an important principle, but not an inviolable one. When determining whether it is appropriate to breach confidentiality, take into account the probability of harm, the magnitude of the expected harm, and alternative methods of avoiding harm that do not require encroaching on confidentiality.

In the previous scenario, factors do not justify breaching confidentiality. The person who called 911 for emergency assistance, however, is under no such obligation. The scenario comes to an end as follows:

> When you inform the guest that you are unable to discuss the case with anyone because of confidentiality, he replies, "Well, you may not be able to do anything about it, but I can. I'm calling the manager!"

Consent

Consider this scenario:

> Bob, a 58-year-old male, has been having crushing substernal pain radiating to his left arm for several hours. He also is pale, sweaty, and nauseated. He denies shortness of breath. His condition remains unchanged after you give him oxygen and nitroglycerin. When you ask Bob which hospital he wants to go to, he tells you, "I'm not going to any hospital." Surprised, you find it difficult to understand why someone in this much pain would not want to go to a hospital. You try to enlist the help of relatives over the telephone (Bob lives alone), but they are unable to persuade the patient. He has no regular physician, so that option is not available to you. Finally, you decide to try on-line medical direction. While you are waiting for the physician to come to the phone, you wonder: If the patient continues to refuse, can you force him to go? How can you act in the best interest of a patient who refuses to accept what you feel certain is best for him?

A competent patient of legal age has the fundamental right to decide what health care he will receive and will not receive. This is at the core of patient autonomy. To exercise this right, a patient must have the information necessary to make an informed decision, the mental faculties to weigh the risks and benefits of various treatment options, and the freedom from restraints that might hamper his ability to exercise his options (such as threats).

It is sometimes appropriate to use the doctrine of implied consent to force the patient to go to the hospital. For the paramedic to use this approach, the patient must be unable to give consent. Typically, the doctrine is invoked when the patient is unable to communicate, but it also can be employed when the patient is incapacitated because of drugs, illness, or injury. In this scenario, however, the patient shows no signs of being incapacitated. He is alert; oriented to person, place, and time; aware of his surroundings; and making judgments and answering questions in a manner completely compatible with competence. The fact that the patient refuses something you recommend does not, in itself, necessarily indicate that he is incompetent.

Before you leave the patient, you must not only do the things you need to do to protect yourself legally, but you must also assure yourself that the patient truly understands the issues at hand and is able to make an informed decision. As difficult as it may be for the paramedic, if the patient is able to do these things, he may have to accept the patient's desires and leave him.

Allocation of Resources

Paramedics do not usually think of themselves as guardians of finite resources, but occasionally they are. The most obvious example of this is when there are more patients present than the paramedic is able to manage, such as in a multiple-casualty incident (MCI). While learning how to provide emergency medical care for multiple patients at the same scene, you might ask: What are the ethics of triage?

There are several possible approaches to consider in parceling out scarce resources. Patients could all receive the same amount of attention and resources (true parity). They could receive resources based on need. Or they could receive what someone has determined they've earned.

The civilian method of triage, where the most seriously injured patients receive the most care, is based on need. This is intended to produce the most good for the most people. However, other methods of triage are in use. Military triage, for example, has traditionally concentrated on helping the least seriously injured because this approach produces the greatest number of soldiers who can return to duty. When the president or vice president visits a town or city, there is typically an ambulance dedicated for the dignitary's use, if needed. The ambulance is not to be used for anyone else. Because these officials are so important and because so many others need them, the typical order of care is changed.

A controversy exists in emergency medicine as to whether or not celebrities should be treated ahead of others. The argument for doing so typically emphasizes the disorder brought to the ED by the presence of a celebrity and the need to get the person out of the ED as quickly as possible to restore normal operation. The argument against takes the position that giving preferential treatment to a celebrity is an affront to justice and fairness.

All these methods have their proponents for different situations. The key to resolving the issue of allocation of scarce resources is to examine the competing theories in light of the circumstances at hand.

Obligation to Provide Care

By virtue of membership in a profession, a paramedic takes on a responsibility to help others. The public, through the government, grants certain privileges to professionals in return for the expectation of professional behavior. As a practitioner of paramedicine, the paramedic has even greater responsibilities. Those who provide emergency care have a special obligation to help all those in need. Many other health care professionals are free to pick and choose their patients, accepting only those who have health insurance or who can themselves pay for the services delivered by the health care professional. This is not the case in emergency medicine.

Paramedics, like other emergency professionals, are obligated to provide medical care for those in need without regard to ability to pay. They also have an ethical obligation to prevent and report instances of patient "dumping," where those without insurance are transferred against their will to public or charity hospitals.

A particular issue arises regarding the patient who is a member of a managed-care organization such as a health maintenance organization (HMO). The HMO may insist that the patient be treated at a particular facility with which the HMO has a contract. This must not be allowed to interfere with the patient's emergency care. The paramedic, like every other member of the EMS system, has an obligation to act in the patient's best interest, even when that goes against the HMO's economic interests.

A very different aspect of providing care has to do with offering assistance when off duty. Although only two states require paramedics, among others, to stop and render help when they come upon someone in need of emergency care, there is still a strong ethical obligation to do so. This does not extend to situations where the paramedic would put himself in danger (such as getting into a car teetering on the edge of a cliff), if assisting would interfere with important duties owed to others (such as leaving young children unattended in a car), or when someone else is already providing assistance. In return, society offers limited liability in the form of Good Samaritan statutes in every state in the United States.

Teaching

Many paramedics act as preceptors or mentors in their EMS systems. Two issues raised by this role are whether or not patients should be informed that a student is working on them and how many attempts a student should be allowed to have in performing critical interventions before the preceptor steps in.

When patients call for EMS, they generally expect to receive care from individuals who have finished their education and who hold credentials qualifying them to work. If a system decides not to inform patients of the presence of students, the system runs the risk of being accused of concealing important information from patients.

To avoid this problem, EMS systems with students working in them should make sure students are clearly identified as such by the uniform they wear. The preceptor should also, when appropriate, inform patients of the presence of a student and request the patient's consent before the student performs a procedure. This sounds more cumbersome than it actually is. Patients who are unable to consent obviously do not fall into this category; implied consent is invoked in this case. And patients who are able to consent are frequently very understanding of the student's need for experience. As long as the preceptor stresses that he is overseeing the student, the vast majority of patients usually give their consent.

Another issue related to students is how many attempts they should be allowed in order to perform procedures such as intravenous placement and endotracheal intubation before the preceptor steps in. Factors to consider include the student's skill level (as determined by classroom practice on mannequins and previous field experience), the anticipated difficulty of the procedure (some patients are obviously going to be more difficult to intubate or start an IV on), and the relative importance of the procedure (not all IVs are equally important). It is important to have a limit, at least initially, for the number of times a student will be allowed to attempt a procedure. Such a number will need to be decided by each system in consultation with the medical director.

Professional Relations

As a health care professional, the paramedic answers to the patient. As a physician extender, the paramedic answers to a physician medical director. As an employee (or volunteer), the paramedic answers to the EMS system. These competing interests can sometimes make life difficult. Each can lead to ethical challenges.

In general, there are three potential sources of conflict between paramedics and physicians. One possibility is a case in which a physician orders something the paramedic believes is contraindicated. For example, suppose a physician ordered a paramedic to transport a critical blunt-trauma patient without attempting any intravenous access, either at the scene or en route during the anticipated 45-minute transport. This order runs counter to standard medical practice. The patient will have spent more than an hour since the trauma without receiving any intravenous fluid or intravenous access.

A different situation arises when the physician orders something the paramedic believes is medically acceptable but not in the patient's best interests. For example, imagine you are transporting a patient with stable vital signs who is complaining of abdominal pain. In accordance with your protocols, you and your partner have each tried twice to start an IV line without success. The patient's veins are some of the worst you have ever seen, and you have no expectation that you will be successful on further attempts. The patient experienced considerable pain with each attempt and is now crying, asking you not to try any more. The physician, however, insists you continue attempts to gain access.

A third potential source of conflict is the situation in which the physician orders something the paramedic believes is medically acceptable, but morally wrong. For example, say you are ordered to stop CPR on a young male found in cardiac arrest after blunt trauma. His initial rhythm of asystole has remained unchanged, and you know it is almost always associated with death. Nonetheless, although there is a very slim chance of recovery for the patient if you continue your resuscitation efforts, you would not be able to live with yourself if you did not at least try.

In each of the three cases, it is certainly appropriate for the paramedic to start by confirming the order and asking the physician to repeat it. If the order is confirmed, the medic would be prudent to ask the physician for an explanation, given the controversial nature of the orders in the first two situations (in the third, the physician's thoughts and goals are fairly clear). The next steps will depend on the physician's explanation, the patient's condition, the need for the intervention in the judgment of the paramedic, the feasibility of performing the intervention (like gaining IV access), and the amount of time available to discuss the issue.

Ultimately, the paramedic must determine for himself how the patient's interests are best served. This typically does not lead to conflict, but on occasion the paramedic may run into situations like the ones previously described. In these cases, the paramedic must consider the competing interests of beneficence, nonmaleficence, autonomy, and justice; the roles of the physician and the paramedic; the relative confidence (or lack thereof) the paramedic has in his own medical and ethical judgment; how far the paramedic is willing to go as an advocate for his patient; and the degree of risk acceptable to the paramedic in contravening physician orders.

It is important for the paramedic to understand that no matter what decision he makes, he will have to defend it. The explanation that he was just following the doctor's orders (or, conversely, just doing what he felt was right) will not be sufficient in and of itself. A paramedic is expected to be more than a robot. He or she is expected to simultaneously be a physician extender, working under a physician's license, and a clinician with the ability and independence to recognize and question inappropriate orders. The paramedic should also understand that he is not expected to act in ways he feels are immoral. However, if the individual's morals are significantly out of step with the expectations of the profession, he needs to reconsider his profession.

Disagreements with physician orders happen rarely. Usually they are the result of poor communication (such as saying one thing while meaning another or static interfering with the radio transmission) or lack of sufficient information. Conflicts with physicians that reach the level in the previous examples are fortunately rare. When they happen, the paramedic must be willing to be an advocate for the patient and act in the patient's best interests.

Research

EMS research is relatively new but absolutely important for the profession to advance. Research is the foundation on which all scientific endeavors, including medicine, are built. Research will help introduce new innovations that improve patient outcomes and remove those that do not. As this occurs, paramedics will become instrumental in implementing research protocols and gathering data. It is essential that a paramedic participating in a research project understand the importance of gaining expressed patient consent or following federal, state, and local regulations regarding implied consent.

The goal of patient care is to improve the patient's condition. The goal of research, however, is to help future patients by gaining knowledge about a specific intervention. The two goals are not the same, so patients must be protected from untoward outcomes as much as possible.

One very important way of protecting the patient is by gaining the patient's expressed consent. There are several difficulties with this. One is the concern that a patient experiencing an emergency may not be able to truly consent because of the emotional pressures he is feeling. This pressure may occur in spite of the paramedic's best efforts to explain matters calmly and impartially.

Another concern is with the patient who is unable to consent. An excellent example of this occurs in cardiac arrest research. By the very nature of the problem being studied, the investigators will be unable to gather consent from the patient. In this case, the federal government has strict rules, for example, about community notification before the study begins and gaining consent from the patient or an appropriate family member as soon as possible after a patient is entered into the study. A paramedic participating in such a study needs to be familiar with these rules and their implications.

Although many interventions have been tested and found to be life saving, there are unfortunately documented instances of patients denied treatment for life-threatening conditions in the name of research in the United States (e.g., the Tuskegee syphilis research project). The paramedic has an obligation to prevent such things from happening in EMS research.

SUMMARY

Should you start CPR or withhold it? Do you allow the patient to refuse essential care or not? These are some of the most challenging and most common ethical challenges seen in EMS.

As a paramedic, you must learn to make ethical decisions that will have an effect on you, your patient, or others. Your decision-making process should always be based on the patient's best interest. Keep in mind that the patient's best interest includes more than lifesaving procedures. Cultural sensitivity should also be included in the decision and respected, even if it is against your personal beliefs. Remember, the patient has autonomy; that is, he has a right to determine what happens to his own body and can legally dictate that. Remember there is a clear distinction between ethics, religion, and law even though there is common ground between them.

At some point in your career you may be called upon to defend a decision you made. The best defense results from being able to state that your actions were legal and within your scope of practice (justice), helpful (beneficence), not harmful (nonmaleficence), and the direct wishes of the patient (autonomy). As long as you can defend your decision using these staples of ethics, your decision is correct.

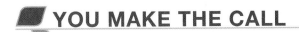

YOU MAKE THE CALL

You are transporting a 32-year-old male, Phil Cornock, who has a long history of kidney stones and has all the classic signs of having another one now. He is in severe pain and is unable to find a comfortable position. You know that although this condition can be excruciating, it is not generally life threatening. He is allergic to the only narcotic analgesic you can administer for pain. He asks you, "Can't you use the lights and sirens to get to the hospital faster?" Your service's policy regarding the use of lights and sirens restricts their use to cases in which the paramedic believes there is a significant threat to life or limb. This patient's condition does not qualify. You wonder, though, whether you should use the lights and sirens to speed up transport since the patient is in severe pain.

1. What potential benefits are there in yielding to the patient's request (beneficence)?

2. What potential harm is there in yielding to the patient's request (nonmaleficence)?

3. How does justice come into play in this situation?

4. How should paramedics in general respond when a patient requests an intervention that is not medically indicated?

See Suggested Responses at the back of this book.

REVIEW QUESTIONS

1. _____ are generally considered to be social, religious, or personal standards of right and wrong.
   a. Ethics
   b. Morals
   c. Standards
   d. Principles

2. _____ means not doing harm.
   a. Autonomy
   b. Maleficence
   c. Nonmaleficence
   d. Beneficence

3. These groups serve to protect the rights of subjects participating in research projects.
   a. IRBs
   b. HMOs
   c. EMS
   d. CQI

4. This quick way to test ethics asks whether you would be willing to undergo a particular procedure or action if you were in the patient's place.
   a. impartiality test
   b. navigation test
   c. universalizability test
   d. interpersonal justifiability test

5. Every state has laws requiring the reporting of certain health facts such as:
   a. births.
   b. deaths.
   c. child neglect and abuse.
   d. all of the above.

See Answers to Review Questions at the back of this book.

REFERENCES

1. Adams, J. G., R. Arnold, L. Siminoff, and A. M. Wolfson. "Ethical Conflicts in the Prehospital Setting." *Ann Emerg Med* 21 (1992): 1259–1265.

2. Hilicser, B., C. Stocking, and M. Siegler. "Ethical Dilemmas in Emergency Medical Services: The Perspective of the Emergency Medical Technician." *Ann Emerg Med* 27 (1996): 239–243.

3. American College of Emergency Physicians. "Code of Ethics for Emergency Physicians." *Ann Emerg Med* 52 (2008): 581–590.

4. Touchstone, M. "Part 3: How to Adhere to a Code of Ethics in EMS." *EMS Magazine* 39 (2010): 75–76.

5. Iserson, K. V., et al. *Ethics in Emergency Medicine.* 2nd ed. Tucson, AZ: Galen Press, 1995.

FURTHER READING

Hope, T. *Medical Ethics: A Very Short Introduction.* Oxford, NY: Oxford University Press, 2004.

Larkin, G. L. and R. L. Fowler. "Essential Ethics for EMS: Cardinal Virtues and Core Principles." *Emerg Med Clin North Am* 20 (2002): 887–911.

9

EMS System Communications

Bryan Bledsoe, DO, FACEP, FAAEM, EMT-P
Kevin McGinnis, MPS, EMT-P

STANDARD
Preparatory (EMS System Communication)

COMPETENCY
Integrates comprehensive knowledge of EMS systems, the safety and well-being of the paramedic, and medical/legal and ethical issues, which is intended to improve the health of EMS personnel, patients, and the community.

OBJECTIVES

Terminal Performance Objective
After reading this chapter you should be able to use technology and knowledge of EMS communications systems and skills to communicate effectively in carrying out your responsibilities as a paramedic.

Enabling Objectives
To accomplish the terminal performance objective, you should be able to:

1. Define key terms introduced in this chapter.
2. Describe the benefit of effective EMS system communication to patient care.
3. Discuss anticipated future trends in EMS system communication.
4. Identify the parties with whom you must communicate in the course of an EMS response and what you must communicate with each.
5. Explain how the basic communication model applies to EMS communications.
6. Describe factors that contribute to effective verbal communications.
7. Follow standard reporting procedures and format when communicating in the EMS system.
8. Identify the uses of written communication in EMS, particularly those of the patient care report (PCR).
9. Explain the purpose of the National EMS Information System (NEMSIS).
10. Depict the sequence of communications in an EMS response.
11. Identify challenges and barriers to effective EMS system communication.
12. Describe the responsibilities of EMS dispatchers.
13. Demonstrate effective communications with dispatch, the medical direction physician, and the hospital staff receiving your hand-off report.
14. Explain how communication and technology can contribute to situational awareness and a common operating picture.
15. Describe the typical equipment, including advantages and disadvantages, and types of frequencies used in EMS system communication.

16. Discuss the regulation of public safety communications.

17. Explain the importance of the ability to communicate effortlessly between multiple agencies and jurisdictions.

KEY TERMS

accelerometers, p. 157

ad hoc database, p. 160

advanced automatic crash notification (AACN), p. 157

automatic crash notification (ACN), p. 156

automatic location information (ALI), p. 156

automatic number identification (ANI), p. 156

bandwidth, p. 165

call routing, p. 156

cells, p. 163

cellular telephone system, p. 163

cognitive radio, p. 165

common operating picture (COP), p. 160

communication, p. 152

communication protocols, p. 153

data dictionary, p. 154

dead spots, p. 159

digital communications, p. 163

duplex, p. 162

echo procedure, p. 154

Emergency Medical Dispatcher (EMD), p. 157

Federal Communications Commission (FCC), p. 168

geographic information system (GIS), p. 160

global positioning systems (GPS), p. 156

hand-off, p. 159

hotspot, p. 163

information communications technology (ICT), p. 160

mission-critical communications, p. 163

mobile data unit (MDU), p. 163

multiband radio, p. 165

multiplex, p. 162

National Emergency Medical Services Information System (NEMSIS), p. 154

prearrival instructions, p. 158

prehospital care report (PCR), p. 154

priority dispatching, p. 157

public safety answering points (PSAPs), p. 156

radio bands, p. 161

radio frequencies, p. 161

repeaters, p. 161

SafeCom, p. 153

semantic, p. 152

simplex, p. 162

situational awareness (SA), p. 160

smart phone, p. 164

10-code, p. 153

terrestrial-based triangulation, p. 156

trunking, p. 162

ultrahigh frequency (UHF), p. 161

very high frequency (VHF), p. 161

voice over Internet protocol (VOIP), p. 157

CASE STUDY

TODAY

On a dry, warm Sunday afternoon, a 31-year-old male loses control of his car at 50 miles per hour and strikes a bridge abutment. Nobody witnesses the incident, as it is on a remote stretch of secondary roadway. The first motorist happens on the crash 20 minutes later and dials 911 on his cell phone. Emergency Medical Dispatcher Vern Holland takes the necessary information and dispatches a basic life support engine company and an advanced life support ambulance. As Holland dispatches the emergency units, his partner, paramedic dispatcher Fred Hughes, instructs the caller in basic emergency care.

The units receive the call via a computer printout of essential information. They arrive at the scene 20 minutes later, initiate the appropriate care, and call for a medical helicopter. Because the patient has a severe head injury, the paramedic performs only a limited assessment and immediately initiates transport to a preplanned remote landing site, where the helicopter will land in 20 minutes. As the ambulance departs, he relays the following by radio to Dr. Doyle, the medical direction physician at the regional trauma center:

Paramedic: Depew Ambulance to Mercy Hospital.

Dr. Doyle: Go ahead, Depew.

Paramedic: We are leaving the scene of a car crash on Route 17 in Mount Vernon. We have one patient, a male who is in his thirties, the driver of a car that went off the roadway and struck a bridge abutment. He responds to pain only, with obvious facial and chest trauma. There is a large laceration above the right eye with an exposed skull fracture. There is also blood draining from the right ear. Vital signs are blood pressure 110/60, pulse 110 and regular, respirations 10 and labored. Pupils are dilated and minimally reactive, yet equal. Palpation of the cervical spine does not reveal any obvious deformity. There is no tracheal deviation. Breath sounds are symmetrical, yet diminished. There is subcutaneous emphysema on the right side of his chest and several palpable rib fractures. The abdomen is soft, and the pelvis appears stable. There may be some lower extremity fractures. A rigid C-collar is in place and the spine has been stabilized. An endotracheal tube has been placed. Respirations are being assisted with a BVM using supplemental oxygen. We will attempt an IV en route to the remote landing site where LifeFlight 2 is 15 minutes out. The patient's ETA to your facility is 40 minutes.

Dr. Doyle: We copy, Depew. Attempt an IV, but expedite transport and notify us of any further problems.

Paramedic: We copy. Attempt an IV and we will notify you with any changes.

Dr. Doyle: The trauma team will be in the ED awaiting the patient's arrival.

Paramedic: Copy that, Mercy. Depew clear.

A rapid transfer to the helicopter and exchange of information with its crew is accomplished. On arrival at the trauma center, the trauma team and a neurosurgeon meet the patient. The time interval from injury to surgical intervention is 1 hour and 40 minutes. Despite comprehensive care, the patient dies as a result of his head injury. At the family's request, the patient's organs are harvested. They are sent to cities more than 1,500 miles away and used in two transplant operations.

THE NOT TOO DISTANT FUTURE

On a dry, warm Sunday afternoon, a 31-year-old male loses control of his car at 50 miles per hour and strikes a bridge abutment. Nobody witnesses the incident, as it is on a remote stretch of secondary roadway. The vehicle's advanced automatic crash notification (AACN) device immediately sends a data burst to the AACN call center where the data message is identified as a crash and is automatically forwarded to the public safety answering point (PSAP) for the global positioning system (GPS)-identified jurisdiction of the crash. Voice and video links are also patched to the PSAP.

The Emergency Medical Dispatcher, Vern Holland, tries the voice and video links, with no voice response or useful pictures from the crashed car, while he reviews the data from the vehicle. He knows, within a minute of the crash, the type of vehicle, its location, speed, and direction of impact. Seeing a "potential major injury" warning displayed, he initiates a response protocol keyed to that warning. He dispatches a heavy rescue/extrication truck, a support engine company, and an advanced life support ambulance. Simultaneously, he requests LifeFlight 2 to launch and puts the Mercy Hospital Trauma Center on alert. The responding vehicle crews have all the AACN data on their mobile data units (MDUs) as they leave their quarters (location data are automatically fed to the onboard GPS and a best route provided by a local transportation authority hourly update). The extrication crew en route views on their MDU a "just in time training" review of the hazards and best entry and cutting points for the identified crash vehicle. The helicopter and trauma center staffs receive the AACN information as well.

The ground units arrive at the scene 20 minutes later. The paramedic performs a primary survey and simultaneously speaks his patient findings into a throat microphone (same report as given in the first, "today," version of the case study), activates the video camera on his safety glasses, and places a wireless multi-vital-sign monitor with probes on the patient's chest. He inserts a flash memory card, the size of a thumbnail and worn by the patient, into his public safety communications device (PSCD—a combined very smart phone and push-to-talk radio device) and downloads the patient's pertinent medical history. The paramedic's patient report is translated to a text file and stored on his PSCD and sent to the ambulance MDU, as are the patient video, multi–vital-sign data, and medical history. Immediately, the MDU sends a signal to dispatcher Holland who notifies LifeFlight 2 and Mercy Hospital of the patient data feed availability. Dr. Doyle taps into the four data feeds from his personal digital assistant (PDA) and sends a message confirming the IV order. The helicopter medical crew reviews the patient feeds and doctor's order, then messages the ground paramedic of their three-minute estimated time of arrival (ETA) and willingness to get the IV going in the air if not already established.

A rapid transfer to the helicopter and exchange of information with its crew are accomplished. On its arrival at the trauma center, the trauma team and a neurosurgeon meet the patient. The time interval from injury to surgical intervention is 50 minutes. The patient leaves the hospital alive with months of intensive rehabilitation ahead but a bright prognosis.

(AACN systems, PSAPs, GPS, smart phones, and MDUs will be discussed in more detail later in the chapter.)

INTRODUCTION

The way people communicate has changed radically in the past 40 years. Coincidentally, this is also the period during which modern EMS went from birth to maturity. Unfortunately, in that same time span, the way we communicate in EMS has remained largely unchanged.

In society, person-to-person communication has evolved from face-to-face, telephoned, telegraphed, radioed, and postal dialogue to face-to-face, telephoned, cell-phoned, radioed, e-mailed, texted, and social-network-messaging dialogue. In EMS, person-to-person communication has typically been face-to-face, telephone, and voice radio dialogue, cycles of telemetry data use, and handwritten records. Cell phones and other voice radio systems (e.g., trunked systems) have augmented these methods, but EMS, by and large, still communicates as it did in the 1970s.

This lag in the development of EMS communications technology has resulted in two impacts on current paramedic practice. First, for the near future, face-to-face, written records (whether handwritten or electronic records), and voice radio or wireless telephone will continue to be the prime methods of communication in EMS. The first part of this chapter focuses on effective verbal and written communications and the sequence of communications on a typical EMS call as they take place today.

Second, the availability of increasingly sophisticated diagnostic and treatment technology and the busier environments in which paramedics, medical direction physicians, and other EMS team members work will soon force changes in the information communications technology used in EMS. The last part of this chapter discusses those changes.

EFFECTIVE COMMUNICATIONS

Knowledge of communications plays an important role in your paramedic training. All aspects of prehospital care require effective, efficient communications. During a routine transfer or a life-threatening emergency run, you will communicate with a wide variety of people, including the following:

- *The Emergency Medical Dispatcher (EMD),* whose job it is to manage an entire system of EMS response and readiness, not just your call. You will transmit administrative information such as "responding," "arrived," "transporting," and "back-in-service." The EMD must know the location of all his resources to manage the system effectively. On a serious emergency call, the EMD can be your best ally by securing for you the resources you need to manage your incident.

- *Your patient, his family, bystanders, and others* who may, at times, not understand what you are doing and become obstructive. Quite often, people misconstrue your actions and words. You must try to keep them well informed.

- *Personnel from other responding agencies,* such as the police department, fire department, or mutual aid ambulances who may not share your priorities at the scene. You must communicate effectively with other responders to coordinate and implement your treatment plan. You will accomplish this face to face, via the radio, and through data messages and other data transmission.

These communications require you to exhibit confidence and authority.

- *Health care staff* from physicians' offices, health care facilities, and nursing homes that frequently do not understand the extent of your training or abilities. Often, uninformed staff may think you are just "ambulance drivers." In these cases, you must exhibit professionalism and a calm demeanor while you ask pertinent questions and discuss the case intelligently.

- *The medical direction physician* who teams with you to interpret patient findings and make medical decisions that will best benefit your patient. The physician's expertise and advice can be a tremendous resource for you during the call. You will need to communicate patient information and scene assessment effectively to him.

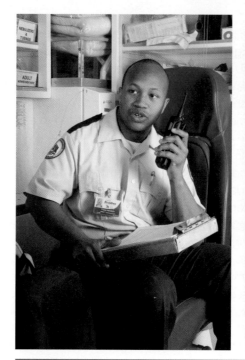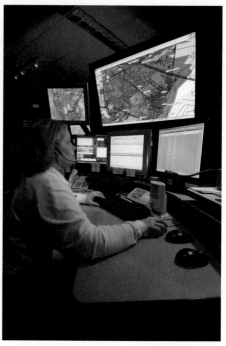

● **Figure 9-1** Communication occur when individuals exchange information through an encoded message.

The medical direction physician can prepare for your arrival if you have communicated to him the needs of your patient. For example, you are transporting a patient with a serious head injury who exhibits a decreasing level of consciousness. By reporting this information, the emergency department can arrange for the trauma team, including a neurosurgeon, to meet you in the ED on arrival. In such cases, good communication results in good patient care.

You must interact effectively with everyone involved in the call to coordinate a unified effort resulting in top-quality patient care. EMS is the ultimate team endeavor. Your performance as a paramedic is just one component in a series of interactions that ensure continuous first-rate care. From the call taker to the rehabilitation specialist, all the players in this continuum are equally important—only their specific roles differ.

Communication is not merely one aspect of an EMS response; it is the key link in the chain that results in the best possible patient outcome. Effective communication optimizes patient care during every phase of the EMS response.

BASIC COMMUNICATION MODEL

Communication is the process of exchanging information between individuals. It begins when you have an idea or message you would like to convey to someone else. You then encode that information in the language best suited for the situation. The language you use might include words, numbers, symbols, or special codes. For instance, if you wanted to describe a patient's condition to the medical direction physician, you would ideally choose medical terminology that is precise and takes less time to convey than a description using nonmedical terms. In some

systems, we communicate using codes. For example, a "Code Blue" might mean a cardiac arrest.

In addition to encoding your message, you must select the medium for sending it. You can speak face to face, send a fax, leave a voice message, send a letter or electronic mail (e-mail), or speak directly by telephone or radio. You might send your encoded message via a paging system that posts words or numbers; some pagers allow you to speak your message. Next, your intended receiver must decode and understand your message. Finally, that person must give you feedback to confirm that he received your message and understood it. You might then confirm his reply and conclude the communication. Consider the following example of an effective radio communication:

Dispatcher: Control to Unit 192, respond high priority to 483 County Route 22, cross street Canfield Road, on a possible heart.

Unit 192: Control, Unit 192 copy, responding high priority to 483 County Route 22.

Dispatcher: Unit 192 responding, 1228 hours.

In this simple example, the sender (dispatcher) encodes his message in a language that he knows the receiver (Unit 192) will understand. Unit 192 receives the message and acknowledges by repeating the key data. Finally, the sender confirms and concludes the communication (Figure 9-1 ●).

VERBAL COMMUNICATION

Factors that can enhance or impede effective communication may be **semantic** (the meaning of words) or technical (communications hardware). Communication requires a mutual language. For example, a city unit and a county unit that use different **10-code** systems will find it difficult to communicate effectively. A "10-10" may mean a working fire in one system and a cardiac emergency in another. Thus, many EMS systems have stopped using 10-codes and changed to plain English. In fact, it is now a standard, embraced by all major public safety associations in an effort through U.S. Department of Homeland Security's **SafeCom** Program, to use plain English emergency radio communications.[1] While regional variations in the use of plain English terminology exist, stopping the practice of enshrouding messages in coded substitutions for plain English is a reasonable start at clarifying communications in an emergency environment.

When reporting your patient's condition to the medical direction physician, you should use terminology that is widely accepted by both the medical and emergency services communities. Telling the medical direction physician that you have a victim of a "MAC 10 drive-by" or "Signal G" (by which you mean "assault with a gun") may be meaningless. Conversely, if the medical direction physician asks you for your pregnant patient's EDC (due date) or her LMP (last menstrual period) and you do not know those abbreviations, you have failed to communicate. The receiver must be able to decode the sender's message.

Reporting Procedures

As a paramedic, you must effectively relay all relevant medical information to the receiving hospital staff. Initially, you might do this over the radio or by cell phone. Later, when you deliver your patient to the emergency department, you can give additional information in person to the appropriate receiving hospital personnel.

One of your most important skills will be gathering essential patient information, organizing it, and relaying it to the medical direction physician. The medical direction physician will then issue appropriate orders for patient care. The amount and type of information you relay to the medical direction physician will depend on the type of technology you use, your patient's priority, and your local **communication protocols**. For example, if communications in your region are not secure (private), you must limit the type of information you can communicate without breaching patient confidentiality. The acuteness of your patient's clinical status and the amount of local radio traffic also may determine the length of your report. For a critical patient you may give a brief report while you tend to your patient's medical needs. For a complicated medical emergency, you may wish to communicate a greater share of the results of your history and physical exam to the medical direction physician.

Standard Format

Communicating patient information to the hospital or to the medical direction physician is a crucial function. Verbal communications by radio or phone give the hospital enough information on your patient's condition so they can prepare for his care. These communications also should elicit the medical orders you need to treat your patient in the field.

A standard format for transmitting patient assessment information helps to achieve those goals in several ways. First, it is efficient. Second, it helps the physician to assimilate information about the patient's condition quickly. Third, it ensures that medical information is complete.

In general, your verbal reports to medical direction should include the following information:

- Identification of unit and provider
- Description of scene
- Patient's age, sex, and approximate weight (for drug orders)
- Patient's chief complaint and severity
- Brief, pertinent history of the present illness or injury
- Pertinent past medical history, medications, and allergies (SAMPLE)
- Pertinent physical exam findings
- Treatment given so far/request for orders
- Estimated time of arrival at the hospital
- Other pertinent information

The formats and contents of reports for medical patients and for trauma patients differ to include only the information relevant to either type of emergency. Reports for medical patients emphasize the history in the beginning of the report; reports for trauma patients emphasize the injuries and the physical exam.

After transmitting your report, you will wait for further questions and orders from the medical direction physician. On arrival, your spoken report will give essential patient information to the provider who is assuming care. It should include a brief history, pertinent physical findings, treatment you have provided, and the patient's responses to that treatment.

General Radio Procedures

All radio transmissions must be clear and crisp, with concise, professional content (Figure 9-2 ●). Always follow these guidelines for effective radio use:

1. Listen to the channel before transmitting to ensure that it is not in use.
2. Press the transmit button for one second before speaking.
3. Speak at close range, approximately 2 to 3 inches, directly into, or across the face of, the microphone.
4. Speak slowly and clearly. Pronounce each word distinctly, avoiding words that are difficult to understand.
5. Speak in a normal pitch, keeping your voice free of emotion.
6. Be brief. Know what you are going to say before you press the transmit button.
7. Avoid codes unless they are part of your EMS system (if they are, work to change to plain English).
8. Do not waste airtime with unnecessary information.
9. Protect your patient's privacy. When appropriate:
   - Use telephone rather than a radio.
   - Turn off the external speaker.
   - Do not use your patient's name; doing so violates FCC regulations (unless your system is considered a closed system by the FCC).

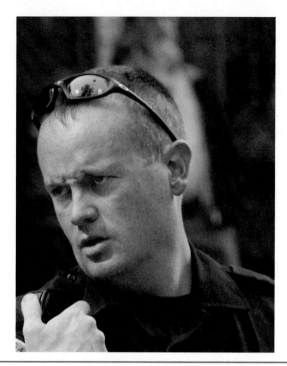

● **Figure 9-2** The professionalism of your communications reflects on the professionalism of your patient care. (© Kevin Link)

10. Use proper unit or hospital numbers and correct names or titles.

11. Do not use slang or profanity.

12. Use standard formats for transmission.

13. Be concise in order to hold the attention of the person receiving your radio report.

14. Use the **echo procedure** when receiving directions from the dispatcher or orders from the physician. Immediately repeating each statement will confirm accurate reception and understanding.

15. Always write down addresses, important dispatch communications, and physician orders.

16. When completing a transmission, obtain confirmation that your message was received and understood.

Occasionally, communications equipment will not function properly. Even a weak battery can disrupt clear communication. If you are far from the base station, particularly if you have a portable radio, try to broadcast from higher terrain. Structures that contain steel and concrete can interfere with radio transmission. Simply moving outside the building or standing near a window may improve communications. If that does not work, try a telephone.

WRITTEN COMMUNICATION

Written records are another important aspect of EMS communications. Your **prehospital care report (PCR)** (also called patient care report) is a written or an electronic, keyboard/mouse-entered record of events. The written report includes

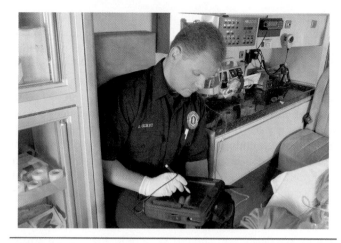

● **Figure 9-3** The prehospital care report is as important as the run itself. Complete it promptly and legibly.

administrative information such as times, location, agency, and crew, as well as medical information. Hospital staff, agency administrators, system quality assurance/improvement committees, insurance and billing departments, researchers, educators, and lawyers will use it. The data collected from your PCR can help to monitor and improve patient care through medical audits, research, education, and system policy changes. Furthermore, your written documentation becomes a legal record of the incident and may become part of your patient's permanent medical record. All legal rules regarding confidentiality and disclosure pertain to your PCR.

Most of the same factors that influence verbal communication also affect written communication. Be objective, write legibly (the written version of speaking clearly), thoroughly document your patient's assessment and care, and use terminology that is widely accepted in the medical community (Figure 9-3 ●). Finally, your PCR illustrates your professionalism. A sloppy, incomplete PCR suggests sloppy, inefficient care. Chapter 10, on documentation, deals with PCRs and other written communications in much greater detail.

The data elements that are collected on the PCR and how they are interpreted are usually defined in a **data dictionary**. All states and territories have agreed to adopt, as soon as is practical for each, the **National Emergency Medical Services Information System (NEMSIS)** data dictionary and to participate in reporting some data to a NEMSIS national database.[2] This will, for the first time, allow national EMS performance to be assessed.

TERMINOLOGY

Every industry develops its own terminology. Doing so makes communication within the industry more clear, concise, and unambiguous for those within that industry. The airline industry, for example, uses the term *payload* to describe the total weight of everything (passengers, fuel, luggage, and other items) on an airplane. Musical composers and arrangers use terms like *allegro, fortissimo,* or *a cappella* to describe a specific tempo or style.

The medical field also uses an extensive list of terms, acronyms, and abbreviations that allow quick, accurate communication of complex information. (Chapter 10 includes an extensive

TABLE 9-1	Common Radio Terminology
Term	**Meaning**
Copy, 10-4, roger	I understand
Affirmative	Yes
Negative	No
Stand by	Please wait
Repeat	Please repeat what you said
Landline	Telephone communications
Rendezvous	Meet with
LZ	Landing zone (helicopter)
ETA	Estimated time of arrival
Over	I am finished with my transmission
Mobile status	On the air, driving around
Stage	Wait before entering a scene
Clear	End of transmission
Unfounded	We cannot find the incident/patient
Be advised	Listen carefully to this

table of standard charting abbreviations.) An emergency physician may request a CBC (complete blood count), ABGs (arterial blood gases), or CMP (comprehensive metabolic panel)—common terms describing diagnostic tests run on patients.

The emergency services industry has developed its own terms for radio communication (Table 9-1). These words or phrases shorten airtime and transmit thoughts and ideas quickly. For example, "copy" means "I heard you and I understand what you said." Using industry terminology appropriately is an important part of effective communication, providing a commonly understood means of communicating with other emergency care professionals. Terminology is considered to be plain English within the discipline in which it is used; its use is not considered to be the same as coded substitutions for plain English (such as 10-codes), which were discussed earlier, and are discouraged.

THE IMPORTANCE OF COMMUNICATIONS IN EMS RESPONSE

Your ability to communicate effectively during a stressful EMS response is very likely to determine the success or failure of your efforts. A brilliant assessment and management plan will be futile if you cannot communicate it to others.

Dealing effectively with your patient and bystanders requires a variety of communication skills, such as empathy, confidence,

self-control, authority, and patience. Your clinical experience will suggest which skills to use in any particular situation. For example, you might display confidence and use an authoritative posture when dealing with unruly bystanders. On the other hand, you would need to be gentle and empathetic with a child or an elderly grandmother. If you were in charge of an incident, you would have to communicate authoritatively within the structure of the emergency scene to providers from other responding agencies. Delegating tasks, listening to initial reports, and coordinating the scene require effective communication and interpersonal skills.

The Sequence of Communications in an EMS Response

The sequence of an EMS response illustrates the importance of communications in prehospital care. A typical EMS response includes the chain of events described next.

Detection and Citizen Access

To begin the response to any emergency, someone must detect the problem and summon EMS (Figure 9-4 ●). Any citizen with an urgent medical need should have a simple and reliable mechanism for accessing the EMS system. In the United States, most people access EMS by telephone; thus, a well-publicized universal telephone number such as 911 provides direct citizen access to the communications center.

The 911 system has been available since the late 1960s. The first 911 system simply provided the common, easy to remember access number and allowed 911 centers to automatically "ring back" a caller's phone if there was a disconnect.

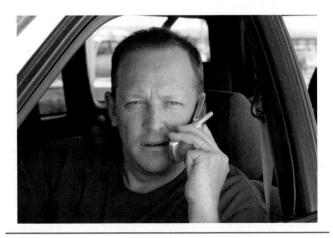

● **Figure 9-4** The EMS response begins when someone detects an emergency and summons EMS assistance.

At newer Enhanced 911 (E911) communication centers, a computer also displays the caller's telephone number (a feature called **automatic number identification** or ANI) and location (a feature called **automatic location information** or ALI).

911

Currently, 99 percent of the population in the United States and 96 percent of the nation's geographic area have a 911 system. Of the geography covered by 911 systems, 93 percent has E911 service. Highway 911 call boxes, citizens band (CB) radio, and amateur radio all provide alternative means of accessing emergency help in some regions.

Increasingly, manual and automatic alerting systems are used by the elderly and those who are incapacitated, such as "Help, I've fallen and I can't get up" devices. Other types of patient home monitoring devices may have automatic alarms as well. Typically, all these types of devices alert a monitoring center which, in turn, calls 911 rather than sending a message directly from the device to 911. **Automatic crash notification** (**ACN**) is another type of automatic event alerting system that may result in EMS dispatch.[3] (A more sophisticated version of ACN—advanced notification (AACN)—will be discussed later.)

Most 911 centers are now called **public safety answering points (PSAPs)**. The PSAP routes the 911 call to the appropriate agency for dispatch and response if it does not also do the dispatching itself. In some systems, the PSAP call taker will elicit the information, determine the nature of the needed response, and dispatch the appropriate responding agencies. In others, the call taker will simply answer with the question "Is this a police, fire, or medical emergency?" and transfer the caller to the appropriate dispatcher, who will then elicit specific information. Many systems use computerized technology at the PSAP to connect the caller automatically with the appropriate agency. Some even provide language translation.

E911 technology has always worked well with landline systems in which there is a wired connection all the way from the caller's phone to the PSAP. The landline connection also allows ANI and ALI (which identify the phone number and location of the caller) to work because of the unique, direct-wired connection to a telephone associated with a physical address to which EMS could respond. This automatic provision of ANI and ALI allows dispatch of an emergency response even while Emergency Medical Dispatch (EMD) prearrival instructions are being given. Few EMS providers would disagree that E911 in connection with landline telephone service saves many lives each year.

By 2010, however, a full third of the 240 million annual 911 calls in the United States (half or more in some communities) come from wireless/cell phones. Without a direct-wired connection to a physical location, ANI and ALI did not work with the early wireless phone systems. An emergency dispatcher who received a call from a cell phone had to rely on the caller's ability to state his location and phone number. In many cases, the caller, who was traveling in an unfamiliar area or had an altered level of consciousness or was incapacitated, could not

provide his location and number and could not be found. These cases were often associated with bad patient outcomes.

Further complicating the problem has been the issue of **call routing**. Typically, wire-line 911 calls are routed via a trunk line and a specialized address database to the nearest 911 center. Wireless 911 calls that do not carry address database data with them cannot be automatically routed to the nearest 911 center. Thus, emergency calls from early wireless telephone systems were often routed out of the caller's location to the location associated with the wireless service provider—which may have been a different city, county, state, region, or even country.

In many cases the caller is simply too excited to provide the emergency dispatcher with the correct information. One such case involved a 19-year-old girl in a rural New York State community who called 911 to report an oven fire. She was cooking dinner at her grandmother's home when the fire began. She assisted her grandmother out of the home and dialed 911 on her wireless phone. When the dispatcher asked her for her address, she gave "her address" and not the address of her grandmother's home. The resulting confusion over the location of the emergency was responsible for total loss of the structure. Cases like this are still not unheard of, even with the increasingly widespread installation of sophisticated E911 systems that can determine the location of a wireless or cell phone (using triangulation or GPS technology, as will be described next). This event happened not that long ago, in the year 2002.

Recognizing the rapidly expanding popularity of cell phones in the last decades of the twentieth century, the Federal Communications Commission (FCC) began phased implementation of rules requiring wireless providers to enable ANI and one of two versions of an ALI application. Public Safety Answering Points would also be required to accommodate the data to enable them to display and use this number and location identification data.

Wireless phones can now be located by **terrestrial-based triangulation**, by **global positioning systems (GPS)**, or by a combination of the two. Triangulation of a wireless signal involves the use of three cell phone towers. Based on the strength of telephone signal and time of signal arrival at each of the towers, the signal location can be calculated to within several meters. This calculated location is identified as a longitude/latitude that is then translated to a map location and street address in a specialized database. Because the call is recognized as having come from a phone with a unique identifier, another specialized database assigns the correct callback number associated with that specific phone. This packet of information—a phone call with a 911 prefix, ALI data, and ANI data—is then transmitted digitally through selective routers and trunk lines to the closest public safety answering point.

Geographic regions, such as individual counties, have had to decide to which PSAP they prefer to have these calls sent. Systems that use global positioning location data require that the individual phones be fitted with hardware and software that allow them access to the GPS system. Emergency 911 calls originating from such phones are still routed in the same manner and require access to the ANI database but not to an ALI database. Location information is transmitted automatically with the packet of data that comes from the phone when a 911 prefix is associated with the call. The data from these phones are transmitted to the appropriate PSAP.

Call takers and dispatchers see the data from wireless/cell phones in the same format as they see for landline E911 calls. In other words, the method of data transmission is inconsequential to the dispatch personnel, because data are provided in identical formats with both methods, ANI/ALI or landline. Putting these new communications technologies in place ensures the reliability of Enhanced 911 as cellular communications continue to increase.

A more recent 911 phenomenon has been the emergency access issue created by **voice over Internet protocol (VOIP)** technology which, like cellular technology, has rapidly gained in popularity. VOIP uses both wired and wireless Internet access technology (e.g., cable, DSL, wireless air card, wireless hotspot) through a computer or mobile Internet access device to provide voice communications that are increasingly of comparable quality to other forms of telephony. Low calling costs through VOIP help drive its popularity. Unfortunately, as with early cell phone systems, VOIP was not designed with ANI, ALI, or best-routing-to-closest-PSAP capabilities. Technology has become available to alleviate these issues, however, and organizations like the National Emergency Number Association (NENA)[4] and the Association of Public Safety Communications Officials-International (APCO)[5] are working to incorporate the capabilities required.

The challenges of new technology with 911 center implications do not end with cell and VOIP phones. The ability to send photos, video, or text messages from a handheld device to a 911 number or to access or interact with social networking systems presents similar issues. As a result, an initiative called Next Generation 911 (NG-911) is under way, spearheaded by NENA, APCO, and the EMS Office in the National Highway Traffic Safety Administration (NHTSA), which has federal responsibility for the program.[6]

Advanced Automatic Crash Notification

The 2009 Centers for Disease Control and Prevention (CDC) report *Recommendations from the Expert Panel: Advanced Automatic Collision Notification and Triage of the Injured Patient*[7] found that **advanced automatic crash notification (AACN)** can improve outcomes among seriously injured patients by:

- Predicting the likelihood of serious injury among vehicle occupants,
- Decreasing response times by prehospital care providers,
- Assisting with field triage destination and transportation decisions, and
- Decreasing the time it takes for patients to receive definitive trauma care.

It further found that systems like AACN may be especially important in rural or isolated areas where there may not be a passerby to report a crash and a Level I trauma center is too far away to treat the kind of injuries sustained in severe crashes. The Case Study at the beginning of this chapter illustrates just this kind of situation.

AACN systems are data collection and transmission mechanisms that may change the way we assess and treat victims of car crashes. As the name implies, AACN systems can automatically contact a national call center or local PSAP and transmit crash-specific data.

For example, imagine a car with a driver and one passenger traveling at 45 miles per hour along a highway. The driver loses control of the vehicle, leaves the roadway, rolls over, and comes to rest against a tree. Because the AACN system in the vehicle contains special sensors called **accelerometers**, it can measure the change in total velocity ("change in velocity" is written as delta V or ΔV), the forces that were applied to the vehicle, the direction in which they were applied, whether or not the car rolled over, whether or not air bags were deployed, and the car's final resting position. The sensor also has a GPS-enabled chip that can transmit the exact location of the vehicle. Other data available from the system may in the future contribute to the determination of whether a severe injury was likely to have occurred.

As in the second Case Study at the beginning of this chapter, protocols can be established for the automatic notification and routing of AACN data to responders and hospitals likely to be involved and for the automatic dispatch of resources rather than waiting for a responder to arrive at the scene and make that determination. In rural responses, this can save minutes to hours in the time required for definitive surgical intervention.

Emergency Medical Dispatch

Once a 911 call is received at a PSAP and determined to have emergency medical consequences, it should be managed from then on by a dispatcher with the special training and resources to do so. This is the **Emergency Medical Dispatcher (EMD)**, who is the public's first contact with the EMS system and who plays a crucial role in every EMS response.

In a coordinated system known as **priority dispatching**, Emergency Medical Dispatchers interrogate a distressed caller using a set of medically approved questions to elicit essential information about the chief complaint (Figure 9-5 ●). Then, the dispatcher follows established guidelines to determine the appropriate level of response (Figure 9-6 ●).

These predetermined guidelines are based on criteria approved by the medical director. For example, an elderly man with a history of heart problems who is complaining of chest pain radiating to his left arm may indicate a high-priority response (life-threatening emergency, lights and siren). In some systems, the appropriate response may include a fire department basic life support first responding unit, a paramedic engine company, and a transporting ambulance. Other systems may require only a paramedic ambulance. Another type of call may result in a nonemergency response, and another call may be transferred to a consulting-nurse advice line because it would not be an appropriate use of EMS resources to respond.

This form of call screening, when done appropriately, saves time and money, because only the necessary resources are sent. It also limits the liability associated with a lights-and-siren response to possible life-threatening incidents by authorizing such responses only when necessary. Because these systems make decisions that may result in a nonemergency response or in no EMS response, they must be undertaken cautiously, using

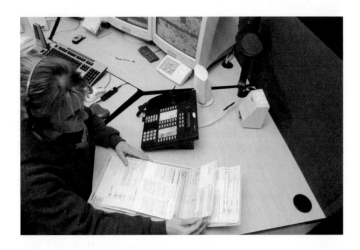

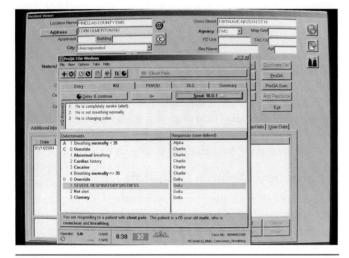

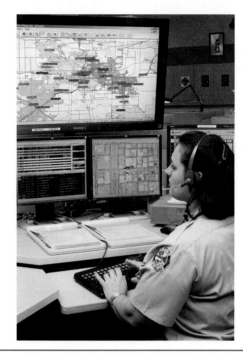

● **Figure 9-6** The dispatcher determines the appropriate level of response according to established guidelines.

● **Figure 9-5** Priority dispatching and prearrival medical instructions are commonly used in EMS. (Top photo: © *Jeff Forster*)

only priority dispatch systems that have been proven to support these decisions effectively. Many private and public EMS systems throughout the United States use the priority dispatching system.[8]

Prearrival Instructions Many EMS systems provide **prearrival instructions**, a service that is considered the standard of care. Prearrival instructions complement the call-screening process in a priority dispatch system and are an essential part of the EMD function. As the dispatcher sends the appropriate response, the caller remains on the line and receives instructions for suitable emergency measures to carry out while waiting for the emergency responders to arrive, such as cardiopulmonary resuscitation or hemorrhage control.

During prearrival instructions, the dispatcher also can obtain further information for the responding units. In the case of cardiac arrest, the dispatcher can relay information concerning the presence of a living will, a "Do Not Resuscitate" (DNR) form, or other advance directives. In another case, paramedics en route to help a baby who had stopped breathing could reduce their response speed if they learned that the child had now started breathing and was conscious.

Prearrival instructions have saved many lives. They also are useful for comforting a distressed caller or providing emotional support to bystanders, family members, or the patient himself.[9]

Call Coordination and Incident Recording After sending the appropriate response and providing prearrival instructions, the Emergency Medical Dispatcher's main duties are support and coordination. He will provide the responding units with any additional resources needed and will record information about the call such as times, locations, and units involved. Your dispatcher can be your best friend. He can assign the resources you need to manage an incident, such as additional medical personnel to help with a cardiac arrest or the fire department to provide specialized rescue. He also may facilitate communication with other agencies, hospitals, communication centers, and support services.

Discussion with the Medical Direction Physician

After conducting your assessment and initiating care as outlined by your local protocols, you will contact the medical direction physician to discuss the case. Following consultation, he may give you further orders for interventions such as medications or other medical procedures. The many ways to conduct this communication today include radio, telephone, and cell phone. Taping these communications for use later is advisable. For example, if a discrepancy arose as to what your orders had been, you could always refer to the tape, which never lies.

After consulting the medical direction physician, you will continue treatment and prepare your patient for transport. You will then contact your dispatcher, who will record the time when you leave the scene and the time when you arrive at your destination.

Your professional relationship with medical direction physicians must be based on trust. Transmission of clear, concise, controlled reports will encourage your medical direction physicians to accept your assessments and on-scene treatment plans. Your ability to communicate effectively on the radio will secure a large part of your professional reputation. The general radio procedures and standard format sections given earlier in this chapter offer guidelines for communicating with the medical direction physician and transmitting patient information (Figure 9-7 ●).[10]

Transfer Communications

As you transfer care of your patient to the receiving facility staff, you must give the receiving nurse or physician a formal verbal briefing (Figure 9-8 ●). This report, commonly called the **hand-off**, should include your patient's vital information, chief complaint and history, physical exam findings, and any treatments that have been rendered.[11] Do not assume that the receiving nurse heard your radio report and knows about your patient or that this information has been given to the physician you may first encounter. Some systems require the receiving nurse to sign the PCR to verify and document the transfer of care. Many systems also require the medical direction physician to sign the PCR for any medications administered by paramedics, especially if they included controlled substances such as morphine or diazepam.

Never leave your patient until you have completed some type of formal transfer of care; otherwise you may be charged with abandonment. In all cases, end your PCR documentation with information about the transfer of care. It may also be appropriate to have a parting chat with your patient, particularly if the patient is not receiving immediate care and has questions or anxiety.

INFORMATION AND COMMUNICATIONS TECHNOLOGY

Modern EMS is approximately 40 years old. Prior to the EMS systems we know today, ambulances were, by and large, "horizontal taxicabs" capable of little more than transportation. Communications from the scene of the injury or illness, or during transport to the receiving hospital, did not exist.

In the early era of modern EMS, radios were installed in ambulances and hospital emergency departments. The 1970s brought the practice of notifying a receiving hospital of an ambulance's impending arrival. The 1970s also saw the widespread development of medical direction systems and the advance of field capabilities. Crews would send voice descriptions of patient condition by VHF radio, and in some cases could send telemetry ECG data by UHF radio, and in exchange receive real-time review and medical orders from an emergency physician. These developments constituted the birth of field medical intervention.

Unfortunately, the majority of EMS communications systems have not kept pace with the blooming sophistication of EMS in general. Nor have they kept pace with concurrent rapid developments in communications technology. With some notable exceptions, often in a pilot project or other experimental form, the methods by which EMS providers are dispatched, communicate with resources as needed for response and patient care, and communicate with hospital medical supervisors and staff are the same as they were 35 to 40 years ago.

If one asks average paramedics if their communications system adequately supports them, their fast answer often will be "yes." They may describe **dead spots** (where communications transmission and reception are poor), but aside from that they can talk to their dispatcher, can talk with other resources (either directly or through a dispatcher), and can talk to the hospital staff as needed.

But pressing those same average paramedics to think about additional pieces of information that would benefit their next response and patient if they could have that information earlier or more easily, and the answer also would probably be "yes." When EMS providers really think about it, they know they are often frustrated by the lack of information they passively "wonder about" as they make their way through an emergency call.

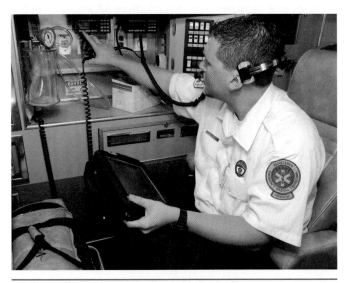

● **Figure 9-7** You may occasionally need to discuss a case with a physician in order to guide further care. (© *Jeff Forster*)

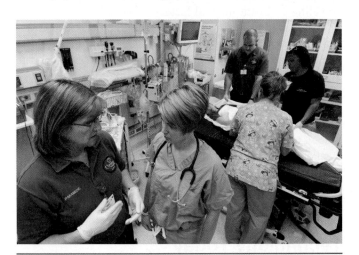

● **Figure 9-8** The patient hand-off is an essential aspect of emergency care and ensures continuity of care between the prehospital and hospital environments.

How often do we know how serious the call is only when we get there, and only then are able to call for additional resources (which may or may not be available)? How often do we wonder, en route to a call 20 minutes away, if a resource will be available if the call turns out to be a "bad one," then take the initiative to ask for it, only to have that resource become unavailable by the time we reach the destination? With the voice, data, and video technology available today, "wondering" should become increasingly unnecessary.

Situational awareness (SA) and **common operating picture (COP)** are important considerations in EMS. These are concepts that address how prepared a paramedic and his team are to perform their jobs effectively at any given moment, particularly when time is a factor. Both awareness and operating procedure are improved by having just the right amount of updated information exactly when it is needed—information about resources the team can bring to bear and events that may impact their current situation (Figure 9-9 ●).

As EMS emergency call volumes continue to grow and medical direction physicians become busier with ED overcrowding, the opportunity for the paramedic in the field and the ED physician providing medical direction to communicate becomes increasingly constrained. The likelihood is rapidly diminishing that a paramedic and physician are going to be available to talk at the same time. Voice communications then become a bottleneck to the emergency patient care process.

Further, there are no generally available systems through which EMS providers can access real-time information concerning events and resource status that may affect their work. For example, an EMS crew may have no information on the number and severity of the patients to whom they are responding until they arrive at the scene, no information about the availability of air medical or extrication resources until they actually call for them, and no information about the availability of the hospital to which they want to transport until they call that hospital.

In the future, it will be necessary to develop networks of databases that contain information about events and resources updated in real-time and accessible through a user friendly, **geographic information system (GIS)** capable of interface

with smart phone/PDA/communication devices carried by responders and physicians, mobile data units in EMS vehicles, and desktop units at responders' bases of operations, dispatch centers, and hospitals.

A GIS-based interface screen would show a rough depiction of an ambulance service's relevant operations area. It would represent the jurisdictions and catchment areas of the user; list information about neighboring services, hospitals, and other resources with which it commonly operates; and detail events occurring within those areas. Selecting an icon and opening a second screen would access information not readily available on the initial screen.

This array of databases (e.g., the status of hospitals, ambulances, helicopter services, and EMS calls in current operation) might be called an EMS Resource and Event Monitoring System (EMREMS). It would be one information communications network that is linked with similar networks for fire, police, departments of transportation, and other responder colleagues. While such a system may seem a thing of dreams, its concept has been repeatedly described in EMS and emergency planning literature as a necessary next step to ensure SA and COP in the paramedic's everyday work.

In the new "EMREMS" systems to be developed, an **ad hoc database** will be created each time a patient is encountered. Multiple vital signs, video, electronic health record, and voice-to-text translation of medic findings will be pushed to those databases and parked until the intended recipient (e.g., an incoming air medical crew or a medical direction physician in the hospital) is available to review them. These recipients can then pull down that data to their own screen and push queries or orders back to the EMS crew for consumption and response when they are available. When an emergency dictates, either party could break into the other's process and revert to voice and data communication as needed.

Some of the capabilities described have been employed in the military. Hospital- and health care-system-based electronic medical-records-sharing networks are being established in many states. These systems allow emergency room and primary care physicians to access the records of patients in the system who present for care. Such systems would have application for providing pertinent medical history information to EMS providers in real time during calls. At least one EMS system, a system based in Indiana, has already implemented this capability.

Modern EMS communications needed to provide adequate SA and COP require both voice and data communications support. This becomes a blending of two systems and sets of professional skills: (1) traditional communications technology that generally involves telecommunications engineers and (2) data systems technology that involves hardware and software development professionals. **Information communications technology (ICT)** is the new concept that blends traditional communications technology (CT) systems and information technology (IT) systems.

Technology Today

Depending on where you practice as a paramedic, you may be living in a communications world of 1970s technology (a VHF simplex voice radio system—with or without access to a UHF

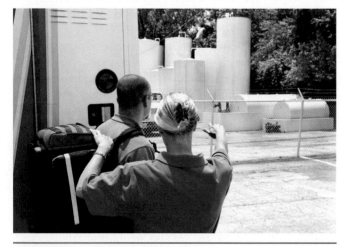

● **Figure 9-9** Situational awareness on the part of EMS providers helps ensure efficient patient care as well as provider and patient safety.

duplex system with biotelemetry capability), or with hints of the 1990s technology (trunked 800 MHz with lots of channels and talk-groups; cell phones used routinely and perhaps transmitting 12-lead ECGs) or hints of future technology (mobile data unit—hardened laptop—that uses an air card access to wireless phone providers and/or hotspot access to the Internet and beyond; video transmission connection to the ED; and multi-vital-sign transmission from your monitors to the ED using one of these connections).

Regardless, your communication network must consist of reliable equipment designed to afford clear communication among all agencies within the system. This becomes a challenge in systems that cover large geographical areas or where terrain interferes with transmission and reception. If you want to communicate with a unit clear across the county but your radio is not powerful enough to transmit that far, communication will be difficult, if not impossible. A system that covers a large geographical expanse can place **repeaters** strategically throughout its service area. These devices receive transmissions from a low-powered source and rebroadcast them at a higher power (Figure 9-10 ●).

Your regional EMS system may consist of many agencies that have conducted business for decades on different **radio bands** and **radio frequencies**. City units may transmit on **ultrahigh frequency (UHF)** radio waves because they penetrate concrete and steel well and are less susceptible to interference. Rural and suburban units may use a lower band frequency— **very high frequency (VHF)**—because those waves travel farther and better over varied terrain. In any event, communicating among agencies will be difficult unless all units share a common frequency. This is rarely the case. Again, the spectrum of communications equipment currently ranges from antiquated radios to mobile data units mounted inside emergency vehicles.

Geographically integrating communications networks would enable routine and reliable communication among EMS, fire, law enforcement, and other public safety agencies. This would in turn facilitate coordinated responses during both routine and large-scale operations. Developing the necessary hardware (equipment and network) and software (language) will be essential to improving emergency communications.

See further discussion in the Public Safety Communication System Planning and Funding section near the end of this chapter.

LEGAL CONSIDERATIONS

EMS and other public safety radio systems operating below 512 MHz (this includes all EMS VHF [generally in the 155 MHz range] and UHF [generally in the 463/468 paired ranges] must go through a process called "narrowbanding" before January 2013 to remain in compliance with FCC regulations. This may require nothing for systems with total equipment and license updates after 1997, or it may mean at least reprogramming of equipment or wholesale replacement of systems. APCO, NENA, the FCC, and the International Municipal Signal Association (IMSA—the FCC-designated frequency coordinator for EMS) all have narrowbanding content and updates on their websites, as do the major police and fire associations. Your EMS agency communications service staff or vendor should have a plan for coordinating your narrowbanding process with other agencies and hospitals with which you work to minimize interference issues as you each transition to narrower bandwidths at the same frequencies.

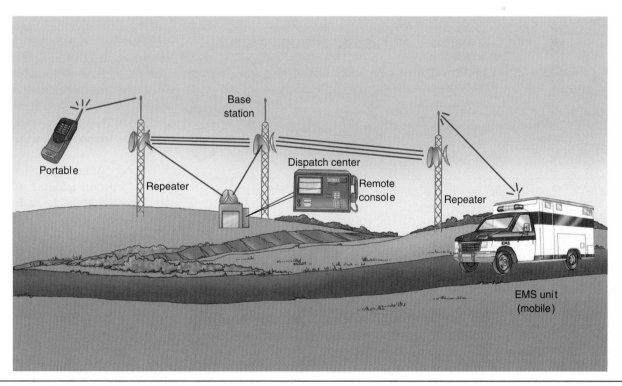

● **Figure 9-10** Example of EMS repeater system.

CONTENT REVIEW

▶ Types of Radio
Communication

• Simplex
• Duplex
• Multiplex
• Trunked
• Digital

Radio Communication

Many types of radio transmission are possible, with new technologies being developed every day. Usage may vary from system to system. This section discusses some of the more common technologies in use today.

Simplex The most basic communications systems use **simplex** transmissions. These systems transmit and receive on the same frequency and thus cannot do both simultaneously (Figure 9-11 ●). After you transmit a message, you must release the transmit button and wait for a response. This slows communication because you have to wait for all traffic to stop before you can speak. It also makes the system more formal and prevents open discussion. Simplex communication systems are most effective on the scene, when the incident commander or EMS dispatcher must transmit orders or directions without interruption. Most dispatch systems and on-scene communications use simplex transmissions.

Duplex **Duplex** transmissions allow simultaneous two-way communications by using two frequencies for each channel (Figure 9-12 ●). Each radio must be able to transmit and receive on each channel. For example, on a UHF radio, a hospital base station might transmit on 468.000 megahertz (MHz) and receive on 478.000 MHz. Field radios would then transmit on 478.000 MHz and receive on 468.000 MHz—just the opposite. Either party could then transmit and receive on the same channel simultaneously.

Duplex systems work like telephone communications. Many areas use them for communications between the field paramedic and the medical direction physician. The duplex system's major advantage is that one party does not have to wait to speak until the other party finishes his transmission. This allows a much freer discussion and consultation between physician and paramedic. For example, the medical direction physician can interrupt your report with an important question or concern. On the other hand, this ability to interrupt can be a disadvantage when abused.

All duplex systems allow you to transmit either voice messages or data such as ECG strips.

Multiplex **Multiplex** systems are duplex systems with the additional capability of transmitting voice and data simultaneously (Figure 9-13 ●). This enables you to carry on a conversation with the medical direction physician while you are transmitting an ECG strip. Speaking while you are transmitting the ECG strip, however, causes much interference on the ECG strip.

Trunking Many communications systems operating in the 800-MHz range use **trunking** to hasten communications. Trunked systems pool all frequencies. When a radio transmission comes in, a computer routes it to the first available frequency. The computer routes the next transmission to the next available frequency, and so on. When a transmission terminates, that frequency becomes available and reenters the pool of unused frequencies. Trunking thus frees the dispatcher or field unit from having to search for an available frequency.

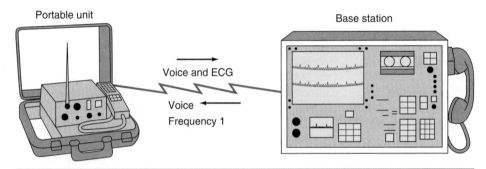

● **Figure 9-11** Simplex communications systems transmit and receive on the same frequency.

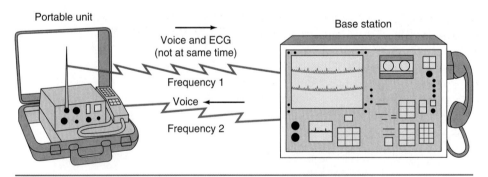

● **Figure 9-12** Duplex communications systems use two frequencies for each channel.

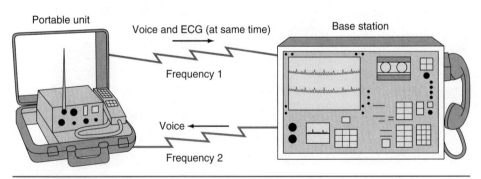

● **Figure 9-13** Multiplex systems can transmit voice and data at the same time.

Trunked 800-MHz systems have been developed over the past 20 years, usually by one sponsoring state system user (e.g., police, transportation). When states began to suffer financial setbacks in the 1990s and more recently, these systems became forced to seek other users, generally at a "per device per month or per year" cost. Trunked systems appeal to potential fire and EMS users because they offer more channels to use and the ability to configure special "talk-groups" (a preselected set of users who can be instantly keyed up and addressed as a group with no others participating).

EMS users now using VHF and UHF systems should be aware of the need to plan, engineer, and coordinate system development if you expect to change to a trunked system. A city jurisdiction that switches to this system and includes all hospitals may create problems for rural EMS units that occasionally transfer patients into those hospitals and use only VHF or UHF frequencies. Suburban and rural users may find that the cost of new antennas needs to be factored in, because transmission distances and coverage will be less with 800-MHz equipment than with UHF and VHF systems. Buyers beware!

Digital Communications   Voice transmission can be time consuming and difficult to understand. The trend toward combining radio technology with computer technology (ICT) has encouraged a shift from analog to **digital communications**. Digital radio equipment is becoming increasingly popular in emergency services communication systems. This technology translates, or encodes, sounds into digital code for broadcast. Digital transmission is much faster and much more accurate than analog transmission. Because the messages are transmitted in condensed form, they help to ease the overcrowding of radio frequencies. Cell phone companies now use digital transmissions. Issues remain with the use of digital communications in certain noise environments, such as fire grounds, that cause distortion of voice transmissions. This may be alleviated with changes in radio technology but may also constrain the abandonment of analog voice communications altogether.

The **mobile data unit (MDU)** in many emergency vehicles (typically a "ruggedized" or "hardened" laptop computer) is a robust form of digital communications. MDUs are mounted in the vehicle cab or patient compartment (depending on use) and wired to the radio, a wireless **hotspot** modem (in urban settings), or through a wireless provider air card. These are replacing mobile data terminals that are radio-based devices (more often used in law enforcement) that have limited applications because they have no broadband capacity. MDUs, however, may be used for receiving dispatch and other information and sending status information such as "en route," "arrived," or "transporting to the hospital" but may also be used to send electronic PCR data to the hospital or back to quarters for processing.

It is a positive step forward to begin to use data communications on a daily basis in EMS. These cutting-edge applications are increasingly widespread, and gaining experience with them is instructive for all of us. Dependence on commercial cellular and other wireless providers (air cards and hotspots) and on unlicensed, municipal hotspot/"mesh" technology (2.4-GHz systems) for **mission-critical communications** (e.g., when the information must get through without fail because a patient's

well-being depends on it) is not recommended. These systems are not built to public safety reliability, security, or infrastructure hardening standards. Further, they are shared with the general public whose use is rapidly increasing, and offer no higher priority of use for EMS. If mission-critical data communications are required, explore the public safety licensed option of 4.9 GHz in urban areas or teaming with transportation colleagues for use of 5.9 GHz intelligent transportation systems (ITS) channels. Another, better solution is under development and that is the FCC's proposed national public safety broadband network at 700 MHz. This solution promises broadband coverage in areas beyond urban centers.

Although means of digital communication are developing rapidly, it is important to remember that voice communications will always have a place in emergency services. Crews will always need to speak to one another, to physicians and nurses, or to dispatchers.

Cell Phones and Mobile Broadband   Many EMS systems have found that a **cellular telephone system** provides a cost-effective way to transmit essential patient information to the hospital (Figure 9-14 ●). Cellular technology is available in even the most remote areas of the country, though availability is wireless provider dependent. A cell phone service is divided into regions called **cells**. These cells are radio base stations that communicate with mobile telephones. When the transmission leaves one cell's range, another cell picks it up immediately, without interruption. Agreements among wireless providers now allow seamless roaming across cell regions and states coast-to-coast. Limitations in any one provider's roaming arrangements, however, can limit access in certain areas of the country.

Handheld cell phone devices still exist with capabilities that do not extend beyond simple voice communications. These can also send limited data such as ECGs when connected to a heart monitor that is set up for this operation. But these devices are "narrowband" and, like the VHF/UHF/800-MHz radio systems we commonly use today (which are also narrowband—and with the VHF/UHF systems, as discussed earlier, getting even narrower by 2013), they support limited data transmission. In fact, they send data more slowly than the first dial-up Internet

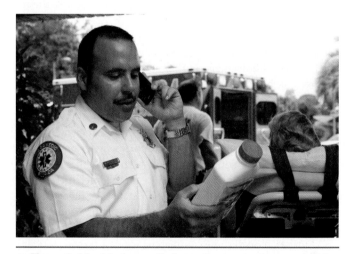

● **Figure 9-14**   Modern cell phones have amazing capabilities and are becoming increasingly more sophisticated.

connections 20 years ago and only about 20 percent as fast as basic dial-up connections today.

More common today are **smart phone** devices in which the voice capability of a basic cell phone is joined by the ability to perform a variety of data messaging functions, like taking and sending photos and video, sending and receiving e-mail and text messages, and connecting with the Internet and its variety of communications options (e.g., using the handheld as a wireless hotspot VOIP device to save cell phone call charges).

Smart phones incorporate broadband data capability to be able to accomplish these functions by, essentially, widening the "pipe" through which data flow, allowing more data to flow faster and increasingly supporting data- and bandwidth-hungry operations (e.g., gaming with multiple players and sophisticated, highly responsive graphics in real time; and the sending of video and higher quality photos in social networking environments while texting/instant messaging among recipients).

Broadband data capabilities are rapidly expanding and becoming more sophisticated as technology moves from second to third and, now, fourth generations ("2G", "3G", "4G") of development. The popularity of smart phones, smart pads/tablets, and netbook devices, added to the data transmission demands of laptop and desktop computer users, creates a real issue of "pipe availability" to send data. It is not uncommon, particularly in urban and suburban environments, to see commercial wireless data sending and receiving rates fluctuate greatly with time of day and day of week. Occasional system "crashes" leave users of some wireless providers without data communications for varying periods of time. As with older-generation, narrowband cell phones, availability of newer generations of data communications varies with the commercial wireless provider company and the area of the country (with large urban areas usually the first to be upgraded).

Like duplex radio transmissions, cell and smart phones make communication less formal, promote discussion, and reduce on-line times. They further allow the medical direction physician to speak directly with the patient and offer the additional advantages of being widely available and highly reliable. The telephones themselves are inexpensive, but commercial wireless providers charge a monthly fee for their use, generally with additional charges for data services and specific data applications.

As with data communications, even simple voice communications are not always reliable in commercial wireless systems. Their major disadvantage is that each cell can handle only a limited number of calls. Geography can interfere with the cell phone's signals, and in large metropolitan areas the cells often fill up and become unavailable, especially during peak hours. Cell congestion frequently occurs in times of disaster when many local, state, and federal response agencies, news media, and citizens all require communications.[12] The National Communications System in the U.S. Department of Homeland Security, however, has programs that local and state EMS agencies can subscribe to that provide priority access to wire line and wireless communications services in emergencies.

Further, though some commercial wireless providers offer a "push to talk" (PTT) feature that resembles that of your mobile EMS radio, no cell or smart phone is capable of communicating directly with another phone even if the callers are standing next to one another. All calls must go through the cell system network. Also, these phones are not capable of "one-to-many" communications as radios are. If a caller wants to get a voice message to several responders, the caller would have to call each individually.

Despite their limitations, commercial wireless phones have become a popular medium for on-scene and medical direction communications. When using wireless phones for on-line medical direction, it is important to contact the base station physician on a recorded line. On-line medical direction recordings have been used as powerful allies in cases of litigation. Be sure to find out how to do this in your system.

Because of all the limitations just described, no paramedic or EMS provider agency should ever rely solely on commercial wireless communications for mission-critical voice communications. This is also true of municipal or other 2.4-GHz unlicensed hotspot systems that are common in urban areas to provide Internet access to residents. (4.9 GHz public safety licensed systems are another matter, have limitations for voice communications, and have good potential for urban hotspot and "mesh"—interconnected hotspot antennae to make citywide or area-wide network operations.)

Expanding Computer Uses Computers have entered every aspect of our daily lives. In emergency services communications, they have revolutionized system management and incident data collection. Most dispatchers no longer enter data by pen and pencil, time-stamping machines, or typewriters. They can make a permanent record of any incident's events in real time. Virtually all new PCR systems are no longer paper based, but rely on the electronic input of patient and call data into ruggedized mobile laptops and/or computers at the ED or EMS quarters.

It is increasingly commonplace for an EMS unit to "dump" its electronic PCR data for recent calls to a central database at its quarters, using an air card in the computer and a commercial wireless provider's network. Crews in the field will be able to use their smart phones, PDAs, or laptops to access regional health care system medical record depositories for medical history data on their current patient in real time. (The first well-publicized system of this kind is in Indiana, but such regional and statewide record systems are in development virtually everywhere following the federal push for universal electronic health records use.)

Computers also make research faster and easier. For example, if you wanted to determine the day of the week when most cardiac calls happen, or what time of day is busiest, or which area of a city needs more coverage, you could retrieve the pertinent data from your computerized records immediately. You can program your system to provide whatever type of data you want, in whatever format you desire. It also eliminates the need to enter retrospective data when conducting research. For example, the times, locations, and particulars of a call will already be in the computer files for immediate retrieval during a research project.

Software-Defined Radio In many areas of the country, it is not unusual for ambulances to have multiple communications devices. These may be required in order to talk with other response agencies that use other bands (e.g., VHF versus

800 MHz), to overcome areas of bad reception, or for other reasons. In rural services it would not be unusual to find a VHF radio (to talk locally), a cell phone, an 800-MHz trunked radio (to talk with hospitals in "the big city"), and a satellite phone for those areas that are totally "dead" for other forms of communications. The trick is knowing which device to use at any given moment in the middle of an emergency.

Now imagine a communications device that combines all these bandwidths, that is smart enough to "sniff" the airwaves covered for strong signals and no competing transmissions, and then obeys a protocol programmed into it for connecting the user with the desired target, say "Hospital A." The feature of combining a wide range of radio bands is called **multiband radio**. The feature of "sniffing" the airwaves for signal strength and clear channels among the bands in the device is called **cognitive radio**. Like trunked radios, it can pick an open, strong frequency without the user knowing which one was selected (they just know they are talking to Hospital A). Finally, the ability exists to combine all these features and then program them with additional operational protocols (e.g., "only select satellite transmission if all other options are unreliable"—because satellite use can be relatively expensive).

Multiband radios are now available that cross bands from high frequency to VHF, UHF, and 800 MHz in one device. These radios can be programmed to jump from channels in one band to another very quickly and to scan channels throughout. Devices that combine the new public safety broadband capability and satellite capability are expected to be produced to give universal public safety interoperable broadband coverage. Cognitive and software-defined radios are widely available and beginning to make inroads in the public safety arena.

New Technology

When planning got under way for a nationwide public safety broadband system, between 2005 and 2010, planners watched popular commercial applications such as the Apple iPhone cause a boom in broadband use that began eating up an increasing share of available **bandwidth**. Consequently, public safety communications planners in the FCC and the emergency services began to investigate how much bandwidth they were going to require.

One of the earliest efforts in this vein was sponsored by the National Public Safety Telecommunications Council (NPSTC), the National Association of State EMS Officials (NASEMSO), and the National Association of EMS Physicians (NAEMSP) and was funded by the federal government. An expert panel was created that produced a report in 2010. The panel was asked to consider "What potential diagnostic and treatment technologies may possibly be used in the next 10 years that have implications for voice and data communications technology and bandwidth use?" The panel's report affirmed some national consensus work by the Intelligent Transportation Society of America (ITSA) in 2008 and the U.S. Department of Homeland Security's SafeCom in their document *Public Safety Communications Statement of Requirements*" in 2006.

The following sections describe some of the new technologies that the expert panel and others have predicted. These predicted technologies are being used by researchers, the FCC, and others to develop various projections of bandwidth that will be needed for a public safety broadband system.

One conclusion is clear. If any of these technologies become used to any great degree by multiple EMS provider agencies in any given area, broadband access will be mandatory. Current communications capabilities in the narrowband frequencies EMS has traditionally used, and continues to use, cannot support these patient care operations.

Medical Quality Video and Imaging

The use of video to send patient images from the scene or ambulance to a physician consultant/medical director is being used currently in Texas, Arizona, and Louisiana.[13] While the utility of video in EMS remains an open question in the national EMS community, it is more likely to have a role in rural settings than in urban settings for two reasons: a lesser call volume and the emerging concept of community paramedicine in rural areas.

Call Volume   First, urban systems have high call volumes, and can afford highly trained EMS personnel (paramedics) who have a high level of patient interaction experience. The combination in urban systems of a large call volume, short transport times to hospitals, and the training and experience of the personnel means that true emergencies are dealt with effectively and that subtleties in signs and symptoms that may become a treatment factor later can be managed by a physician in the ED after a few minutes' transport.

Rural areas often do not have the call volume to be able to afford the cost of paramedic-level personnel or to provide sufficient experience to maintain an effective emergency practice. Transport times are relatively long, and subtle signs and symptoms that may not be appreciated by personnel with a lesser amount of training and experience may become a treatment factor before arrival at the hospital.

Therefore, in urban areas, injecting the expense and process of video transmission may not be as value-added as it could be in rural areas. In the rural areas, the interpretive eye of an emergency physician able to view the patient, or see portable CT images (e.g., to determine the type of stroke a patient is suffering), or review portable ultrasound video/images of the patient (e.g., to determine the presence of internal bleeding) may make a critical difference in treatment and how and where the patient is transported.

Today, satellite-based and wired broadband audio/video/imaging systems operate in military and civilian applications to link remote and rural medical facilities with specialists in urban centers to provide intensive care monitoring, treatment, and "tele-trauma" consultation. The public safety broadband network, including satellite backup and node links to telemedicine and other fiber networks, could wirelessly provide these capabilities to ambulance and rural hospital/clinic personnel to effectively intervene in life-threatening situations that they would otherwise not be adequately trained or experienced to accomplish.

Community Paramedicine   Second, an emerging concept in rural EMS and health care is community paramedicine. Under a widely discussed "medical home" concept of implementation and financing, paramedics and other EMTs could become affordable in rural communities because they not only provide advanced life support services but also help to fill gaps in primary health care services. Working in and out of rural clinics and hospitals, paramedics and other EMTs could provide preventive care services in the community and other primary care and follow-up services in patient homes. They would be responsible for patient remote monitoring and for visiting patients in their homes, thereby reducing the need for clinic visits and catching incipient problems before they necessitate an ambulance call or a clinic or ED visit.

Paramedics would be able to respond to some emergency calls and be able to address the patient's needs without transport to a hospital. (One study suggests that transports could be reduced by 15 percent with such a system in an urban setting.)[14] Because it would not be cost-effective to train these EMS providers at a level to make them independent practitioners, the ability to wirelessly video consult with physicians and mid-level practitioners in rural clinics and hospitals will become crucial for the benefits of community paramedicine to be robustly realized.

This concept projects a need for ongoing and frequent broadband use by EMS in rural areas in years to come.

Other EMS Applications

The following are other technology applications with broadband implications that the national EMS communications initiatives have suggested:

- *Patient Multi-Vital-Signs Monitoring.* The ability to attach one or more micro-monitors to a patient to wirelessly receive and transmit electrocardiograph, capnography, blood pressure, and other vital signs packaged for display in a database.

- *Responder Multi-Vital-Signs Monitoring.* Similar to the patient multi-vital-sign monitoring but intended for use by EMS responders monitoring fire, police, and other responders in hazardous circumstances (e.g., firefighters inside a burning building, SWAT team members inside a building in a hostage-taking scenario). This could also be used to detect chemicals, gases, radioactivity, and other hazards being encountered by monitored responders.

- *Stand-Off Vital-Signs Monitoring.* The ability to wirelessly detect, receive, and transmit multiple vital signs to a database without physically touching the patient.

- *Infrared Crowd Disease Detection.* The ability to wirelessly scan, receive, and transmit to a database the body temperatures (and body area temperatures) of individuals in crowds that suggest illness.

- *Wireless Speech-to-Text Translation.* The ability to speak into a microphone in a noisy emergency scene environment and have that speech translated and wirelessly transmitted into an ad hoc patient-event database for real-time review by others on the scene, coming to the scene, or in a hospital ED supervising care at the scene.

- *Receipt of Electronic Patient Records in Real Time.* The ability of on-scene EMS staff to receive and potentially manipulate (to focus on pertinent records only) medical

history for their patients either wirelessly from a regional health care medical record system or by patient-carried data records.

- *Creation of Ad Hoc Multi-Component Patient Databases.* This is simply transmission of electronic patient care reports to hospitals before the patient arrives, augmented by separate transmissions of 12-lead electrocardiography and simple vital sign transmission. Using technologies already described, the ability to create, in a single-user interface window, data sent wirelessly from the scene that includes video, multi-vital-signs, voice-to-text translated patient notes, and pertinent patient history components. This database could be made available in real time to authorized responders (e.g., incoming airmedical crews who will transport the patient), specialists guiding care remotely (e.g., trauma surgeons directing a specialized procedure in the field), and emergency physicians routinely supervising EMS calls.

- *EMS-Mediated Remote Patient-Monitoring Systems and "Just in Time" Patient Warning and Reference Guidance.* In community paramedicine and other settings, patients with post-hospital-discharge and/or chronic-health-monitoring needs can be remotely followed through the use of multi-vital-signs monitors (as described earlier), video, or specialized monitors appropriate to their condition. These could be monitored at EMS dispatch and/or nurse advice service centers and would have alarms should the vital signs monitored go outside a preset range.

While this kind of monitoring could be done by wireline service in most settings, though less so in rural areas, the ability to rebroadcast the monitoring device transmissions to responding EMS crews would need to be wireless. In addition, based on the patient history and current monitoring results, care warnings pertinent to the particular patient and condition, along with other relevant reference or medical protocol guidance, could automatically be sent to EMS responders in real time. In a similar fashion, "I've fallen and I can't get up" emergency alerting systems, currently wireline dependent and plaguing responders as a common source of false alarms, could be set up with audio-video and vital-signs-monitoring interfaces with not only wireline support but wireless retransmission to responding EMS crews.

- *Advanced Automatic Crash Notification (AACN) Data Rebroadcasting and "Just in Time" Training and Reference Material Rebroadcasting.* AACN has the potential to significantly reduce death and disability in rural car crashes by eliminating the time now required to "discover" that the crash has occurred, the time required to determine the physical location of the crash, and the time now required to respond to a crash and determine that specialty response (e.g., extrication, special resources) is needed.

To take optimum advantage of these potential time savings, the AACN data should be simultaneously transmitted to all potential responders and to hospital and specialty care facilities that have requested to be notified of crashes exceeding a certain severity in a specific geographic area. In addition, certain crash data need to be automatically assessed and resulting information transmitted to responders and facilities based on the assessment. For example, speed/rollover/impact-vector data may be among data used to determine the severity of the crash and result in automatic dispatch of airmedical and other specialty responders and notification of trauma centers.

Other vehicle data such as vehicle type and year/speed/rollover/impact-vector could be used to send an electronic vehicle access manual to responding extrication crews with diagrams and methods for best accessing patients and avoiding hazards in that vehicle.

○ *Closed Circuit Television (CCTV) Scene Transmission.* Wireless receipt of live video feeds of an emergency scene from traffic, police, homeland security, and other public monitoring CCTV systems by responding crews will help plan approach and vehicle staging at the scene.

○ *Robotic Remote Hazard Suppression and Patient Extrication.* The use of remotely controlled robots to defuse/suppress hazards and remove patients from hazardous settings. This application requires audio, video, and robot-control data transmission.

○ *Wireless Vehicle Systems, Equipment and Supply Monitoring.* The ability now exists to monitor virtually every critical system of a public safety vehicle. Radio frequency identification (RFID) and other tagging device technology make it possible to track the inventory of equipment and supplies in a vehicle. Wirelessly transmitting this information to the vehicle operator's communications unit, with event-linked special warnings (e.g., sending a "leaving scene to transport to hospital" message while a critical patient care device is registered as not having been returned to the vehicle; transmitting an "en route to scene" message with a critically low air pressure in a tire or low inventory of a critical supply) would reduce delays in restocking and inventorying vehicles and medical errors caused by missing equipment or supplies.

○ *Syndromic Surveillance and Quick Alerting to Specific Populations.* Real-time transmission of dispatch and ePCR data to monitoring systems that assess for specific patterns of patient complaints, signs, and symptoms in specific geographic areas. Transmission of these assessments to EMS responders and public health authorities when specific outbreak or hazardous event occurrence is predicted.

PUBLIC SAFETY COMMUNICATIONS SYSTEM PLANNING AND FUNDING

Since 9/11, the need for statewide systems with nationwide capability for interoperability has changed the ways public safety communications systems are planned and implemented.

No longer can EMS communications systems be planned as a "stovepipe" activity. Today, they must be part of larger local, regional, statewide, and national interoperable public safety and health care communications systems. To that end, and because EMS has a poor track record of participating in and benefitting from federal and state planning and funding initiatives, compared with the success of fire and law enforcement, today's paramedic and agency officials should be aware of opportunities to be a part of communications system planning and funding initiatives.

Under the auspices of the U.S. Department of Homeland Security's Office of Emergency Communications (OEC), much progress has been made in ensuring well-planned development of interoperable public safety communications systems on the national, state, regional, and local levels. In 2009, for the first time ever, a National Emergency Communications Plan (NECP) was developed by OEC. Also, for the first time ever, virtually every state and territory developed a statewide communications interoperability plan (SCIP) under the leadership of a statewide, multidisciplinary public safety committee (generically referred to as a statewide interoperability executive committee [SIEC] but given different names in various states). States are now developing statewide interoperability coordinator (SWIC) positions as a single point of responsibility for system development and funding disbursement. All states are encouraged by OEC, and by grant incentives, to have SCIPs, SIECs, and SWICs. (The funding initiatives through which OEC provides funding generally require the states to pass 80 percent of the funds to local agency providers.) It is up to local paramedics and agencies to take advantage of these opportunities to be heard and to have projects funded.

PUBLIC SAFETY COMMUNICATIONS REGULATION

The **Federal Communications Commission (FCC)** controls and regulates all nongovernmental communications in the United States. This includes AM and FM radio, television, aircraft, marine, and mobile land-frequency ranges. The FCC has designated frequencies within each radio band for special use. They include public safety frequencies in all bandwidths. The FCC, in 2008, established a new office to handle public safety issues, the Public Safety and Homeland Security Bureau. The FCC's primary functions include:

- Licensing and allocating radio frequencies
- Establishing technical standards for radio equipment
- Licensing and regulating the technical personnel who repair and operate radio equipment
- Monitoring frequencies to ensure appropriate usage
- Spot-checking base stations and dispatch centers for appropriate licenses and records

The FCC requires all EMS communications systems to follow appropriate governmental regulations and laws. In licensing activities, the FCC requires public safety agencies to use frequency coordinators. For EMS this is the International Municipal Signal Association (IMSA). You must stay abreast of and obey any FCC regulations that apply to your communications.

SUMMARY

This is an extremely exciting time to be involved in EMS. Advances in communications technology are dramatically improving the communications among patients, paramedics, and physicians. As systems improve and technology becomes more affordable, paramedics will be able to arrive on scene of an injury within just a few minutes and, with the click of a button, obtain all the necessary medical information from the patient. As they load and transport the patient, the satellite communications system will link streaming video and audio with the emergency room doctor.

As one of the fundamental aspects of prehospital care, accurate and effective communications help ensure an EMS system's efficiency and improve a patient's survivability. Communications includes not only your radio traffic but also your spoken and nonspoken (body language) messages. All your communications must be concise, professional, and complete and must conform to national and local protocols. As communications systems and technology continue to advance, so will patient care and survival rates. The paramedic will be able to quickly gain access to the appropriate facility and medical direction, allowing for a much quicker and more seamless treatment plan through discharge at the hospital.

YOU MAKE THE CALL

A call comes into your unit for a "possible heart attack" on State Route 11. You and your partner climb into Palermo Rescue, a nontransport first-response vehicle. Your response time is about 10 minutes. On arrival, a family member meets you. He leads you into the den of a small farmhouse. Here you see your patient sitting in an overstuffed chair. You note that your patient is a 69-year-old male in obvious distress.

You begin questioning your patient to develop a history. As he speaks, you immediately notice that he has difficulty breathing. He complains of severe chest pain, which began about 30 minutes ago. With his hand, he indicates that the pain is pressure-like and substernal. He also indicates that it radiates to his left arm and jaw. He describes a history of heart disease, including two prior heart attacks. Three years ago, he had cardiac bypass surgery. He currently takes Lanoxin, Lasix, Capoten, and an aspirin a day. He is allergic to Mellaril.

You and your partner complete your assessment. Your patient says he weighs about 250 pounds. He is alert, but anxious. He exhibits jugular venous distention and bibasilar crackles. His abdomen is nontender. His distal pulses are good. Vital signs include blood pressure 210/110 mmHg, pulse of 70 per minute and regular, and respirations of 20 breaths per minute and mildly labored. Pulse oximetry is 93 percent on supplemental oxygen. During your assessment, your patient becomes progressively more dyspneic. The transporting ambulance arrives and the paramedic asks you to give a radio report to the receiving hospital based on your assessment while she prepares her patient for transport.

- Based on the information provided, organize and prepare your radio report to inform the receiving hospital of your patient's condition.

See Suggested Responses at the back of this book.

REVIEW QUESTIONS

1. The process of exchanging information from one individual to another is:
   a. encoding.   c. communication.
   b. decoding.   d. communion.

2. General radio procedures include all of the following except:
   a. listen for traffic before speaking.
   b. press the transmit button for 1 second before speaking.
   c. speak slowly and clearly.
   d. describe in detail your needs and the situations before releasing the transmit button.

3. When receiving orders from a dispatcher or physician you should:
   a. use the echo procedure.
   b. confirm the order.
   c. write the order down.
   d. none of the above.

4. A recent report entitled "Recommendations from the Expert Panel: Advanced Automatic Collision Notification and Triage of the Injured Patient" shows that _____ shows promise in improving outcomes among severely injured crash patients.
   a. ACANN   c. ANCCA
   b. AACN   d. NCAS

5. A recent report entitled "Recommendations from the Expert Panel: Advanced Automatic Collision Notification and Triage of the Injured Patient" found that Advanced Collision Notification can improve outcomes among seriously injured patients by:
   a. predicting the likelihood of serious injury among vehicle occupants.
   b. decreasing response times by prehospital care providers.

   c. assisting with field triage destination and transportation decisions.
   d. decreasing the time it takes for patients to receive definitive trauma care.
   e. all of the above.

6. _____ frequencies may be used by cities and municipalities for their ability to better transmit through concrete and steel.
   a. UHF   c. 800-mHz
   b. VHF   d. none of the above

7. _____ frequencies are typically used by county and suburban agencies due to their ability to transmit over various terrain and longer distances.
   a. UHF   c. 800-mHz
   b. VHF   d. none of the above

8. The most basic form of communications systems uses _____ transmissions, which use the same frequency to both transmit and receive.
   a. multiplex   c. simplex
   b. duplex   d. complex

9. A communications system that uses a different transmit and receive frequency, allowing for freer communications between two parties, is called _____.
   a. multiplex   c. simplex
   b. duplex   d. complex

10. _____ systems have the additional capacity to transmit both data and voice simultaneously.
    a. Multiplex   c. Simplex
    b. Duplex   d. Complex

See answers to Review Questions at the back of this book.

REFERENCES

1. Department of Homeland Security. SAFECOM [Available at: http://www.safecomprogram.gov/default.aspx]

2. National EMS Information System (NEMSIS). The NEMSI Technical Assistance Center (TAC) . . . [Available at: http://www.nemsis.org/]

3. American College of Emergency Physicians (ACEP). "Automatic crash notification and intelligent transportation systems." *Ann Emerg Med* 55 (2010): 397.

4. National Emergency Number Association (NENA). National Emergency Number Association. [Available at: http://www.nena.org/]

5. Association of Public-Safety Communications Officials (APCO). [Available at: http://www.apco911.org/]

6. Department of Transportation, Research and Innovative Technology Administration. Next Generation 911. [Available at: http://www.apco911.org/]

7. Centers for Disease Control and Prevention. Recommendations from the Expert Panel: Advanced Automatic Collision Notification and Triage of the Injured Patient. [Available at: http://www.cdcfoundation.org/sitefiles/AACNReport.pdf]

8. Wilson, S., M. Cooke, R. Morrell et al. "A Systematic Review of the Evidence Supporting the Use of Priority Dispatch of Emergency Ambulances." *Prehosp Emerg Care* 6 (2002): 42–49.

9. Billittier, A. J., 4th, E. B. Lerner, W. Tucker, and J. Lee. "The Lay Public's Expectations of Prearrival Instructions When Dialing 911." *Prehosp Emerg Care* 4 (2000): 234–237.

10. Munk, M. D., S. D. White, M. L. Perry et al. "Physician Medical Direction and Clinical Performance at an Established Emergency Medical Services System." *Prehosp Emerg Care* 13 (2009): 185–192.

11. Cheung, D. S., J. J. Kelly, C. Beach et al. "Improving Handoffs in the Emergency Department." *Ann Emerg Med* 55 (2010): 171–180.

12. Chan, T. C., J. Killeen, W. Griswold, and L. Lenert. "Information Technology and Emergency Medical Care during Disasters." *Acad Emerg Med* 11 (2004): 1229–1236.

13. DREAMS Ambulance Project. [Available at: http://tees.tamu.edu/index.jsp?page=feature_dreams]

14. Haskins, P. A., D. G. Ellis, and J. Mayrose. "Predicted Utilization of Emergency Medical Services Telemedicine in Decreasing Ambulance Transports." *Prehosp Emerg Care* 6 (2002): 445–448.

FURTHER READING

Bass, R., J. Potter, K. McGinnis, and T. Miyahara. "Surveying Emerging Trends in Emergency-related Information Delivery for the EMS Profession." *Topics in Emergency Medicine* 26 (April–June 2004): 2, 93–102.

Fitch, J. "Benchmarking Your Comm Center." *JEMS* 2006: 98–112.

McGinnis, K. K. "The Future of Emergency Medical Services Communications Systems: Time for a Change." *N C Med J* 68 (2007): 283–285.

McGinnis, K. K. *Future EMS Technologies: Predicting Communications Implications*. National Public Safety Telecommunications Council, National Association of State EMS Officials, National Association of EMS Physicians: June, 2010.

McGinnis, K. K. "The Future Is Now: Emergency Medical Services (EMS) Communications Advances Can Be as Important as Medical Treatment Advances When It Comes to Saving Lives." *Interoperability Today* (SafeCom, U.S. Department of Homeland Security), Volume 3, 2005.

McGinnis, K. K. *Rural and Frontier Emergency Medical Services Agenda for the Future*. National Rural Health Association Press: October, 2004.

McGinnis, K. K., et al. *Guide to Information Communications Technology for EMS Officials*. NASEMSO/NHTSA: July, 2008-07-08.

10

Documentation

Bryan Bledsoe, DO, FACEP, FAAEM, EMT-P
Jeff Brosious, EMT-P

STANDARD
Preparatory (Documentation)

COMPETENCY
Integrates comprehensive knowledge of EMS systems, the safety and well-being of the paramedic, and medical/legal and ethical issues, which is intended to improve the health of EMS personnel, patients, and the community.

OBJECTIVES

Terminal Performance Objective
After reading this chapter you should be able to create complete, well-written patient care reports.

Enabling Objectives
To accomplish the terminal performance objective, you should be able to:

1. Define key terms introduced in this chapter.

2. Explain the purposes and goals of the patient care report in EMS.

3. Explain the importance of proper spelling, terminology, abbreviations, and acronyms, or as an alternative, plain English, in written documentation.

4. Discuss the importance of accurate documentation of times and radio communications.

5. Given a series of patient care reports, identify the elements of good documentation.

6. Given a variety of patient care scenarios, write effective patient care narratives using a standard format.

7. Discuss the differences in documentation for special situations such as refusals of care and mass-casualty incidents.

8. Predict the consequences of inappropriate documentation.

9. Discuss the benefits and drawbacks of electronic patient care reports as compared to paper patient care reports.

KEY TERMS
addendum, p. 184
against medical advice (AMA),
  p. 188
bubble sheets, p. 174
field diagnosis, p. 186

jargon, p. 185
libel, p. 185
prehospital care report (PCR),
  p. 172
response time, p. 173

slander, p. 185
triage tags, p. 190

Tom Brewster is nervous. He has never been to a deposition before, and though everyone has assured him that he is not the target of any legal action, he has to wonder what the lawyers want from him.

As he sits outside the conference room, he goes over the call in his head. It was about 2:30 in the morning. He and Eric Billings, his partner, had just finished cleaning up from a GI bleeder when they were dispatched to the single-vehicle crash. The driver had gone off the left side of the road, crossed a ditch, and smashed into a tree. He had been lucky. He was out of the car, standing on the side of the road, and did not seem to have any serious injuries. He told Tom and Eric, "I think I'm fine, I just fell asleep and ran off the road." Still, they had performed a primary assessment followed by a rapid trauma assessment, immobilized the man, administered oxygen, and transported him to the emergency department. Tom rode in the back with the patient. On the way to the hospital he checked the glucose level, started an IV as a precaution, and applied a cardiac monitor.

"Everything was normal," Tom now thinks. "What did I miss?" He has reread his prehospital care report a hundred times. Though it has been three years, he now remembers almost every detail of the call. Until two weeks ago, he had almost completely forgotten about it.

All too soon, the lawyers call Tom into the conference room, introduce themselves, and swear him to honesty. One of the lawyers begins. "Do you recall the crash that occurred on the evening in question?"

"Yes, I do," Tom replies. He recounts that upon their arrival at the scene, the driver was out of the vehicle. Tom states that they managed him like any other trauma patient, and he had no obvious injuries or indications of illness.

"Did the gentleman tell you he is diabetic?"

"No," Tom answers, "but we checked his blood sugar, and it was normal."

"Did he tell you he has heart problems?"

"No," Tom says again, "but we did put him on the heart monitor, and his rhythm was normal."

"Did he tell you he ran off the road because he passed out?"

"No, he told me he fell asleep." Tom feels better. He has the answer to every question, and he has the PCR to back him up.

After a few more questions, the lawyers dismiss Tom and allow him to leave. He has no idea what they were getting at, but he does know that he answered every question honestly. He wonders if he would have had all the answers if the case had been from six or eight years ago. He has really worked on his documentation in the last few years, and he knows he would have never remembered all those details without the help of his PCR.

Six weeks later Tom gets a letter from the lawyer thanking him for his testimony. It turns out the patient was suing his private doctor for not "recognizing his obvious diabetes and heart problems. He claimed these illnesses caused him to be involved in the motor vehicle accident, and it resulted in serious injury." Tom's testimony—and his PCR—have been pivotal in getting the case dismissed.

INTRODUCTION

The **prehospital care report (PCR)** is a factual record of events that occur during an EMS call or other patient contact. When written correctly it accurately describes your assessment and care throughout the emergency call. It documents exactly what you did, when you did it, and the effects of your interventions.

It can be your best friend or your worst enemy in a court proceeding.

Your PCR is your sole permanent, complete written record of events during the ambulance call. The dispatch center may have a record of the call times and audiotapes of radio transmissions, and your patient will have his memory of the call. You and other responders also may have some recollections about the call. However, your PCR will always be considered the most comprehensive and reliable record of the event. In addition, it reflects your professionalism. A well-written, thorough PCR suggests a thorough, efficient assessment and quality care. A sloppy, incomplete PCR suggests sloppy, inefficient care.

You will often be the first member of the health care system with whom the patient interacts. At the very least, the results of patients' interaction with you and other EMS personnel will affect their opinion of the health care system in general. EMS is a profession in which you can make a difference. Every call and every patient interaction can literally mean the difference between life and death for the patient. Few professions carry such awesome responsibility.

The PCR has three major goals:

- *To provide information to subsequent health care professionals about the patient and treatments provided in the prehospital setting.* This information helps the nursing staff, emergency physicians, and even physicians who will be caring for the patient in the hospital.

- *To provide essential information for proper billing of the patient.* There is a direct correlation between the detail of the report and the level of reimbursement subsequently provided for care and transport of the patient.

- *To provide a legal record of the call's circumstances.* There have been many cases where poor documentation was a factor in EMS personnel losing a lawsuit and many cases where good documentation has resulted in EMS personnel winning a lawsuit—or, more likely, not being sued in the first place.

USES FOR DOCUMENTATION

Your PCR will be a valuable resource for a variety of people. They include medical professionals, EMS administrators, researchers, and occasionally, lawyers.

Medical

Hospital staff (nurses and physicians) may need more information from you than they can get before you have to take another call. For example, they may want a chronological account of your patient's mental status from the time you arrived on the scene. Your PCR can tell the emergency department staff of your patient's condition before he arrived at the hospital. It serves as a baseline for comparing assessment findings and detecting trends that indicate improvement or deterioration.

● **Figure 10-1** The run data in a prehospital care report is vital to your agency's efforts to improve patient care.

The surgical staff will want to know the mechanism of injury and other pertinent findings during your primary assessment of your patient and the scene.

If your patient is admitted to the hospital, the floor or intensive care unit staff may need more information about his original condition than he can remember. In addition, your PCR provides them with information from people at the scene to whom they might not have access—family, bystanders, first responders, or other witnesses. Knowing about the circumstances that led to the event or the mechanism of injury may also help rehabilitation specialists to provide better therapy. Your PCR becomes an important document that helps ensure your patient's continuous effective care (Figure 10-1 ●).

Administrative

EMS administrators must gather information for quality improvement and system management. Information regarding **response times**, call location, the use of lights and siren, and date and time is vital to evaluating your system's readiness to respond to life-threatening emergencies. It also is essential to providing information about community needs. The quality improvement or quality assurance committee will use PCRs to identify problems with individual paramedics or with the EMS system. In some agencies, the billing department will need to determine which services are billable. Insurance carriers may need to know more about the illness or injury to process the claim. Some states will use your PCR data to allocate funding for regional systems.

Research

Your PCR may give researchers useful data about many aspects of the EMS call. For example, they may analyze your recorded data to determine the efficacy of certain medical devices or interventions such as drugs and invasive procedures. They also may use the data to cut costs, alter staffing, and shorten response times. Some systems use computerized or electronic PCRs and a computerized database to analyze the data (Figure 10-2 ●).

▶ Uses for PCRs

CONTENT REVIEW
▶ Uses for PCRs
- Medical
- Administrative
- Research
- Legal

Prehospital Care Report

Agency Name	ARLINGTON RESCUE				
Dispatch Information	CARDIAC				
Call Location	124 CYPRUS ST 2nd FLOOR				

MILEAGE
END 2 4 4 9 6
BEGIN 2 4 4 7 6
TOTAL 0 0 0 2 0

LOCATION CODE
0 1 2 4

CHECK ONE: ☑ Residence ☐ Health Facility ☐ Farm ☐ Indus. Facility ☐ Other Work Loc. ☐ Roadway ☐ Recreational ☐ Other

CALL TYPE AS REC'D
☑ Emergency
☐ Non-Emergency
☐ Stand-by

MECHANISM OF INJURY
☐ MVA (✓ seat belt used) N/A
☐ Fall of _____ feet N/A
☐ Unarmed assault
☐ GSW
☐ Knife
☐ Machinery
☐ _____

USE MILITARY TIMES
CALL REC'D 0 7 0 5
ENROUTE 0 7 0 7
ARRIVED AT SCENE 0 7 1 9
FROM SCENE 0 7 3 8
AT DESTIN 0 7 5 4
IN SERVICE 0 8 1 0
IN QUARTERS 0 8 3 2

CONTENT REVIEW

▶ Characteristics of a Well-Written PCR

- Appropriate medical terminology
- Correct abbreviations and acronyms
- Accurate, consistent times
- Thoroughly documented communications
- Pertinent negatives
- Relevant oral statements of witnesses, bystanders, and patient
- Complete identification of all additional resources and personnel

Regardless of the method you use, your written documentation provides the basis for continuously improving patient care in your EMS system.

Legal

Your PCR becomes a permanent part of your patient's medical record. Lawyers may refer to it when preparing court actions, and in a legal proceeding it might be your sole source of information about the case. You may be called on to testify in a case where your PCR becomes the central piece of evidence in your testimony. Or your PCR may serve as evidence in a criminal case and help determine the accused's innocence or guilt. Each state has its own laws regarding the length of time the hospital must keep its records.

Always write your PCR as if you know you will have to refer to it someday in a court proceeding. Describe your patient's condition when you arrived and during your care, and note his status on arrival at the hospital. Always document his condition before and after any interventions, and avoid writing any subjective opinions such as "the patient is intoxicated, obnoxious, and looks like a crack-addict." After your PCR is written, ask your partner to review it for completeness and accuracy. A complete, accurate, and objective account of the emergency call may be your best and only defense against a plaintiff's attorney who will try to find inconsistencies and ambiguities in your account.

GENERAL CONSIDERATIONS

Every EMS system has its own specific requirements for documentation. The type of call record used also varies from system to system. Some systems use reports with check boxes, whereas some use **bubble sheets**, computer-scannable reports on which you record patient information by filling in boxes or "bubbles" (Figure 10-3 ●). Still others may use computerized documentation. The particular type of operational data collected, such as time intervals, will also differ among systems. For example, proprietary EMS agencies may require more billing information than community-based volunteer agencies. The general characteristics of a well-written PCR, though, remain constant among all agencies and systems.

Medical Terminology

An essential component of good documentation is the appropriate use of medical terminology. Medical terms, though sometimes difficult to spell, transform your report into a

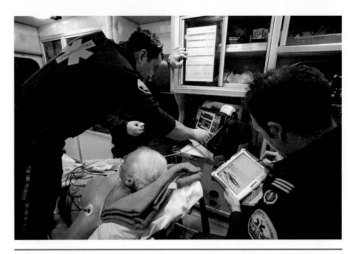

● **Figure 10-2** The handheld electronic clipboard enables you to enter your prehospital care report directly into a computer. (© Kevin Link)

universally accepted medical document. Learning the meanings and correct spellings of the medical terms that you will use in your PCRs is essential. Misused or misspelled words reflect poorly on your professionalism and may confuse the report's readers.

If you do not know how to spell a word, look it up or use another word. Many paramedics carry pocket-size medical dictionaries in their ambulances for this purpose. Using "plain English" is acceptable when you do not know the appropriate medical term or its correct spelling. *Chest* is just as accurate as *thorax* and better than "thoracks." *Belly* is not as professional as *abdomen*, but it is still better than "abodemin."

Do Not Staple or Fold

AGENCY CODE | **UNIT #** | **UNIT TYPE**

UNIT TYPE: Ambulance, Rescue, Other

DATE: Jan, Feb, Mar, Apr, May, Jun, Jul, Aug, Sep, Oct, Nov, Dec — DAY / YR (91, 92, 93, 94, 95 RPT)

PERSONNEL INFORMATION — ATTENDANT #1, ATTENDANT #2, ATTENDANT #3 (F, B, P, N, Q)

RESPONSE/TRANSPORT MODE
To Scene: (1) Non-Emerg, (3) Emergency
From Scene: (2) Non-Emerg, (3) Emergency

RESPONSE OUTCOME
Transported By This Unit
Care Transfer/Another Unit
Cancelled Enroute
Cancelled On Scene
False Call/No Patient Found
Dead on Scene
Refused Treatment
Treated, Refused Transport
P.O.V.
Standby
Unknown
Other

CALL RECEIVED | **ENROUTE** | **ARRIVE SCENE** | **DEPART SCENE** | **ARRIVE HOSPITAL** | **RETURN TO SERVICE** (MILITARY TIME)

INCIDENT LOCATION
Residence, Interstate, Highway, Street/Road, Public Access, Industrial/Off., HMO/Clinic/Doctors Office, Hospital, Other

DISPATCH/INCIDENT TYPE
Abdominal Pain, Asphyxiation/Choke, Chest Pain, Diff. Breathing, Drowning, Heat/Cold Problems, Ill Person, OB/GYN, OD/Poison, Person Down/Unconsc., Psych/Behavioral, Seizures, Other Medical
MVA, MVA - Motorcycle, MVA - Ped/Bike, Assault, Assault - Sexual, Bite/Sting, Burn/Elect., Fall, Person Trapped, Stab/Gunshot, Other Trauma, Standby, InterFacility Transfer

SUSPECTED MEDICAL ILLNESS (None)
P/S: Abdom. Pain, Airway Obstr, Allergic React, Cancer Compli, Cardiac Arrest, Cardiac Sympt., Chest Pain, Childbirth, COPD, Diabetes Comp., Drug Reaction, Heat/Cold Problems
Inhalation, OD/Poison, Psych/Behv, Resp. Arrest, Resp. Dist, Seizures, Stroke, Syncope, Unconscious, Other
P=Primary S=Secondary

INJURY SITE/TYPE
Amputate, Bite/Sting, Blunt-Major, Burn-Elec., Frac/Disloc., Penetrate, Soft-Closed, Soft-Open
None, Head, Face, Eye, Neck, Chest, Back, Upper Ext, Abdomen, Pelvis, Lower Ext

MECHANISM OF INJURY
Flail Chest, Burns 10+%/face/arwy, Fall 20+ feet, Speed 40+ mph, 20+ speed change, Deformity 20+", Intrusion 12+", Rollover, Ejection, Death same MV, Pedest. vs. MV 5+mph, Pedst. thrown/run over, Mtcycle 20+mph/sep., Extrication >15 min.

GLASGOW COMA SCALE
EYES: (4) Spontaneous, (3) To Voice, (2) To Pain, (1) Unresponsive
VERBAL: (5) Oriented, (4) Confused, (3) Inappropriate, (2) Garbled, (1) None
MOTOR: (6) Obeys Comm., (5) Pain-Local., (4) Pain-Withdraws, (3) Pain-Flexion, (2) Pain-Extends, (1) None

PRIOR AID: None, CPR, Extricate, Wound Mgmt — Fire, Police, 1st Resp., Rescue, Bystander

THIS PATIENT LOCATION/PROTECTION
Driver, Front Pass, Rear Pass, Other, Unknown
Shldr/Lap Belt, Shoulder Belt, Lap Belt, Safety Seat, Helmet
Not Used, Not Available, Unknown
Airbag (Deployed) Yes

SEX: F / M
AGE: Months, Approx.
This Patient Resident of: City, County, Arizona, Out of State, Unknown

INITIAL VITAL SIGNS: Unable to Take, Not Taken, Pt. Refused
SYSTOLIC, DIASTOLIC, PULSE, RESP, PUPILS (L/R: NR NR)

BLS TREATMENT (A1 A2 A3 O)
Assessment, C-Spine Precautions, Oxygen, CPR, Crisis Intervention, Defibrillation (AUTO), Extrication, Fracture Stabilize, Hemorrhage Control, Ipecac/Charcoal Admin.
MAST Application, MAST Inflation, Monitor IV, Oral Care/Airway, Oral Glucose, Restraints Applied, Suction, Traction Splint, Wound Management, Other

ALS TREATMENT (A1 A2 A3 O)
Cardiac Monitoring, Cardioversion, Cricothyroidotomy, Defibrillation, EOA
Intubation - Nasal, Intubation - Oral, IV-Central, IV-Peripheral, Medication Admin
NG Tube, Needle Thoracostomy, Phlebotomy, SVN, Other
ATTEMPTS: IV, ET, OTH (1 2 3 U)

CPR INFORMATION
Time: Minutes <4 4-10 >10 Unk
Arrest to CPR, Arrest to Defib, Arrest to ALS
Witnessed Arrest? Y N Unk
Pulse/Rhythm Restored? Y N
Traumatic Cardiac Arrest? Y N

MEDICATIONS
Albuterol, Aminoph., Atropine 1/10, Atropine 8/20, Bretylium, Calcium Chl., D50, Diazepam, Diphenhydram., Dopamine, Epi 1:1000, Epi 1:10,000, Furosemide, Isoetharine, Isoproteranol
Lidocaine-Bolus, Lidocaine Drip, Methylprednisone, Morphine, Naloxone, Nifedipine, Nitrostat. Tab., Nitrous Oxide, Oxytocin, Phenobarbital, Sodium Bicarbonate, Thiamine, Verapamil, Other, HAZMAT

EKG INITIAL/LAST
Nrml Sinus, Sinus Tach, Sinus Brady, Asystole, AV Block, Atrial Fib, Atrial Flut, EMD, Junctional, Paced, SV Tach, Vent Tach, Vent Fib, Other, PVC's

IV TYPE/RATE: TKO, Bolus, Wide, Other
D5W, Normal Saline, Ringers Lact., Other
Peripheral (1 2 3 4), # Central (1 2 3 4)

MEDICAL CONTROL: First / Hospital
Radio/Good, Radio/Poor, Protocol, Telephone, Radio/Phone Patch, Cellular, Phys On-Scene, None Required, Unable
ORDERS BY: Protocol, Standing, Verbal

PATIENT DISPOSITION
Improved, Worsened, Unchanged, Died in ER

 # LINES / **PT. RECEIVED BY** / **RESEARCH CODE**

MISCELLANEOUS
If Multiple Pts On Scene, How Many?
If Transport to Level 1 Receiving Facility, Due to: Pt. Condition, Mechanism

PLEASE DO NOT MARK IN THIS AREA — 2002094

EMS FIRST CARE FORM - ARIZONA DEPARTMENT OF HEALTH SERVICES
Return to State EMS Office

SCANTRON® FORM NO. F-3087-EMS   0792-C 671-5 4 3 2 1
© 1992 EMS DATA SYSTEMS

● **Figure 10-3** This prehospital care report's format can be scanned into a computer. *(© 1992 EMS Data Systems)*

Abbreviations and Acronyms

Both abbreviations and acronyms are formed from the initial letters of the words they stand for. An acronym, however, is an abbreviation you can pronounce as a word. For example, *CPR*, for *cardiopulmonary resuscitation,* is an abbreviation. *AIDS*, for *acquired immune deficiency syndrome*, is an acronym.

Medical abbreviations and acronyms allow you to increase the amount of information you can write quickly on your report (Table 10-1). They also pose problems, however, because they can have multiple meanings. For instance, their meanings can vary in different areas of medicine. Is *CP* chest pain, cardiovascular perfusion, or cerebral palsy? Is *CO* cardiac output or carbon monoxide? Is *BLS* basic life support or burns, lacerations, and swelling? These are all common abbreviations with more than one accepted meaning. Furthermore, many abbreviations are specific to one community. You must be familiar with those used in your local EMS system.

Abbreviations and acronyms can cause considerable confusion when someone unfamiliar with the call reads your report. Health care professionals who are not familiar with local customs or with emergency medicine might not understand them. One way to clarify the meaning of a new abbreviation or acronym is to write it out the first time you use it, followed by the abbreviation or acronym in parentheses. After that, you can use the abbreviation alone throughout the report. The following examples illustrate how abbreviations and acronyms can shorten your narratives. In standard English the report might be written:

> The patient is a 54-year-old conscious and alert male who complains of sudden onset of chest pain and shortness of breath that started 20 minutes ago. He has taken two nitroglycerin with no relief. He denies any nausea, vomiting, or dizziness. He has a past history of coronary artery disease, a heart attack three years ago, and high blood pressure. He takes nitroglycerin as needed, Procardia XL, hydrochlorothiazide, and potassium. He has no known drug allergies.

Using abbreviations and acronyms, the same report might be written:

> Pt. is 54 y/o CAO male c/o sudden onset CP/SOB × 20 min. Pt took NTG × 2 Ø relief. n/v, dizziness. PH: CAD, AMI × 3y, HTN. Meds: NTG prn, Procardia XL, HCTZ and K$^+$; NKDA.

Times

Incident times are another important but perilous part of the PCR. The times you record on your PCR are considered the official times of the incident. For medical and legal purposes, you must ensure their accuracy.[1]

The PCR typically has spaces for the time the call was received, the dispatch time, the time of arrival at the scene, time of departure from the scene, time of arrival at the hospital, and time back in service (refer to Figure 10-1). Other time intervals are important as well. The time you and your crew arrived at the patient's side is often very different from the time the ambulance arrived at the scene—when your patient is on the fourth

floor of a building without an elevator, for example, or in a field several hundred yards from the road. Whatever the reason, document in your report any significant discrepancies between your arrival at the scene and your arrival at the patient. The times of vital signs assessment, medication administration, certain medical procedures as local protocols require, and changes in patient condition are also important and require accurate documentation.

One common problem with documenting times is inconsistencies among the dispatch center clock, the ambulance clock, and your watch. Imagine a report that documents that the ambulance arrived on scene at 20:32 according to the dispatch time, that CPR was started at 20:29 according to your watch, and the first defibrillation was administered at 20:43 according to the defibrillator's internal clock. While we may recognize this phenomenon and tend to discount the accuracy of the recorded times, they are nonetheless the official, legal times. Whenever possible, therefore, record all times from the same clock. When that is not possible, be sure that all the clocks and watches you use are synchronized. If they cannot be synchronized and the documented times seem to conflict with each other, explain this in your narrative. A simple statement such as the following will suffice: "All time intervals on the scene were documented using my watch, all other times are those reported by the dispatch center."

Communications

Your communications with the hospital are another important item to document. Though your system may make voice recordings of those communications, the recordings are usually not kept indefinitely. Again, the PCR will likely be the only permanent record of your discussion with the medical direction physician. Specifically, you should document any medical advice or orders you receive and the results of implementing that advice and those orders. In some situations you might need to document what you reported to the physician and/or discussed with him, so the reader will be able to understand the decision-making process. Finally, always document the physician's name on your PCR and, if possible, have him sign it to verify your treatments.

Pertinent Negatives

The patient assessment and medical interventions are the essence of the EMS event and become the core of your PCR. We will discuss specific approaches to documenting assessment and interventions later in this chapter, but some general rules apply regardless of the method.

Document all findings of your assessment, even those that are normal. Although the positive findings are usually of most interest, some negative findings—known as *pertinent negatives*—are also important. For example, if your respiratory distress patient does not have swollen ankles or crackles, that helps rule out a field diagnosis of congestive heart failure. Or if your patient with a broken leg does not have loss of sensory or motor function, it suggests he has no serious neurologic injury. You should include such information in your report.

TABLE 10-1 | Standard Charting Abbreviations

Patient Information/Categories

Asian	A	Medications	Med
Black	B	Newborn	NB
Chief complaint	CC	Occupational history	OH
Complains of	c/o	Past history	PH
Current health status	CHS	Patient	Pt
Date of birth	DOB	Physical exam	PE
Differential diagnosis	DDx	Private medical doctor	PMD
Estimated date of confinement	EDC	Review of systems	ROS
Family history	FH	Signs and symptoms	S/S
Female	♀	Social history	SH
Hispanic	H	Visual acuity	VA
History	Hx	Vital signs	VS
History and physical	H&P	Weight	Wt
History of present illness	HPI	White	W
Impression	IMP	Year-old	y/o
Male	♂		

Body Systems

Abdomen	Abd	Gynecological	GYN
Cardiovascular	CV	Head, eyes, ears, nose, and throat	HEENT
Central nervous system	CNS	Musculoskeletal	M/S
Ear, nose, and throat	ENT	Obstetric	OB
Gastrointestinal	GI	Peripheral nervous system	PNS
Genitourinary	GU	Respiratory	Resp

Common Complaints

Abdominal pain	abd pn	Lower back pain	LBP
Chest pain	CP	Nausea/vomiting	n/v
Dyspnea on exertion	DOE	No apparent distress	NAD
Fever of unknown origin	FUO	Pain	pn
Gunshot wound	GSW	Shortness of breath	SOB
Headache	H/A	Substernal chest pain	sscp

Diagnoses

Abdominal aortic aneurysm	AAA	Adult respiratory distress syndrome	ARDS
Abortion	Ab	Alcohol	ETOH
Acute myocardial infarction	AMI	Atherosclerotic heart disease	ASHD

(Continued)

TABLE 10-1 | Standard Charting Abbreviations *Continued*

Chronic obstructive pulmonary disease	COPD	Mass-casualty incident	MCI
Chronic renal failure	CRF	Mitral valve prolapse	MVP
Congestive heart failure	CHF	Motor vehicle crash	MVC
Coronary artery bypass graft	CABG	Multiple sclerosis	MS
Coronary artery disease	CAD	Non-insulin-dependent diabetes mellitus	NIDDM
Cystic fibrosis	CF	Organic brain syndrome	OBS
Dead on arrival	DOA	Otitis media	OM
Deep vein thrombosis	DVT	Overdose	OD
Delirium tremens	DTs	Paroxysmal nocturnal dyspnea	PND
Diabetes mellitus	DM	Pelvic inflammatory disease	PID
Dilation and curettage	D&C	Peptic ulcer disease	PUD
Duodenal ulcer	DU	Pregnancies/births (*gravida/para*)	G/P
End-stage renal failure	ESRF	Pregnancy-induced hypertension	PIH
Epstein-Barr virus	EBV	Pulmonary embolism	PE
Foreign body obstruction	FBO	Rheumatic heart disease	RHD
Hepatitis B virus	HBV	Sexually transmitted disease	STD
Hiatal hernia	HH	Transient ischemic attack	TIA
Hypertension	HTN	Tuberculosis	TB
Infectious disease	ID	Upper respiratory infection	URI
Inferior wall myocardial infarction	IWMI	Urinary tract infection	UTI
Insulin-dependent diabetes mellitus	IDDM	Venereal disease	VD
Intracranial pressure	ICP	Wolff-Parkinson-White syndrome (disease)	WPW

Medications

Angiotensin-converting enzyme	ACE	Lactated Ringer's, Ringer's lactate	LR, RL
Aspirin	ASA	Magnesium sulfate	$MgSO_4$
Bicarbonate	HCO_3^-	Morphine sulfate	MS
Birth control pills	BCP	Nitroglycerin	NTG
Calcium	Ca^{2+}	Nonsteroidal anti-inflammatory agent	NSAID
Calcium channel blocker	CCB	Normal saline	NS
Calcium chloride	$CaCl_2$	Penicillin	PCN
Chloride	Cl^-	Phenobarbital	PB
Digoxin	Dig	Potassium	K^+
Dilantin (diphenylhydantoin)	DPH	Sodium bicarbonate	$NaHCO_3$
Diphendydramine	DPHM	Sodium chloride	NaCl

(Continued)

TABLE 10-1 | Standard Charting Abbreviations *Continued*

Diphtheria-pertussis-tetanus	DPT	Tylenol (acetaminophen)	APAP
Hydrochlorothiazide	HCTZ		

Anatomy/Landmarks

Abdomen	Abd	Lymph node	LN
Antecubital	AC	Medial collateral ligament	MCL
Anterior axillary line	AAL	Metacarpophalangeal (joint)	MCP
Anterior cruciate ligament	ACL	Metatarsophalangeal (joint)	MTP
Anterior-posterior	A/P	Midaxillary line	MAL
Distal interphalangeal (joint)	DIP	Posterior axillary line	PAL
Dorsalis pedis (pulse)	DP	Posterior cruciate ligament	PCL
Gallbladder	GB	Proximal interphalangeal (joint)	PIP
Intercostal space	ICS	Right lower lobe	RLL
Lateral collateral ligament	LCL	Right lower quadrant	RLQ
Left lower lobe	LLL	Right middle lobe	RML
Left lower quadrant	LLQ	Right upper lobe	RUL
Left upper lobe	LUL	Right upper quadrant	RUQ
Left upper quadrant	LUQ	Temporomandibular joint	TMJ
Left ventricle	LV	Tympanic membrane	TM
Liver, spleen, and kidneys	LSK		

Physical Exam/Findings

Arterial blood gas	ABG	Electroencephalogram	EEG
Bilateral breath sounds	BBS	Expiratory	Exp
Blood sugar	BS	Extraocular movements (intact)	EOMI
Breath sounds	BS	Fetal heart tones	FHT
Cardiac injury profile	CIP	Full range of motion	FROM
Central venous pressure	CVP	Full-term normal delivery	FTND
Cerebrospinal fluid	CSF	Heart rate	HR
Chest X-ray	CXR	Heart sounds	HS
Complete blood count	CBC	Heel-to-shin (cerebellar test)	$H \rightarrow S$
Computerized tomography	CT	Hemoglobin	Hgb
Conscious, alert, and oriented	CAO	Inspiratory	Insp
Costovertebral angle	CVA	Jugular venous distention	JVD
Deep tendon reflexes	DTR	Laceration	Lac
Dorsalis pedis (pulse)	DP	Level of consciousness	LOC
Electrocardiogram	EKG, ECG	Moves all extremities well	MAEW

(Continued)

TABLE 10-1 | Standard Charting Abbreviations *Continued*

Nontender	NT	Pupils equal, round, reactive to light and accommodation	PERRLA
Normal range of motion	NROM	Range of motion	ROM
Palpation	Palp	Respirations	R
Passive range of motion	PROM	Tactile vocal fremitus	TVF
Point of maximal impulse	PMI	Temperature	T
Posterior tibial (pulse)	PT	Unconscious	Unc
Pulse	P	Urinary incontinence	UI
Pupils equal and reactive to light	PEARL		

Miscellaneous Descriptors

After (post-)	$\bar{p}$	Not applicable	n/a
After eating	pc	Number	No or #
Alert and oriented	A/O	Occasional	Occ
Anterior	ant.	Pack years	pk/yrs, p/y
Approximate	≈	Per	/
As needed	prn	Positive	+
Before (ante-)	$\bar{a}$	Posterior	post.
Before eating (*ante cibum*, before meal)	a.c.	Postoperative	PO
		Prior to arrival	PTA
Body surface area (%)	BSA	Radiates to	→
Celsius	C	Right	®
Change	Δ	Rule out	R/O
Decreased	↓	Secondary to	2°
Equal	=	Superior	sup.
Fahrenheit	F	Times (for 3 hours)	× (×3h)
Immediately	stat	Unequal, not equal	≠
Increased	↑	Warm and dry	W/D
Inferior	inf.	While awake	WA
Left	L	With (*cum*)	$\bar{c}$
Less than	<	Within normal limits	WNL
Moderate	mod.	Without (*sine*)	$\bar{s}$
More than	>	Zero	0
Negative	−		
No, not, none, null	Ø		

Treatments/Dispositions

Advanced cardiac life support	ACLS	Against medical advice	AMA
Advanced life support	ALS	Automated external defibrillator	AED

(Continued)

TABLE 10-1 | Standard Charting Abbreviations *Continued*

Bag-valve mask	BVM	No transport—refusal	NTR
Basic life support	BLS	Nonrebreather mask	NRM
Cardiopulmonary resuscitation	CPR	Nothing by mouth	NPO
Carotid sinus massage	CSM	Occupational therapy	OT
Continuous positive airway pressure	CPAP	Oropharyngeal airway	OPA
Do not resuscitate	DNR	Oxygen	O_2
Endotracheal tube	ETT	Per square inch	psi
Estimated time of arrival	ETA	Physical therapy	PT
External cardiac pacing	ECP	Positive end-expiratory pressure	PEEP
Intermittent positive-pressure ventilation	IPPV	Short spine board	SSB
Long spine board	LSB	Therapy	Rx
Nasal cannula	LSB	Treatment	Tx
Nasogastric	NG	Turned over to	TOT
Nasopharyngeal airway	NPA	Verbal order	VO

Medication Administration/Metrics

Centimeter	cm	Keep vein open	KVO
Cubic centimeter	cc	Kilogram	kg
Deciliter	dL	Liter	L
Drop(s)	gtt(s)	Liters per minute	LPM, L/min, liters/min
Drops per minute	gtts/min		
Every	Q	Microgram	mcg
Grain	gr	Milliequivalent	mEq
Gram	g, gm	Milligram	mg
Hour	h, hr, or °	Milliliter	mL
Hydrogen-ion concentration	pH	Millimeter	mm
Intracardiac	IC	Millimeters of mercury	mmHg
Intramuscular	IM	Minute	min
Intraosseous	IO	Orally	PO
Intravenous	IV	Subcutaneous	SC, SQ
Intravenous push	IVP	Sublingual	SL
Joules	J	To keep open	TKO

Cardiology

Atrial fibrillation	AF	Atrioventricular	AV
Atrial tachycardia	AT	Bundle branch block	BBB

(Continued)

TABLE 10-1 | Standard Charting Abbreviations *Continued*

Complete heart block	CHB	Premature atrial contraction	PAC
Electromechanical dissociation	EMD	Premature junctional contraction	PJC
Idioventricular rhythm	IVR	Premature ventricular contraction	PVC
Junctional rhythm	JR	Pulseless electrical activity	PEA
Modified chest lead	MCL	Supraventricular tachycardia	SVT
Normal sinus rhythm	NSR	Ventricular fibrillation	VF
Paroxysmal atrial tachycardia	PAT	Ventricular tachycardia	VT
Paroxysmal supraventricular tachycardia	PSVT	Wandering atrial pacemaker	WAP

The pertinent negatives vary for each chief complaint. In general, if a positive assessment finding for any given chief complaint would be important, a negative finding probably is pertinent. Even though these findings do not warrant medical care or intervention, your seeking them demonstrates the thoroughness of your examination and history of the event.

Oral Statements

Also essential to every PCR, regardless of approach, are the statements of witnesses, bystanders, and your patient. They help to document the mechanism of injury, your patient's behavior, the events leading up to the emergency, and any first aid or medical care others rendered before you arrived. They also may include information regarding the disposition of personal items such as wallets or purses. At crime scenes, document safety-related information such as weapons disposition. Your PCR may be the only written report of what happened to a murder weapon. Other details such as where you first saw a victim, what position he was in, and the time you arrived on the scene may someday be crucial evidence in a criminal proceeding.

Whenever possible, quote the patient—or other source of information—directly. Clearly identify the quotation with quotation marks, and identify its source. For example:

Bystanders state the patient was "acting bizarre and threatening to jump in front of the next passing car."

Additional Resources

Document all the resources involved in the event. If an air-medical service transported your patient, your documentation should include your assessment and all interventions up to the point when you transferred care. Identify the air-medical service and your patient's ultimate destination, if you know it. If other EMS, fire, rescue/extrication, or law enforcement agencies were involved in the call, document their roles. This can be particularly important in mutual aid calls, when many different agencies cooperate in your patient's care. Also include information about personnel from law enforcement and the coroner's or medical examiner's office for dead-on-arrival (DOA) scenes.

If a physician stops to help, identify him by name and document his qualifying credentials. If one of your medical direction physicians is on the scene and directs care, document his activities. Likewise document the names, credentials, and activities of any other medically qualified personnel present who offer to help. Your clinical experience and local protocols will determine how you integrate qualified health care workers into your emergency scene. Document that integration carefully.

ELEMENTS OF GOOD DOCUMENTATION

A well-written PCR is accurate, legible, timely, unaltered, and professional. Each of these traits is essential.

Completeness and Accuracy

The accurate PCR should be precise but comprehensive.[2] Include all the relevant information that anyone might be expected to want later, and exclude superfluous information. For example, if your patient's foot was run over by a lawn mower, reporting that his great toe on that foot had been amputated six years ago would be important; documenting that he had his tonsils removed when he was three years old probably would not. That you applied direct pressure to the bleeding foot is pertinent; that the lawn mower was a John Deere model 6354 is not.

Many PCRs provide check boxes and a space for written narratives (Figure 10-4 ●). You should complete both the narrative and check-box sections of every PCR. All check-box sections of a document must show that you attended to them, even if you did not use a given section on a call. The check boxes can help to ensure that routine, common information is recorded for every call, but no PCR has a check box for every possible chief complaint, assessment finding, or intervention.

The narrative is the core of the documentation. Even if you document something in a check box, repeating that information in the narrative might be worthwhile. By doing so, you can expand on the yes-or-no limitations of the check box

Prehospital Care Report

FOR BLS FR USE ONLY

M | D | Y — DATE OF CALL
RUN NO.
AGENCY CODE
VEH. ID.

Name
Address
Ph #
AGE
DOB M D Y
SEX M ☐ F ☐
Physician

Agency Name
Dispatch Information
Call Location
CHECK ONE ☐ Residence ☐ Health Facility ☐ Farm ☐ Indus. Facility ☐ Other Work Loc. ☐ Roadway ☐ Recreational ☐ Other

MILEAGE: END / BEGIN / TOTAL
LOCATION CODE

USE MILITARY TIMES
CALL REC'D
ENROUTE
ARRIVED AT SCENE
FROM SCENE
AT DESTIN
IN SERVICE
IN QUARTERS

CALL TYPE AS REC'D.
☐ Emergency
☐ Non-Emergency
☐ Stand-by

COMPLETE FOR TRANSFERS ONLY
Transferred from
☐ No Previous PCR
☐ Unknown if Previous PCR
Previous PCR Number

CARE IN PROGRESS ON ARRIVAL:
☐ None ☐ Citizen ☐ PD/FD/Other First Responder ☐ Other EMS

MECHANISM OF INJURY
☐ MVA (✓ seat belt used ⟶) ☐ Struck by vehicle ☐ Fall of ____ feet ☐ Unarmed assault ☐ GSW ☐ Knife ☐ Machinery ☐ ______
☐ Extrication required ______ minutes
Seat belt used? ☐ Yes ☐ No ☐ Unknown
Seat Belt Use Reported By ☐ Crew ☐ Police ☐ Patient ☐ Other

CHIEF COMPLAINT
SUBJECTIVE ASSESSMENT

PRESENTING PROBLEM
If more than one checked, circle primary
☐ Airway Obstruction
☐ Respiratory Arrest
☐ Respiratory Distress
☐ Cardiac Related (Potential)
☐ Cardiac Arrest
☐ Allergic Reaction
☐ Syncope
☐ Stroke/CVA
☐ General Illness/Malaise
☐ Gastro-Intestinal Distress
☐ Diabetic Related (Potential)
☐ Pain ______
☐ Unconscious/Unresp.
☐ Seizure
☐ Behavioral Disorder
☐ Substance Abuse (Potential)
☐ Poisoning (Accidental)
☐ Shock
☐ Head Injury
☐ Spinal Injury
☐ Fracture/Dislocation
☐ Amputation
☐ Other ______
☐ Major Trauma
☐ Trauma-Blunt
☐ Trauma-Penetrating
☐ Soft Tissue Injury
☐ Bleeding/Hemorrhage
☐ OB/GYN
☐ Burns
Environmental
☐ Heat
☐ Cold
☐ Hazardous Materials
☐ Obvious Death

PAST MEDICAL HISTORY
☐ None
☐ Allergy to ______
☐ Hypertension ☐ Stroke
☐ Seizures ☐ Diabetes
☐ COPD ☐ Cardiac
☐ Other (List) ☐ Asthma
Current Medications (List)

VITAL SIGNS

TIME	RESP	PULSE	B.P.	LEVEL OF CONSCIOUSNESS	GCS	R PUPILS L	SKIN	STATUS
	Rate: ☐ Regular ☐ Shallow ☐ Labored	Rate: ☐ Regular ☐ Irregular		☐ Alert ☐ Voice ☐ Pain ☐ Unresp.		☐ Normal ☐ ☐ Dilated ☐ ☐ Constricted ☐ ☐ Sluggish ☐ ☐ No-Reaction ☐	☐ Unremarkable ☐ Cool ☐ Pale ☐ Warm ☐ Cyanotic ☐ Moist ☐ Flushed ☐ Dry ☐ Jaundiced	☐ C ☐ U ☐ P ☐ S
	Rate: ☐ Regular ☐ Shallow ☐ Labored	Rate: ☐ Regular ☐ Irregular		☐ Alert ☐ Voice ☐ Pain ☐ Unresp.		☐ Normal ☐ ☐ Dilated ☐ ☐ Constricted ☐ ☐ Sluggish ☐ ☐ No-Reaction ☐	☐ Unremarkable ☐ Cool ☐ Pale ☐ Warm ☐ Cyanotic ☐ Moist ☐ Flushed ☐ Dry ☐ Jaundiced	☐ C ☐ U ☐ P ☐ S
	Rate: ☐ Regular ☐ Shallow ☐ Labored	Rate: ☐ Regular ☐ Irregular		☐ Alert ☐ Voice ☐ Pain ☐ Unresp.		☐ Normal ☐ ☐ Dilated ☐ ☐ Constricted ☐ ☐ Sluggish ☐ ☐ No-Reaction ☐	☐ Unremarkable ☐ Cool ☐ Pale ☐ Warm ☐ Cyanotic ☐ Moist ☐ Flushed ☐ Dry ☐ Jaundiced	☐ C ☐ U ☐ P ☐ S

OBJECTIVE PHYSICAL ASSESSMENT

COMMENTS

TREATMENT GIVEN
☐ Moved to ambulance on stretcher/backboard
☐ Moved to ambulance on stair chair
☐ Walked to ambulance
☐ Airway Cleared
☐ Oral/Nasal Airway
☐ Esophageal Obturator Airway/Esophageal Gastric Tube Airway (EOA/EGTA)
☐ EndoTracheal Tube (E/T)
☐ Oxygen Administered @ ____ L.P.M., Method ______
☐ Suction Used
☐ Artificial Ventilation Method ______
☐ C.P.R. in progress on arrival by: ☐ Citizen ☐ PD/FD/Other First Responder ☐ Other
☐ C.P.R. Started @ Time ▶ ____ Time from Arrest Until C.P.R. ▶ ____ Minutes
☐ EKG Monitored (Attach Tracing) [Rhythm(s)______]
☐ Defibrillation/Cardioversion No. Times ____ ☐ Manual ☐ Semi-automatic
☐ Medication Administered (Use Continuation Form)
☐ IV Established Fluid ______ Cath. Gauge
☐ Mast Inflated @ Time ______)
☐ Bleeding/Hemorrhage Controlled (Method Used: ______)
☐ Spinal Immobilization Neck and Back
☐ Limb Immobilized by ☐ Fixation ☐ Traction
☐ (Heat) or (Cold) Applied
☐ Vomiting Induced @ Time ____ Method ______
☐ Restraints Applied, Type ______
☐ Baby Delivered @ Time ____ In County ______
☐ Alive ☐ Stillborn ☐ Male ☐ Female
☐ Transported in Trendelenburg position
☐ Transported in left lateral recumbent position
☐ Transported with head elevated
☐ Other ______

DISPOSITION (See list)
DISP. CODE
CONTINUATION FORM USED YES ⟵

CREW
IN CHARGE ☐ EMT ☐ AEMT #
DRIVER'S NAME ☐ CFR ☐ EMT ☐ AEMT #
NAME ☐ CFR ☐ EMT ☐ AEMT #
NAME ☐ CFR ☐ EMT ☐ AEMT #

AGENCY COPY/WHITE
EMS 100 (11/86) provided by NYS-EMS PROGRAM
DOH 3822 (6/94)

● **Figure 10-4** Complete both the narrative and check-box sections of every PCR. *(NYS Department of Health Bureau of EMS)*

CONTENT REVIEW

► Elements of Good
Documentation

- Complete
- Accurate
- Legible
- Timely
- Without alterations
- Professional

► (Document exactly what
you did, when you did it,
and the effects of your
interventions.)

to explain the timing, the assessment findings, the circumstances, or the changes in patient condition associated with the indicated action. Always make sure that the information in your checked boxes and in your narrative are consistent. Inconsistencies will be extremely difficult to explain later on, especially in front of a jury.

Remember that proper spelling, approved abbreviations, and proper acronyms also affect your PCR's accuracy. Misspelled words lose their meaning, many abbreviations are not universally recognized, and several acronyms have more than one meaning. Make sure that the meaning of any abbreviation or acronym is clear.

Legibility

Poor penmanship and illegible reports lead to poor documentation. Some EMS providers say, "I wrote it, and I can read it. That's all that matters." This is simply not true. The PCR does not exist solely for its author's reference. It is a permanent record that many different people use. Your handwriting must be neat enough that other people can read and understand the report, especially the narrative. It must also be neat enough that you can read and understand it yourself many years from now, long after the event has faded from your memory. Your writing must be heavy enough to transfer to any carbon copies. Using a ballpoint pen whenever possible makes carbon copies more legible and makes it difficult for someone to tamper with the document. Clearly mark the check boxes to eliminate any doubt that a check mark is not just a meaningless scratch. Always remember that other members of the health care team may use the report for medical information, research, or quality improvement.

Timeliness

As a rule, you should avoid writing your report in the ambulance during transport of your patient for two reasons. First, the bumpy ride makes it difficult to write neatly. More importantly, your time is better spent communicating with your patient and conducting ongoing assessments. Most hospitals have an area where you can sit and complete your paperwork once patient care has been transferred.

Ideally, you should complete your report immediately after you complete the emergency call, when the information is fresh in your mind and you can check with your partner or patient if you have any questions about the events. At times you may be too busy to complete the entire documentation immediately following a call. If so, make notes on scratch paper and write enough of the report that you will be able to finish it completely and accurately later. The sooner you finish it, the more details you are likely to recall and the better the report will be.

Absence of Alterations

Mistakes happen. During a busy shift or in the middle of the night you will check the wrong box, misspell a word, or omit important information. You will be thinking of one medication and write another's name on your report. If you make a mistake writing your report, simply cross through the error with one line and initial it (Figure 10-5 ●). Some systems may expect you to date the correction as well. Do not scribble over or blacken out any area of the call report. Never try to hide an error. Such foolish tactics only raise the reader's curiosity about what you wrote originally. After crossing out the error, continue with the correct information. If you find the error after you've already written several more sentences, submit an **addendum**.

Whenever possible, have everyone involved in the call read or reread the PCR before you submit it. Make all corrections before you submit the report to the hospital or to the EMS administrative offices. Do not make changes on the original report after you have submitted it. If for any reason you need to make corrections after you have submitted the report, or some portion of it, place an addendum. Simply note on the original report, "See addendum," and attach the addendum to the original report. Write the addendum on a separate sheet of paper or on an official form if one exists. Likewise, if more information comes to your attention after you have submitted the report, write a supplemental narrative on a separate report form.

Write any addendum to your report as soon as you realize that you made an error or that additional information is needed. Note the purpose of the revision and why the information did not appear on your original report. The addendum should document the date and time that it was written, the reason it was written, and the pertinent information. Only the original author of a report should attach an addendum, as it is part of the official call record. Agencies should have separate forms for other EMS personnel, supervisors, or citizens who, for some reason, want to contribute to the documentation.

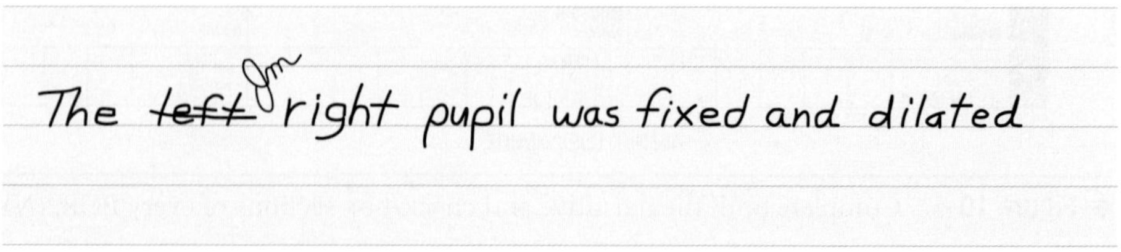

● **Figure 10-5** The proper way to correct a prehospital care report is to draw a single line through the error, write the correct information beside it, and initial the change.

The ~~left~~ right pupil was fixed and dilated

Professionalism

Write your report in a professional manner. Remember that someday it may be scrutinized by hospital staff, quality improvement committees, supervisors, lawyers, and the news media. Your patient's family may request, and is entitled to, a copy of your report from your agency. Write cautiously and avoid any remarks that might be construed as derogatory. **Jargon** can be confusing and does little to enhance your image. Do not describe a patient well known to EMS providers as a "frequent flyer." Never include slang, biased statements, or irrelevant opinions. Include only objective information. "The patient smelled of beer and had slurred speech and difficulty walking" are factual statements. "The patient was very drunk" is an inference; even if accurate, it is still just your opinion. **Libel** and **slander** are, respectively, writing or speaking false and malicious words intended to damage a person's character. Always write and speak carefully. A seemingly innocent phrase or comment can come back to haunt you.

NARRATIVE WRITING

The narrative is the part of the written report in which you depict the call at length. Less structured than the check-box or fill-in sections of your report, the narrative allows you the freedom to describe your assessment findings in detail. When other people read your report, they usually will rely on your written narrative for the most relevant information. For example, as you transfer care to the emergency nurse, she will usually scan your PCR for information concerning your patient's history, vital signs, and physical exam.

Narrative Sections

Any patient documentation includes three sections of importance: the subjective narrative, the objective narrative, and the assessment/management plan.

Subjective Narrative

The subjective part of your narrative typically comprises any information that you elicit during your patient's history. This includes the chief complaint (CC), the history of present illness (HPI), the past history (PH), the current health status (CHS), and the review of systems (ROS). In trauma, this also includes the mechanism of injury (MOI), as told to you by your patient or bystanders. The following is a typical subjective narrative on a patient complaining of shortness of breath:

CC	The patient is a 74-year-old conscious black female who complains, "I can't catch my breath."
HPI	Gradual onset of severe shortness of breath for the past 3 hours; began while sitting in living room watching television; nothing provokes or relieves the dyspnea; her son states this is worse than usual for her. She has had a three-day history of some vague chest discomfort. She denies any chest pressure, nausea, or dizziness.

PH	She has a five-year history of heart problems and congestive heart failure; hospitalized for this problem three times in the past five years; no surgeries.
CHS	Meds: Isosorbide, nitroglycerin, furosemide, digoxin, potassium; no known drug allergies; 50 pack/year smoker; nondrinker; non-drug abuser.
ROS	Resp: Unproductive cough for one day; audible wheezing; no hx of COPD or asthma; last chest X-ray one year ago. Card: no palpitations, pressure, or pain; + orthopnea; + paroxysmal nocturnal dyspnea; + edema for past few days; past ECG one year ago. GU: No changes in urinary patterns. Per. Vasc: + pitting edema for few days; cold feet.

Objective Narrative

The objective part of your narrative usually includes your general impression and any data that you derive through inspection, palpation, auscultation, percussion, and diagnostic testing. This includes vital signs, physical exam, and tests such as cardiac monitoring, pulse oximetry, and blood glucose determination.

To document your physical exam, you can use either of two approaches: head-to-toe or body systems. Although the medical community accepts both extensively, emergency medical services more often use the head-to-toe approach.

Head-to-Toe Approach The head-to-toe approach is well suited for any call when you perform an entire physical exam, because you document your findings in the same order in which you conducted the exam—from head to toe. However, even though you may have conducted your pediatric assessment from toe to head, you should document it in head-to-toe order. This style encourages you to be systematic and thorough. It is appropriate for major trauma and serious medical emergencies, when you examine every body area and system. Include all circulatory and neurologic findings within the body area you are documenting. For example, when recording findings in the extremities, include distal neurovascular function. When documenting the head, include the results of cranial nerve testing. The following illustrates the head-to-toe approach for a patient who has been in a collision:

General	The patient presents in the front seat of the car, in moderate distress with bruises to his forehead and some facial lacerations. Pt. is alert and oriented to self, time, and place.
Vital signs	Pulse—100 strong, regular radial; BP—110/88; resp—24 nonlabored; skin pale and cool.

HEENT	Depression to right frontal bone, minor bleeding controlled prior to arrival; no drainage from ears, nose. No periorbital ecchymosis or Battle's sign; pupils equal and reactive to light; extraocular movements intact, cranial nerves II–XII intact.
Neck	Trachea midline; no jugular vein distention; + cervical spine tenderness.
Chest	Equal expansion; bruises across the chest wall; no deformities; equal bilateral breath sounds.
Abdomen	Soft, nontender, nondistended.
Pelvis	Unstable pelvic ring; pain upon palpation.
Extremities	+ Circulation, sensory, and motor function in all four extremities; no deformities noted.
Posterior	No obvious injuries noted.
Labs	Sinus tachycardia, no ectopy, pulse oximetry 97% on supplemental oxygen.

Body Systems Approach   The body systems approach, as the name indicates, focuses on body systems instead of body areas. It is best suited to screening and preadmission exams in which you conduct a comprehensive exam involving all body systems. Each body system has different key components that you should assess and document.

When you use the body systems approach in emergency medicine, you usually will focus only on the system, or systems, involved in the current illness or injury. For example, a patient having an asthma attack would require an in-depth evaluation of the respiratory system. Another patient with lower abdominal pain would need a close examination of the gastrointestinal system. Neither patient would require a full head-to-toe physical exam but, instead, intensive documentation of the affected body system or systems. The body systems approach can be one of the most comprehensive approaches to documentation. The following illustrates a body systems approach for a patient with chest pain and shortness of breath:

General	Patient is a healthy-looking female who presents sitting upright in her chair, able to speak in phrases only.
Vital Signs	Pulse—irregular, 90; BP—170/80; resp—28 labored; skin—warm and diaphoretic.
HEENT	+ Lip cyanosis and pursing; some nasal flaring; pink, frothy sputum; jugular veins distended.
Respiratory	Labored respiratory effort; accessory neck muscle use; trachea midline; + intercostal, supraclavicular, suprasternal retractions;
	= chest expansion; diffuse crackles and wheezing in all lung fields, decreased breath sounds.

Per. Vasc.	+ Ascites fluid wave; + 2 pitting edema in lower extremities; strong peripheral pulses.
Labs	Sinus tachycardia with occasional unifocal premature ventricular contractions. Pulse oximetry—92% room air; 97% on supplemental oxygen.

Assessment/Management Plan

In the assessment/management section, you document what you believe to be your patient's problem. This is also known as your **field diagnosis**, or impression. For example, your field diagnosis for a patient with chest pain may be "possible angina or rule out myocardial infarction." You do not have to make an exact diagnosis. When you are not sure, simply document what you suspect is the general problem. Sometimes, for instance, your field impression might be "rule out acute abdomen, or seizures." *Rule out* identifies possible diagnoses that you believe the emergency physician should evaluate.

Record your complete management plan from start to finish. This includes how you packaged and moved your patient to the ambulance. Did you carry him on a stair-chair or on a backboard fully immobilized or did he walk? List any interventions you completed before contacting your medical control physician. For example, did you control bleeding with direct pressure? Did you start an IV? Then describe any orders from the medical control physician, and always include his name. Describe how you transported your patient and the effects of any interventions such as drug administration or other invasive procedures. Include the results of ongoing assessments and any changes in your patient's condition. Finally, describe your patient's condition when you transferred care to the emergency staff. The following example is a management plan for a trauma patient with a pelvic fracture whose condition deteriorates en route to the hospital:

On-Scene

Extrication	Rapid extrication from vehicle, placed supine on backboard
Airway	Airway cleared with suctioning, nasopharyngeal airway inserted
Breathing	Oxygen @ 15 liters/min via nonrebreather mask
Circulation	Foot of stretcher raised 30°; bleeding from arm laceration controlled with dry sterile dressing and direct pressure; PASG applied; IV—16 ga. left antecubital area—normal saline run KVO per Dr. Johnson.

Transport

Transported by ground ambulance to University Hospital with full body immobilization supine on long spine board; ETA 10 minutes.

Ongoing	Patient becomes restless and anxious; VS: pulse—120 weak carotid only, BP—50 palpated, resp—28, skin: cool, pale, clammy

| | with some mottling; PASG inflated; initial IV run wide open; second IV 16 ga. right antecubital normal saline—run wide open. |

Arrival

Patient transferred to ED staff; restless; VS: pulse 120, BP—80 palpated, resp—26, skin—mottled and cool.

General Formats

The acronyms SOAP and CHART are memory aids that identify two common patterns for organizing a narrative report. These acronyms provide templates that can be used for most medical and trauma reports. They help you to arrange your history, physical exam, and management plan into a logical, readable structure. They are widely used because they group information in categories that differentiate between subjective and objective information. For example, someone wanting only to determine your patient's medications can find that list easily in history or current health status segments of either the SOAP or the CHART format. Either pattern is acceptable and effective when used consistently.

SOAP Format

SOAP stands for *S*ubjective, *O*bjective, *A*ssessment, and *P*lan. The detailed SOAP format includes:

Subjective	• Chief complaint • History of present illness • Past history • Current health status • Family history • Psychosocial history • Review of systems
Objective	• Vital signs • General impression • Physical exam • Diagnostic tests
Assessment	• Field diagnosis
Plan	• Standing orders • Physician orders • Effects of interventions • Mode of transportation • Ongoing assessment

CHART Format

CHART stands for *C*hief complaint, *H*istory, *A*ssessment, *R*x (treatment), and *T*ransport. The detailed CHART format includes:

Chief complaint	• Primary problem or complaint
History	• History of present illness • Past history • Current health status • Review of systems
Assessment	• Vital signs • General impression • Physical exam • Diagnostic tests • Field diagnosis
Rx	• Standing orders • Physician orders
Transport	• Effects of interventions • Mode of transportation • Ongoing assessment

Other Formats

Like patient assessment itself, documentation is not "one-size-fits-all." No one narrative format is ideal for all situations. Two additional formats—patient management and call incident—are appropriate in certain circumstances.

Patient Management   The patient management format is preferred for some critical patients, such as those in cardiac arrest, when you focus on immediately managing a variety of patient problems and not on conducting a thorough history and physical exam. This format is a chronological account from the time you arrived on the scene until you transferred care to someone else. It emphasizes your assessment and management of the conditions you found. Simply begin your chart with a description of the event and any other pertinent information and then document your management, starting with your airway, breathing, and circulation (ABC) assessment. Record everything in real time and in absolute chronological order, and always include the results of your interventions. A patient management chart would look like this:

Patient is an 89-year-old Hispanic male who was found by his wife unconscious on the floor immediately after collapsing. He presents pulseless and apneic.

Time	Intervention
1320	Immediate CPR while monitor applied.
1322	Quick look—ventricular fibrillation.
1322	Defibrillation @ 200 joules—no change.
1323	CPR resumed; IV access 18 gauge left antecubital area—normal saline KVO; epinephrine 1:10,000 1 mg IVP.
1325	Defibrillation @ 200 joules—no change.
1326	CPR resumed; amiodarone 300 mg IVP.
1328	Defibrillation @ 260 joules—patient converts to normal sinus rhythm rate of 72 with strong peripheral pulses, BP—110/76, no spontaneous respirations. ET tube inserted. + lung sounds bilaterally with BVM.
1330	Ventilation continued @ 12/min via BVM.
1332	Patient transferred to ambulance on stretcher—transported to University Hospital.

Time	Intervention
1335	Patient has spontaneous respirations @ 20/min, + bilateral breath sounds; becoming more awake; HR—72, BP—120/76.
1340	Arrived at UH—Patient is conscious, alert, and oriented with retrograde amnesia.

Call Incident   The call incident approach simply emphasizes the mechanism of injury, the surrounding circumstances, and how the incident occurred. Use this approach to begin documenting a trauma call with a significant mechanism of injury. It is most suitable when the events surrounding the call might be significant. It would be inappropriate for a man sitting in his living room with chest pain or for someone who simply cut his finger with a carving knife. You may use this style in both the subjective and objective sections of your PCR. The following example shows call incident documentation for a motor vehicle crash:

Subjective	The patient is a 46-year-old conscious and alert white male who was an unrestrained driver in a low-speed, head-on, two-car motor vehicle crash, moderate front-end damage, no passenger compartment intrusion, deformity to windshield, dashboard, and steering wheel. Patient states he "reached for cigarette on floor and when he looked up, there was another vehicle in front of him." He denies any loss of consciousness and can recall all details prior to and immediately following the crash. Patient complains of pain to the head, neck, chest, and hip from being thrown against the dashboard and windshield.
Objective	The patient presents in the front seat of the car, appears in moderate distress with bruises to his forehead, facial lacerations, and a deformed left leg. His left leg is pinned underneath the dashboard with his left foot hooked around the brake pedal. Upon arrival, fire department rescue personnel were holding manual stabilization of his head and neck and stabilizing the vehicle.

These are not the only systems of documentation. Indeed, you may use some combination of these systems or develop a unique format for your regional system. The important thing is for your documentation to be complete, accurate, and consistent. By using the same system to document every call, you will be less likely to accidentally overlook or omit something.

SPECIAL CONSIDERATIONS

Some circumstances create special problems for EMS documentation. Patient refusals, calls where transport is unnecessary, multiple patients, and mass casualties are among the more common examples. In these and other unusual circumstances, take extra care to document everything that happened during the call.

Patient Refusals

Two types of patients might refuse care. The first type is the person who is not seriously ill or injured and simply does not want to go to the hospital. For example, the belted driver of a minor automobile crash has an abrasion on his knee from striking the dashboard. He is alert and oriented, has no other injuries, and claims he will seek medical attention if it bothers him later. This type of patient usually signs your PCR in a special place marked "Refusal of Care," and you return to service.[3]

The second type of patient is more worrisome. This patient refuses care even though you feel he needs it. This is known as **against medical advice (AMA)**. Some legal experts regard AMA as your failure to convince your patient to accept necessary treatment and transport. Such patient refusals are particularly troublesome because they have the most potential to end badly. Still, patients retain the right to refuse treatment or transportation if they are competent to make that decision and are not actively suicidal.

Although you cannot make a legal determination of competence (sometimes it takes a court decision), document that you believe your patient was competent to refuse care. Though specific laws vary from state to state, your patient will demonstrate competence by his understanding of the circumstances and the risks associated with refusing care and by accepting those risks and the responsibility for refusing care. Assess your patient as thoroughly as possible, with special emphasis on his mental status and behavior. Pay extra attention to any patient suspected of being under the influence of drugs or alcohol. Clearly document that your patient has an adequate mental status and understands your field diagnosis, alternative treatments, and the consequences of refusing care. Also record his reason for refusing care (Table 10-2).

Even after you document your patient's competence, most patient refusals require more thorough documentation than the typical EMS run because the opportunity for and consequences of abandonment charges are tremendous. Simply having your patient sign your PCR is not sufficient. Again, document that you described your patient's injuries to him and that he understood the risks of refusing treatment and transport. Inform him of potential complications from injuries that might not be obvious. Discuss those associated risks also, and document this discussion. Also document any involvement of your patient's family or friends.

Because ruling out serious injury is all but impossible in the field, you may need to make clear the possibility of your patient's dying. Although this might seem extreme, it plainly conveys that the risks are serious. A patient who was informed that he was at risk of dying, refused care, and subsequently had his leg amputated because of an infection would have a hard time convincing a jury that he did not think the risks were serious.

In many systems, you must contact the medical direction physician before allowing a patient to refuse transport. If you confer with a physician, document any information, advice,

TABLE 10-2 | Refusal of Care Documentation Checklist

- Thorough patient assessment
- Competency of patient
- Your recommendation for care and transport
- Explanation to the patient about possible consequences of refusing care, including possibility of death, if appropriate
- Other suggestions for accessing care
- Willingness to return if patient changes mind
- Patient's understanding of statements and suggestions and apparent competence to refuse care based on that understanding

or orders that the physician gives you. If your patient speaks directly to the physician, document that as well. Once more, document that your patient understands the circumstances and the risks and still chooses to refuse transport. Note that you instructed him to call an ambulance or go to the emergency department if his condition worsens, or if he just changes his mind. You can ask a bystander or law enforcement officer to witness the patient refusal, although this is not always required.[4]

Your documentation also should include a complete narrative with quotations and statements from others on the scene. For example, if your patient's wife and son plead with him to go to the hospital, include their comments in your report. If your system uses a specific form for patient refusals, complete that paperwork as well (Figure 10-6 ●). The additional form, however, is not a substitute for a complete documentation of the circumstances.

have occurred. When this happens, first responders such as the fire department rescue unit or a police agency might cancel the ambulance. If the ambulance is canceled en route, document the canceling authority and the time of notification. If you arrive on the scene and find no patients, document that. If, when you arrive, you are canceled by on-scene personnel, document that you made no patient contact and record the person and agency who canceled you. The difference is considerable between "no patients found" and "only minor injuries, patients refusing transport." Although they might refuse transport, evaluate people with even the most minor injuries. Consider them patients and document them accurately.

Multiple Casualty Incidents

Multiple patients, mass casualties, and disasters all present special documentation problems. The number of patients

Services Not Needed

Some systems allow you to determine that your patient does not need ambulance transport. Although such policies help to reduce ambulance utilization rates, the risks of denying transport are even greater than those of patient refusals. In these cases, the documentation must clearly demonstrate that transport was unnecessary. As with patient refusals, document any discussion you have with the emergency physician and any advice you give to your patient.

Transportation may not be needed for other reasons as well. Ambulances are often called to minor accidents where no injuries

RELEASE FROM RESPONSIBILITY

DATE _____ 19 _____ TIME _____ a.m. p.m.

This is to certify that _____

is refusing ☐ TREATMENT ☐ TRANSPORTATION

against the advice of the attending Emergency Medical Technician and of the Phoenix Fire Department, and when applicable, the base hospital and the base hospital physician.

I acknowledge that I have been informed of the following:

1. The nature and potential of the illness or injuries.
2. The potential risks of delaying treatment and transportation, up to and including death.
3. The availability of ambulance transportation to a hospital for treatment.

Nevertheless, I assume all risks and consequences of my decision, including further physical deterioration, loss of limb, paralysis, and even death, and hereby release the attending Emergency Medical Technician and the Phoenix Fire Department, and when applicable, the base hospital and the base hospital physician from any ill effects which may result from my refusal.

Witness _____ Signed: **X** _____

Witness _____ Relationship to Patient _____

Refusal must be signed by the patient; or by the nearest relative or legal guardian in the case of a minor, or when patient is physically or mentally incompetent.

☐ Patient refuses to sign release despite efforts of attending Emergency Medical Technician to obtain such signature after informing patient of concerns listed in numbers 1, 2, and 3 above.

GUIDELINES — Patient Refusal Documentation

In addition to those items normally documented (chief complaint, history of present illness, mechanism of injury, physical assessment, etc.) the following items should be recorded, regardless of patient's cooperation:

- Mental Status (orientation, speech, etc.)
- Suspected presence of alcohol or drugs
- Patient's exact words (as much as possible) in the refusal of care OR the signing of the release form
- Circumstances or reasons (including exact words of patient, if possible) for INCOMPLETE ADVISEMENT (risk of injury, abusiveness, unruliness, risk of injury other than from patient, etc.)
- Advice given to patients' guardian(s)

● **Figure 10-6** One example of a refusal of care form.

CONTENT REVIEW

▶ Narrative Formats

• SOAP
• CHART
• Patient management
• Call incident

needing care and transport during such situations may overwhelm you. Often, more than one ambulance crew cares for the many patients. Some EMS personnel may fill only support roles and never actually provide patient care. Obtaining complete patient information might be impossible, and completing documentation for one patient before going on to care for others might be impractical.[5]

In these situations, you must weigh your patients' needs against the demand for complete documentation. Document as much as possible—as quickly as possible—on your PCR. You can complete the documentation later as an addendum. If you cannot remember the particulars of a specific patient or transport, do not guess. Document only what you know to be factual and accurate. A simple note at the end of the documentation explaining the circumstances will account for any missing information.

Some EMS agencies use special forms for multiple patient events, and most provide a general incident report form or record that anyone connected with the call may complete. You should become familiar with local policies and procedures for documenting these situations. Many systems use **triage tags** to record vital information on each patient quickly (Figure 10-7 ●). A triage tag has just enough room for your patient's vital information—name, major injuries, vital signs, treatment, and priority (urgent, nonurgent). You affix it to your patient, and it remains there throughout the event; you can transfer its information to your PCR later. Whatever your local policies, document as completely and accurately as possible without detracting from patient care.

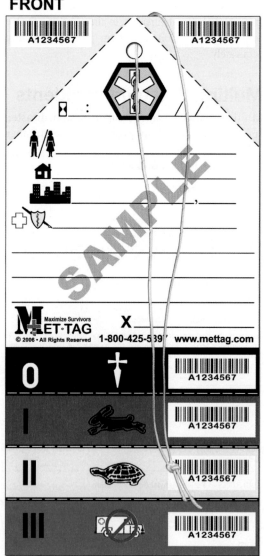

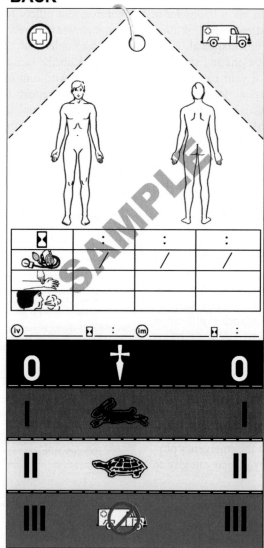

● **Figure 10-7**   A triage tag offers a quick way to record vital information. (*Reprinted with permission of The American Civil Defense Association*)

CONSEQUENCES OF INAPPROPRIATE DOCUMENTATION

Inappropriate documentation can have both medical and legal consequences.[6] The medical consequences of inadequate documentation are potentially the most serious. Health care providers across several disciplines may refer to your PCR in planning their care for a patient. Do not guess about your patient's medical problems if you are not certain. An inaccurate or incomplete report can affect patient care for many hours, even days, after the ambulance call ends. Failing to document a medication allergy or documenting an incorrect medical history could have grave effects. If no one can read your sloppy report, it is useless despite the importance of its information. Good documentation now enables good care later.[7]

The potential legal consequences of inadequate documentation are enormous. If poor documentation results in inappropriate care, you may be held responsible. Or if the documentation does not make it clear that you informed a patient of the risks when he refused transport, you may be legally accountable for any harmful consequences. If the documentation does not explicitly say the patient in ventricular fibrillation was defibrillated immediately, you might be accused of providing inadequate care. Even though you did everything appropriately, poor, incomplete, or inaccurate documentation will encourage anyone who is pursuing a frivolous lawsuit. Good documentation discourages such actions. Always remember that if it is not documented, you did not do it.

Inaccurate, incomplete, illegible documentation also reflects poorly on the EMS provider writing the report. Missing information, misspelled words, and poor penmanship give the impression of a sloppy, incompetent provider. Good documentation, on the other hand, enhances the EMS provider's professional stature.

ELECTRONIC PATIENT CARE RECORDS

A growing trend in EMS is the use of computerized patient recordkeeping software, also known as electronic patient care records, or ePCRs.[8] These platforms offer some advantages over the traditional paper chart; however, they also carry some drawbacks.[9] Multiple ePCR systems are available.

The benefits of electronic PCR systems are numerous. The following is a partial list of ePCR benefits:

- *Greater ease of data collection and analysis.* These systems are built on a database platform, and this makes data analysis and reporting significantly faster than trying to read through hundreds of paper charts, looking for a specific key word.

- *A consistent, uniform, easily read patient chart,* which can be a benefit to hospitals, nurses, and physicians.

- *The reduction of poor penmanship and spelling errors* common to handwritten charts.

- *The opportunity for an EMS Administrator to configure and alter the software* to best suit that service's particular operational model, needs, and requirements. Because different states use different mandatory data sets for reporting, different fields may be required.

- *Integration with dispatch software, billing services, and regulatory agencies.*

- *Interface with medical devices.* For example, cardiac monitor data can be uploaded into the ePCR software.

- *Better Quality Assurance processes, chart reviews, and feedback to the EMT or paramedic.*

Data within the ePCR software can be collected in several different ways. Some fields may include a simple "pick from" list, where acceptable values are presented and the EMT selects the appropriate item or items from the list (Figure 10-8 ●).

Other parts of the ePCR software may include a graphic interface. For example, patient body surveys are often collected using a picture of a person and a list of clinical findings. To record the proper findings, the EMT would select the body part and then the appropriate finding: "right lower leg—amputation," as an example (Figure 10-9 ●).

Another means for entering data is manual entry, where the EMT types in the correct value. This is most commonly seen in the "Vital Signs" or "Times" sections, where most values are numeric (Figure 10-10 ●).

While there are many benefits to implementation and use of an ePCR system, as already noted, there are drawbacks as well. First, and most obvious, is the cost. Such programs vary in price, but all of them have a price tag that some EMS agencies might

CONTENT REVIEW

► SOAP
- Subjective
- Objective
- Assessment
- Plan

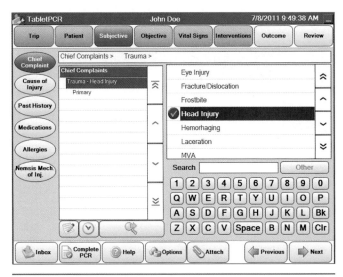

● **Figure 10-8**   A sample screen snap from ePCR. (© *Zoll Medical Corporation*)

CONTENT REVIEW

► CHART

- Chief complaint
- History
- Assessment
- Rx (treatment)
- Transport

find prohibitive. Once past the initial cost, there may be yearly fees for technical support, upgrades, and continued support from the software vendor. Additionally, as with any advanced software program, ePCR systems require that one or more people within the organization are technically savvy enough to administer and deal with any day-to-day issues. Finally, there is often an institutional reluctance or push-back from the field crews, who may be resistant to change: "We've always done paper charts, so why do we need to change now?" or "We're too busy to take time to get used to some new system." The positives, negatives, costs, and benefits of ePCR software must be individually evaluated by each EMS operation.

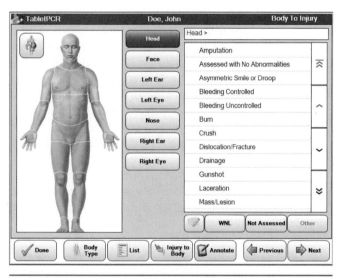

● **Figure 10-9**   A graphic interface on ePCR.
(*© Zoll Medical Corporation*)

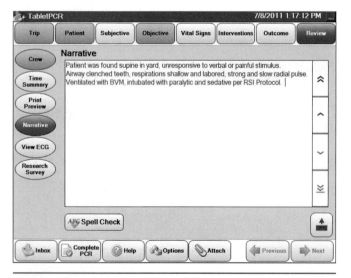

● **Figure 10-10**   Example of an ePCR manual entry screen.
(*© Zoll Medical Corporation*)

LEGAL CONSIDERATIONS

The PCR: Your Best Friend or Your Worst Enemy. *It is often difficult to sit and write a prehospital care report (PCR) after a long and difficult call. However, the importance of this record cannot be overemphasized. Years later, when the call is nothing but a distant memory, the PCR will be there to provide the facts and details of the patient encounter. Thus, for accuracy and clarity, the PCR must be completed as soon as possible after the call when all the facts are known. Waiting even a few hours may result in a PCR that is less than complete or inaccurate.*

The PCR is a valuable document. Not only does it provide medical personnel with the details of care provided in the prehospital setting, but it can also protect prehospital providers from negligence claims and malpractice allegations. In a court of law, it has been said, what is not documented in the patient record was not performed. Although this may not always be the case, it is difficult to prove that a certain prehospital procedure was performed if it was not documented in the PCR.

Although still relatively uncommon, malpractice suits against EMS personnel are on the rise. Most claims of negligence include such things as failure to secure and maintain an airway, failure to follow accepted protocols, failure to transport when care was necessary, and failure to properly restrain a combative or dangerous patient. You should be aware of the various aspects of EMS practice that can result in allegations of negligence and document these accurately. For example, proper placement of an endotracheal tube should be verified by at least three methods and documented in the PCR. In addition, you should document that the tube remained in proper position by repeated patient evaluations and through use of monitoring systems such as capnography and pulse oximetry. Also you must document care to show that you followed appropriate protocols and standing orders. If you deviated from these, you must document in detail why this occurred and whether medical direction was contacted.

Patient refusal is a difficult area for EMS. Competent patients have the right to refuse medical care, even when the failure to obtain medical care may result in harm. However, paramedics cannot adequately determine which patients are competent and which are not (competency is a finding of law). Thus, when faced with a nontransport situation, document the circumstances well and obtain a statement from a third-party witness to the refusal.

Patient restraint poses a significant risk for both the patient and rescuers. Always follow local protocols regarding patient restraint and document that these were followed. Try to involve law enforcement personnel in any situation where restraint may be needed.

In the event you are sued for negligence, the PCR can be either your best friend or your worst enemy. If you prepared it well and documented details of the call, then you have little to worry about. If you prepared it sloppily or incompletely, then be prepared to answer a lot of difficult questions. Always take the time to prepare an accurate patient report—you will not regret it when it is needed.

CLOSING

As a paramedic you will assume responsibility for your documentation. Although documentation is often a begrudged task, it is one of the most important parts of an EMS call. Ensuring that your documentation is complete, accurate, legible, and appropriate is one of your professional responsibilities. As a professional, you should recognize this responsibility and set a positive example for others as you fulfill it.

Your report's confidentiality cannot be overemphasized. Confidentiality is your patient's legal right. Do not discuss your report with anyone not medically connected directly with the case. Generally, you are allowed to share patient information with another health care provider who will continue care, with third-party billing companies, with the police if it is relevant to a criminal investigation, and with the court if it issues a subpoena.

Your report also may be used for quality assurance or research. In these cases, block out the patient's name.

Electronic charting will certainly become common in the future. Several systems now on the market allow you to enter data electronically, transmit that information to the receiving facility, and immediately receive a printed report. When you use such systems, remember that the principles of effective documentation still apply.

 ## SUMMARY

Regardless of the system you use for documentation, all EMS records should possess the same basic attributes. Appropriate terminology, proper spelling, accepted abbreviations and acronyms, and accurate times are essential. A description of the patient assessment and interventions, including pertinent negatives and communications with on-line physicians, is equally important. Finally, all the personnel and resources involved in a call must be documented. The record must be accurate and precise, free of jargon, and neatly written. Corrections should be made properly, including the use of an addendum when appropriate.

Prehospital care providers may use many systems of documentation, including the CHART and SOAP formats. Whatever system you use, it is best if you use the same one consistently. This results in more reliable, complete documentation and reduces the chances of omitting important information. Any of the existing documentation systems can incorporate a head-to-toe assessment of the patient. Special situations such as multiple patients and refusals of transportation require extra attention. They are often the most difficult calls to document, yet they are also the calls for which good documentation can be most valuable. A complete narrative—in addition to any check boxes—is the best way to ensure that all the necessary information is documented.

Although EMS providers frequently dislike documentation, it is one of the most important parts of the EMS call. Ensuring that the documentation is complete, accurate, legible, and appropriate is one of an EMS provider's professional responsibilities. Your PCR, whether written or electronic, is the only permanent record of the ambulance call and the only permanent reflection of your professionalism.

 ## YOU MAKE THE CALL

While helping the quality assurance officer in your agency, you come across the following narrative: "We were dispatched to a 10-48, coroner Main/Spice. Vehicle is upside down. PMD on scene reports no serious injuries. Patient is nasty and abusive. Looks like a drug abuser. Is walking around acting abnoctious. Minor injuries identified and treated per protocol. Police arrested patient. EMS transport not needed."

1. What is wrong with this narrative? (You should be able to identify at least ten faults.)

2. What will you do to make sure your documentation is better than this?

See Suggested Responses at the back of this book.

REVIEW QUESTIONS

1. Your prehospital care report will be a valuable resource for:
   a. medical professionals.
   b. EMS administrators.
   c. researchers.
   d. all of the above.

2. You should always attempt to complete your PCR:
   a. at the scene.
   b. en route to the hospital.
   c. immediately after the call.
   d. at the end of your duty shift.

3. The proper way to correct an error in your prehospital care report is to:
   a. completely and immediately blacken out the error.
   b. draw a single line through the error, correct, and initial.
   c. highlight the error and place quotation marks around it.
   d. erase the error completely and enter the correct information.

4. The call incident approach to documentation emphasizes:
   a. the mechanisms of injury.
   b. the surrounding circumstances.
   c. how the incident occurred.
   d. all of the above.

5. If your patient refuses transport and care, simply having him sign your PCR is not sufficient.
   a. true
   b. false

6. Of the following abbreviations, which one means "drops"?
   a. Gtts
   b. Dps
   c. Drps
   d. Gms

7. The medical abbreviation that means "hypertension" is _____.
   a. HBV
   b. H/A
   c. HPI
   d. HTN

8. The medical abbreviation that means your patient has difficulty breathing during exertion is _____.
   a. CHF
   b. MOI
   c. DOE
   d. DOA

See Answers to Review Questions at the back of this book.

 REFERENCES

1. Frisch, A. N., M. W. Dailey, D. Heeren, and M. Stern. "Precision of Time Devices Used by Prehospital Providers." *Prehosp Emerg Care* 13 (2009): 247–250.

2. Brice, J. H., K. D. Friend, and T. R. Delbridge. "Accuracy of EMS-Recorded Patient Demographic Data." *Prehosp Emerg Care* 12 (2008): 470–478.

3. Graham, D. H. "Documenting Patient Refusals." *Emerg Med Serv* 30 (2001): 56–60.

4. Weaver, J., K. H. Brinsfield, and D. Dalphond. "Prehospital Refusal-of-Transport Policies: Adequate Legal Protection?" *Prehosp Emerg Care* 4 (2000): 53–56.

5. Barnhart, S., P. M. Cody, and D. E. Hogan. "Multiple Information Sources in the Analysis of Disaster." *Am J Disaster Med* 4 (2009): 41–47.

6. Wesley, K. "Write It Right: Keeping Your PCR Clinical and Factual." *JEMS* 24 (2008): 190–196.

7. Laudermilch, D. J., M. A. Schiff, A. B. Nathens, and M. R. Rosengart. "Lack of Emergency Medical Services Documentation Is Associated with Poor Patient Outcomes: A Validation of Audit Filters for Prehospital Trauma Care." *J Am Coll Surg* 210 (2010): 220–227.

8. Taigman, M. "Ending the Paper Trail. Electronic Documentation in EMS." *Emerg Med Serv* 31 (2002): 65–68.

9. Kuisma, M., T. Varynen, T. Hiltunen, K. Porthan, and J. Aaltonen. "Effect of Introduction of Electronic Patient Reporting on the Duration of Ambulance Calls." *Am J Emerg Med* 27 (2009): 948–955.

 FURTHER READING

Snyder, J. *EMS Documentation*. Upper Saddle River, NJ: Pearson/Brady, 2007.

PRECAUTIONS ON BLOODBORNE PATHOGENS AND INFECTIOUS DISEASES

Prehospital emergency personnel, like all health care workers, are at risk for exposure to blood-borne pathogens and infectious diseases. In emergency situations it is often difficult to take or enforce proper infection control measures. However, as a paramedic, you must recognize your high-risk status. Study the following information on infection control carefully.

Infection control is designed to protect emergency personnel, their families, and their patients from unnecessary exposure to communicable diseases. Laws, regulations, and standards regarding infection control include:

- *Centers for Disease Control and Prevention (CDC) Guidelines.* The CDC has published extensive guidelines on infection control. Proper equipment and techniques that should be used by emergency response personnel to prevent or minimize risk of exposure are defined.
- *The Ryan White Act.* The Ryan White Act of 1990 allows emergency personnel to find out if they were exposed to an infectious disease while rendering patient care. Employers are required to name a "designated officer" to coordinate communications with the treating hospital.
- *Americans with Disabilities Act.* This act prohibits discrimination against individuals with disabilities, including those with contagious diseases. It guarantees equal employment opportunities and job protection if the infected individual can perform essential job functions and does not pose a threat to the safety and health of patients and coworkers.
- *Occupational Safety and Health Administration (OSHA) Regulations.* OSHA has enacted a regulation entitled Occupational Exposure to Bloodborne Pathogens that classifies emergency response personnel as being at the greatest risk of occupational exposure to communicable diseases. This regulation requires employers to provide hepatitis B (HBV) vaccinations free of charge, maintain a written exposure control plan, and provide personal protective equipment. These requirements primarily apply to private employers. Applicability to local and state governmental employees varies by locality. Many states have developed their own OSHA plans.
- *National Fire Protection Association (NFPA) Guidelines.* This is a national organization that has established specific guidelines and requirements regarding infection control for emergency response agencies, particularly fire departments and EMS services.

STANDARD PRECAUTIONS AND PERSONAL PROTECTIVE EQUIPMENT

Emergency response personnel should practice Standard Precautions by which ALL body substances are considered to be potentially infectious. To practice Standard Precautions, all emergency personnel should utilize personal protective equipment (PPE). Appropriate PPE should be available on every emergency vehicle. The minimum recommended PPE includes the following:

- *Gloves.* Disposable gloves should be donned by all emergency response personnel BEFORE initiating any emergency care. When an emergency incident involves more than one patient, you should attempt to change gloves between patients. When gloves have been contaminated, they should be removed as soon as possible. To properly remove contaminated gloves, grasp one glove approximately 1 inch from the wrist. Without touching the inside of the glove, pull the glove halfway off and stop. With that half-gloved hand, pull the glove on the opposite hand completely off. Place the removed glove in the palm of the other glove, with the inside of the removed glove exposed. Pull the second glove completely off with the ungloved hand, only touching the inside of the glove. Always wash hands after gloves are removed, even when the gloves appear intact.
- *Masks and Protective Eyewear.* Masks and protective eyewear should be present on all emergency vehicles and used in accordance with the level of exposure encountered. Masks and protective eyewear should be worn together whenever blood spatter is likely to occur, such as during arterial bleeding, childbirth, endotracheal intubation, invasive procedures, oral

suctioning, and cleanup of equipment that requires heavy scrubbing or brushing. Both you and the patient should wear masks whenever the potential for airborne transmission of disease exists.

- *HEPA and N-95 Respirators.* Due to the resurgence of tuberculosis (TB), prehospital personnel should protect themselves from TB infection through use of an N-95 or a high-efficiency particulate air (HEPA) respirator, as approved by the National Institute of Occupational Safety and Health (NIOSH). It should fit snugly and be capable of filtering out the tuberculosis bacillus. An N-95 or HEPA respirator should be worn when caring for patients with confirmed or suspected TB. This is especially true when performing "high-hazard" procedures such as administration of nebulized medications, endotracheal intubation, or suctioning on such a patient.
- *Gowns.* Gowns protect clothing from blood splashes. If large splashes of blood are expected, such as with childbirth, wear impervious gowns.
- *Resuscitation Equipment.* Disposable resuscitation equipment should be the primary means of artificial ventilation in emergency care. Such items should be used once, then disposed of.

Remember, the proper use of personal protective equipment ensures effective infection control and minimizes risk. Use ALL protective equipment recommended for any particular situation to ensure maximum protection.

Consider ALL body substances potentially infectious and ALWAYS practice Standard Precautions.

The following are suggested responses to the "You Make the Call" scenarios presented in each chapter of Volume 1, Introduction to Paramedicine. Each represents an acceptable response to the scenario but should not be interpreted as the only correct response.

Chapter 1—Introduction to Paramedicine

1. *Discuss the vast differences between EMS and paramedic care in the United States, Canada, and other economically developed nations compared with those that exist in some less-developed countries of the world. How should awareness of such differences affect your attitude about your work?*

   While people in the United States, Canada, and other developed countries consider EMS a necessity and benefit from high standards of emergency care, people in some poorer or less-developed countries often do not expect anything more than a ride to the hospital. Rather than feeling smug about our "superiority," however, North American paramedics should feel both privileged and determined to work hard to live up to the high standards we enjoy. There is also an obligation to take part in any opportunities to participate in programs in which information is exchanged between nations and EMS systems in the ongoing effort to raise standards both in the United States and around the world. From those to whom much is given, much is expected.

Chapter 2—EMS Systems

1. *Which of the "ten system elements" identified by NHTSA are mentioned in this scenario?*
   - Transportation—two modes of transportation were used in this incident, air and ground.
   - Facilities—by designating special referral centers, prehospital personnel can make transport decisions to medical facilities based on specific patient's needs.
   - Communications—without a single system of communication, which allows all EMS personnel to communicate with each other, efficiently managing this type of incident would be impossible.
   - Trauma systems—by having a system of specialized care for trauma patients, patients involved in this incident can be assured of the appropriate care.
   - Medical direction—an active physician medical director provided on-line guidance to EMS providers.

2. *For what possible reason was the top-priority patient sent so far from the scene?*

   The top-priority patient was likely sent so far away because of the extent of injuries and/or need for specialty care. Local hospitals may not be the most effective facility to receive a patient when specialty care (burn care, trauma care, stroke, cardiac, etc.) is required. Sometimes it is in the patient's best interest to bypass a local facility for another facility that is better prepared to handle the situation/care.

3. *How important was the role played by the emergency medical dispatcher in this scenario? Explain.*

   The role the 911 dispatcher played was extremely important. He put the mass-casualty plan into effect and sent the appropriate law enforcement and fire personnel. That is, as a key member of a centralized communications system, he directed the movement of resources within the system, while maintaining enough available resources to provide for the rest of the community.

4. *How might the EMS system benefit from an evaluation of this incident?*

   Even if this incident went smoothly, the QI process should review it. If nothing else, the review of the event will prove to be a good opportunity to provide continuing education on how such an event should be handled. It is unlikely that the event was handled so perfectly that there is nothing to learn from it. It could be something as simple as a better staging location for the ambulances or landing zone for the helicopter. Either way, by reviewing the event in QI, the agency will be able to identify and improve areas that may have been overlooked during the heat of the moment.

Chapter 3—Roles and Responsibilities of the Paramedic

1. *What were your key responsibilities in the previously detailed scenario?*

Your primary responsibilities in this scenario, just like any other, are safety for you and your partner followed by patient care and safety of the patient and bystanders. After ensuring that neither you nor your partner are in any danger, assessment and treatment of the patient is your next responsibility. This scenario is complicated by the family's ignorance of the capabilities and roles of EMS within the health care system. If possible, your partner can use this teaching moment to briefly educate the family to your capabilities. Maintaining a professional demeanor and going out of the way to make sure the family is made aware of the patient's status are diplomacy skills used by a true professional.

Additionally, you have the responsibility to transport the patient to the most appropriate facility, notify medical control of the situation, and ensure the continuity of care by reporting and turning the patient over to someone of equal or higher training. Your final responsibilities with continuity of care involve timely and accurate documentation of your assessment and treatment for the patient and being sure the documentation has been submitted to the patient's chart at the receiving hospital. Finally, you must ensure your unit has been placed back in service as quickly as possible and made available for any additional calls.

2. *How should you have prepared yourself mentally and physically for this call?*

Preparing yourself for this call involves physical and mental fitness preparation. A good exercise and diet program helps to ensure good health which, in turn, helps you to deal with stressors of the job. Clearly, this situation is a stressful situation and one that is all too familiar. Mental preparation involves staying up to date with continuing education and familiarizing yourself with your protocols. When you are confident in your actions and care, stressors such as family or bystanders yelling at you will not sway your treatment or confidence.* People will pick up on the slightest signal that you are not confident, which in turn can possibly escalate the situation.

*Confidence and arrogance (cockiness) are close cousins. It is imperative that you learn to be confident without being arrogant. Arrogance breeds dissention between you and coworkers, first responders, hospital personnel, and the public. On the other hand, self-confidence can be calming and build a sense of trust.

3. *Did you and your partner act professionally? If so, explain how.*

Yes, the paramedics acted professionally. Initially, they had to respond to the patient, his wife, and his son. Although the family was being difficult, that did not change the patient-care routine. They did not become rude with the family, or take out their frustrations on the patient. They were self-confident, and showed inner strength, self-control, excellent communication skills, and excellent decision-making skills.

Chapter 4—Workforce Safety and Wellness

1. *Are your stress levels inappropriately high? What are the indications?*

Yes, your stress levels are inappropriately high. This is evidenced by your irritability and sour stomach. Your stress is compounded by a poor diet, financial and home troubles, and the death of a young person. Even worse, you knew this person, and you will see the continued effects of the loss. In this situation, you are not handling the stress appropriately. Instead of spending your time off doing stress-relieving activities such as exercise, hobbies, sports, or other relaxation activities, you took on yet another overtime shift.

2. *Might it be a good idea for you to go to the funeral? Why or why not?*

The answer to this question depends on the individual. Some individuals need to have final closure and can only find this by attending the funeral or at least visiting the family at the funeral home. Other people choose to avoid the funeral home and services, claiming that the lack of closure is easier to deal with. In any event, you should be aware of which method works best to help you deal with stressful events and follow through with them.

3. *How can you improve stress management in the future?*

Methods to manage stress include following through with a healthy diet, regular exercise (30+ minutes a day), avoiding additional stress when possible, relaxation exercises, and finding a hobby to relieve stress. Suggest and attend discussion meetings following any critical events such as the one mentioned in the scenario. Don't hesitate to contact a mental health professional and make an appointment.

Chapter 5—EMS Research

1. What is your study's hypothesis?

The incidence of narcotic overdoses in our EMS system is low.

2. Did you prove or disprove your hypothesis?

Although the term "incidence" is not precise, overall the number of narcotic overdoses in the system is relatively low. To get a better handle on the issue, it would be appropriate, if possible, to compare your system's incidence of narcotic overdoses to systems of similar size and demographics.

3. What was the derived benefit from the study?

The increased awareness of the low incidence of narcotic overdoses in the system resulted in, at least temporarily, decreased overall usage of naloxone.

Chapter 6—Public Health

1. How will you counter the arguments the two paramedics made?

The fire service has been doing prevention and safety programs for years now, and they still have jobs. As long as there are people, there will always be a need for EMS. By doing prevention programs, we are offering another public service and making our community safer. Not to mention, if we can prevent slips, trips, falls, and other minor injuries, we will be more available for the truly life-threatening emergencies. The scope of practice for paramedics is constantly being expanded, but patient care and safety are still our number one priorities.

2. Why is prevention an important responsibility of being a paramedic?

As paramedics, we are part of the medical community. In order for us to be recognized as a profession within the medical community, we need to fully participate in the medical community. Part of medicine is preventive medicine, health education, and controlling communicable diseases. These are the basic principles of public health and an under-addressed area of EMS. Prevention strategies help prevent the spread of communicable diseases through Standard Precautions training. Additional prevention strategies help reduce injuries and long-term disability from injuries.

3. List ten ideas for an illness and injury prevention program that may be appropriate in your area. (Answers might include any of the following suggestions or others.)

1. Seat belt campaigns
2. First aid & CPR classes
3. Swimming lessons
4. Car seat safety classes
5. Helmet and protective padding initiatives for kids
6. Home assessments for the elderly
7. Carbon monoxide detector installing
8. Environmental assessments of homes of the elderly (heat or cold assessment)
9. Vial of life/file of life or other medical information programs
10. Stroke and heart attack awareness programs

Chapter 7—Medical/Legal Aspects of Prehospital Care

1. You believe that the child needs emergency care, but the child's parents are unavailable. What should you do?

Begin emergency care under the doctrine of implied consent.

2. If you decide to treat the child without consent, can you be sued for doing so?

You can be sued for anything. But, in this case, assuming a responsible family member could not be located, you would be rendering care for an apparent life-threatening injury or illness under the doctrine of implied consent.

3. What would you do if the parents returned home and refused to grant permission for treatment?

Make multiple and sincere attempts to convince the parents to accept care for their child; make certain that they are fully informed about the implications of their decision and the potential risks of refusing care; consult with on-line medical direction; have them and a disinterested witness, such as a police officer, sign a "release-from-liability" form; advise them that they may call you again for help if necessary; document the entire situation thoroughly on your patient care report.

Chapter 8—Ethics in Paramedicine

1. What potential benefits are there in yielding to the patient's request (beneficence)?

The potential benefits in yielding to the patient's request are those involving doing good (beneficence). In this case, that would mean possibly getting to the hospital faster and thereby lessening the time the patient has to suffer severe pain.

2. What potential harm is there in yielding to the patient's request (nonmaleficence)?

Nonmaleficence refers to the paramedic's obligation to "first, do no harm." In this case, staying within the service's policy restrictions could be described as causing the patient to suffer pain longer than may be necessary. However, if you consider why the policy restricts the use of lights and siren (because they increase the risk of vehicle collision), perhaps the obligation to do no harm is better met by staying within those restrictions and avoiding the risk of further injury or further delay.

3. How does justice come into play in this situation?

Justice refers to the paramedic's obligation to treat all patients fairly. If the paramedic were to use the emergency lights and siren for Phil Cornock, he would be making an exception to a policy restriction. If he makes this exception, and there are other patients who might benefit by getting to the hospital faster but do not because the paramedics are following the rules, then those patients are not being treated fairly.

4. How should paramedics in general respond when a patient requests an intervention that is not medically indicated?

In the absence of standards or protocols that fit the situation, the paramedic needs to reason out the problem. He must first state the action in a universal form, then consider the implications or consequences of the action and, finally, compare them to relevant values.

Chapter 9—EMS System Communications

1. Based on the information provided, organize and prepare your radio report to inform the receiving hospital of your patient's condition.

Rescue: Palermo Rescue to Davidson Medical Center.

Hospital: Davidson Medical, Doctor Stowe here, go ahead.

Rescue: Davidson Medical, this is Paramedic Kirk inbound to your facility with a 69-year-old male patient complaining of chest pain. How do you copy?

Hospital: I copy a 69-year-old male complaining of chest pain, go ahead.

Rescue: Doctor Stowe, this patient's pain began about 30 minutes ago while he was at rest. He describes it as a substernal pressure-type pain radiating into his arm and jaw. He has a history of heart disease and two prior MIs with bypass surgery two years ago. His current meds are Lanoxin, Lasix, Capoten, and aspirin, and he is allergic to Mellaril. His blood pressure is 210/110, pulse of 70, respirations of 20 mildly labored with a pulse oximetry of 93 percent with supplemental oxygen. He has become progressively more dyspneic in our presence. We have an ETA to your facility of 10 minutes. Do you have any further orders at this time?

Chapter 10—Documentation

1. What is wrong with this narrative?

What is a "10-48"? Is this the same in every EMS system?

Was the ambulance dispatched to the corner of Main and Spice?

Was the ambulance dispatched to the coroner, at Main and Spice?

Was the ambulance dispatched to the main coroner, whose name is Spice?

What is "PMD"?

"Patient is nasty and abusive" is judgmental.

"Looks like a drug abuser" is judgmental.

"Abnoctious" should be spelled "obnoxious."

"Obnoxious" is judgmental.

What exactly are the injuries?

Exactly what treatment, if any, was rendered?

Was EMS transport not needed because the patient was not hurt, or because the police transported him?

Did the patient go to the hospital or to jail?

2. *What will you do to make sure your documentation is better than this?*

Avoid using codes.

Practice spelling and use only words you can spell correctly.

Do not use abbreviations that are unclear; spell out terms the first time you use them, followed by the abbreviation in parentheses.

Do not be judgmental.

Describe the head-to-toe assessment completely.

Be particularly careful and complete in no-transport situations.

ANSWERS TO REVIEW QUESTIONS

Below are answers to the Review Questions presented in each chapter of Volume 1.

CHAPTER 1—INTRODUCTION TO PARAMEDICINE

1. c
2. d
3. a
4. d
5. c

CHAPTER 2—EMS SYSTEMS

1. b
2. b
3. b
4. b
5. b
6. d
7. c
8. b
9. b
10. d

CHAPTER 3—ROLES AND RESPONSIBILITIES OF THE PARAMEDIC

1. b
2. c
3. d
4. a
5. d
6. d
7. c
8. a

CHAPTER 4—WORKFORCE SAFETY AND WELLNESS

1. c
2. c
3. c
4. d
5. d
6. c
7. b
8. b
9. a
10. d

CHAPTER 5—EMS RESEARCH

1. b
2. b
3. a
4. b
5. a
6. d
7. a

CHAPTER 6—PUBLIC HEALTH

1. c
2. b
3. b
4. c
5. b
6. b

CHAPTER 7—MEDICAL/LEGAL ASPECTS OF PREHOSPITAL CARE

1. a
2. d
3. b
4. a
5. c
6. c
7. d
8. c
9. d
10. d

CHAPTER 8—ETHICS IN PARAMEDICINE

1. b
2. c
3. a
4. a
5. d

CHAPTER 9—EMS SYSTEM COMMUNICATIONS

1. c
2. d
3. a
4. b
5. e
6. a
7. b
8. c
9. b
10. a

CHAPTER 10—DOCUMENTATION

1. d
2. c
3. b
4. d
5. a
6. a
7. d
8. c

abandonment termination of the paramedic-patient relationship without assurance that an equal or greater level of care will continue.

abstract a written summary of the key points, especially of a scientific paper; a report presented before publication of the entire paper.

accelerometers sensors in a vehicle that can measure a change in total velocity, forces applied to the vehicle, direction forces were applied, whether the vehicle rolled over, whether air bags were deployed, and the vehicle's final resting position.

accreditation a system ensuring that education programs for paramedics and other EMS personnel levels meet minimal guidelines for faculty, facilities, equipment, medical oversight, clinical affiliations, and financial stability.

actual damages compensable physical, psychological, or financial harm.

ad hoc **database** database created each time a patient is encountered to include information about that patient such as vital signs, video, electronic health record, and voice-to-text medical findings that can be stored and then accessed as needed by rescuers, helicopter crew, and hospital physicians.

addendum addition or supplement to the original report.

administrative law law that is enacted by governmental agencies at either the federal or state level. Also called regulatory law.

advance directive a document created to ensure that certain treatment choices are honored when a patient is unconscious or otherwise unable to express his choice of treatment.

advanced automatic crash notification (AACN) data collection and transmission system that can automatically contact a national call center or local public safety answering point and transmit detailed crash data, such as the type of vehicle, speed and direction of impact, and probable severity of injury to occupants. The AACN call center can simultaneously dispatch a variety of responders, including rescue/extrication crews, fire service, and medical helicopter transport, and advise the most appropriate hospital or trauma center to prepare for arrival of patients.

Advanced Emergency Medical Technician (AEMT) the level of EMS practitioner who performs the responsibilities of an EMT with the addition of limited advanced emergency medical care.

advanced life support (ALS) advanced lifesaving procedures such as intravenous therapy, drug therapy, intubation, and defibrillation.

against medical advice (AMA) your patient refuses care even though you feel he needs it.

allied health professions ancillary health care professions apart from physicians and nurses, such as paramedics, respiratory therapists, and physical therapists.

analysis of variance (ANOVA) parametric statistic used to ascertain the extent to which significant group differences can be inferred to the population.

anchor time set of hours when a night-shift worker can reliably expect to rest without interruption.

assault an act that unlawfully places a person in apprehension of immediate bodily harm without his consent.

automatic crash notification (ACN) data collection and transmission system that can automatically contact a national call center or local public safety answering point and transmit limited specific crash data, such as that a crash has taken place and where it is located.

automatic location information (ALI) in computers at enhanced 911 communication centers, the ability to display the location of a caller's phone.

automatic number identification (ANI) in computers at enhanced 911 communication centers, the ability to display a caller's telephone number.

autonomy a competent adult patient's right to determine what happens to his own body.

bandwidth (1) the width of a range of frequencies, measured in hertz; (2) a rate of data transmission, measured in bits per second (bps).

basic life support (BLS) basic lifesaving procedures such as artificial ventilation and cardiopulmonary resuscitation (CPR).

battery the unlawful touching of another individual without his consent.

bench research research done in a controlled laboratory setting using nonhuman subjects.

beneficence the principle of doing good for the patient.

bias potential unintended or unavoidable effect on study outcomes.

breach of duty an action or inaction that violates the standard of care expected from a paramedic.

bubble sheet scannable run sheet on which you fill in boxes or "bubbles" to record assessment and care information.

burnout when coping mechanisms no longer buffer job stressors, which can compromise personal health and well-being.

bystander a family member, friend, or stranger to the patient who is present at the patient's medical emergency.

call routing the process of transferring an emergency call to the nearest 911 center; occasionally technical problems cause such a call to be routed out of the call area.

case report a structured study of a single unit, subject, event, or patient.

case series observational study that tracks patients with a known exposure or examines their medical records for exposure and outcome.

cells regions into which a cell phone service is divided.

cellular telephone system   A type of wireless communication, called "cellular" because it is based on a complex of separate base stations, each covering one "cell" or geographic area. As a cell phone user travels, calls are transferred from base station to base station.

certification   the process by which an agency or association grants recognition to an individual who has met its qualifications.

chain of survival   As defined by the American Heart Association, the five most important factors affecting survival of a cardiac arrest patient: (1) immediate recognition and activation of EMS; (2) early CPR; (3) rapid defibrillation; (4) effective advanced life support; (5) integrated post–cardiac arrest care.

chi square test   nonparametric statistic used with nominal data to test group differences.

circadian rhythms   physiologic phenomena that occur at approximately 24-hour intervals.

civil law   division of the legal system that deals with non-criminal issues and conflicts between two or more parties.

civil rights   the rights of personal liberty guaranteed to American citizens by the 13th and 14th amendments to the United States Constitution and by certain acts of Congress.

cleaning   washing an object with cleaners such as soap and water.

clinical protocols   the policies and procedures established by a medical director for all components of an EMS system, such as medical treatment protocols.

cognitive radio   a "smart" device that is able to search the airwaves it covers for strong signals with no competing transmissions to provide the best possible channel of communication.

cohort study   study of a group of subjects initially identified as having one or more characteristics in common who are followed over time.

common law   law that is derived from society's acceptance of customs and norms over time. Also called case law or judge-made law.

common operating picture (COP)   a single display of operational information, such as data about a traffic crash and emergency responses to it, that is simultaneously shared by all units involved in responding to the emergency so that all those involved are working with the same information.

communication   the process of exchanging information between individuals.

communication protocols   predetermined, written guidelines for the type of information you may communicate by various means of communication without breaching patient confidentiality and privacy.

competent   able to make an informed decision about medical care.

confidence interval   allows statisticians to express how closely the sample estimate matches the true value in the whole population.

confidentiality   principle of law that prohibits the release of medical or other personal information about a patient without the patient's consent.

consent   the patient's granting of permission for treatment.

constitutional law   law based on the U.S. Constitution.

control group   an experimental study group that does not receive a treatment or intervention that is given to the experimental group.

convenience sampling   sampling in which the subjects or patients are selected, in part or in whole, at the convenience of the researcher.

criminal law   division of the legal system that deals with wrongs committed against society or its members.

critical care transport   the transport of critically ill or injured patients.

cross-sectional study   a study in which a statistically significant sample of a population is used to estimate the relationship between an outcome of interest and population variables as they exist at one particular time.

data dictionary   a source of information about a specific set of data that provides definitions of terms, explanations of interrelations among the separate data, and similar information.

data dredging   the inappropriate (sometimes deliberately so) use of data mining to uncover relationships in data that may be misleading.

data mining   the process of searching large amounts of data for patterns or relationships.

dead spot   an area where transmission and reception of a radio or other signal is poor.

defamation   an intentional false communication that injures another person's reputation or good name.

Department of Homeland Security (DHS)   a department of the United States government charged with the protection of the country from threats and attacks.

dependent variable   variable assessed by the experimenter to determine whether there is a difference in it that is due to the independent variable.

descriptive statistics   statistics that summarize research data.

digital communications   data or sounds translated into a digital code for transmission, usually a binary code consisting of 1 and 0, the numbers corresponding to voltage values.

disinfection   cleaning with an agent that can kill some microorganisms on the surface of an object.

Do Not Resuscitate (DNR) order   legal document, usually signed by the patient and his physician, that indicates to medical personnel which, if any, life-sustaining measures should be taken when the patient's heart and respiratory functions have ceased.

double blind study   study comparing two or more treatments in which neither the investigators nor the subjects know which treatment group individual subjects have been assigned to.

duplex   communications system that allows simultaneous two-way communications by using two frequencies for each channel.

duty to act   a formal contractual or informal legal obligation to provide care.

echo procedure   immediately repeating each transmission received during radio communications.

emancipated minor   a person under 18 years of age who is married, pregnant, a parent, a member of the armed forces, or financially independent and living away from home.

Emergency Medical Dispatcher (EMD)   the person who manages an EMS system's response and readiness and is responsible for assignment of emergency medical resources to a medical emergency.

Emergency Medical Responder (EMR)   the level of EMS practitioner who is likely to be the first person on the scene with emergency care training and the ability to initiate immediate lifesaving care.

Emergency Medical Services (EMS) system   a comprehensive network of personnel, equipment, and resources established for the purpose of delivering aid and emergency medical care to the community.

Emergency Medical Technician (EMT)   the level of EMS practitioner who provides basic emergency medical care and transportation.

employment law   laws that address employee/employer relationships.

epidemiology   the study of factors that influence the frequency, distribution, and causes of injury, disease, and other health-related events in a population.

ethics   the rules or standards that govern the conduct of members of a particular group or profession.

evidence-based medicine (EMB)   the conscientious, explicit, and judicious use of scientific evidence of effectiveness in decisions about the care of a patient or patients.

excited delirium syndrome (ExDS)   a condition that may result from abuse of stimulant drugs, typically presenting as a triad of effects: delirium, psychomotor agitation, and physiologic excitation.

experiment   study in which the researcher has control over some of the conditions in which the study takes place and control over some aspects of the independent variables being studied.

experimental group   the group in experimental design that receives the experimental condition or treatment.

experimental study   study in which subjects are randomly assigned to groups that experience carefully controlled interventions manipulated by the investigator according to a strict logic that allows causal inference about the effects of the interventions under investigation.

exposure   any occurrence of blood or body fluids coming in contact with nonintact skin, mucous membranes, or parenteral contact (e.g., a needlestick).

expressed consent   verbal, nonverbal, or written communication by a patient that he wishes to receive medical care.

external validity   the extent to which the findings of a study are relevant to subjects and settings beyond those in the study; a synonym for *generalizability*.

false imprisonment   intentional and unjustifiable detention of a person without his consent or other legal authority.

Federal Communications Commission (FCC)   agency that controls all nongovernmental communications in the United States.

field diagnosis   what you believe to be your patient's problem, based on the patient's history and physical exam.

geographic information system (GIS)   an information system that stores and analyzes information about or within a specific geographic area for the purpose of aiding decision making within an organization or group for which the specific GIS has been developed.

global positioning system (GPS)   a global navigational satellite system in which satellites orbiting the earth provide specific time and location information.

Good Samaritan laws   laws that provide immunity to certain people who assist at the scene of a medical emergency.

hand-off   the process of transferring patient care to receiving facility staff; the verbal report given by an EMT or paramedic to the receiving nurse or physician.

Health Insurance Portability and Accountability Act (HIPAA)   enacted by the United States Congress in 1996, includes provisions for protecting the security and privacy of a person's health information.

helicopter EMS (HEMS)   emergency care provided by EMS personnel and helicopter flight crews who are trained in the preparation of patients for and the care of patients during helicopter transport.

hotspot   relating to Internet access that is provided over a wireless local area network through a router to an Internet service provider.

hypothesis   testable statement that indicates what the researcher expects to find, based on theory and knowledge of the literature.

immunity   exemption from legal liability.

implied consent   consent for treatment that is presumed for a patient who is mentally, physically, or emotionally unable to grant consent. Also called emergency doctrine.

in vitro   descriptive term for processes that are carried out outside the living body, usually in the laboratory, as distinguished from *in vivo* processes.

in vivo   descriptive term for processes that are carried out within a living body.

incubation period   the time between contact with a disease organism and the appearance of first symptoms.

independent variable   presumed cause of the dependent variable.

infectious disease   any disease caused by the growth of pathogenic microorganisms that may be spread from person to person.

inferential statistics   statistics used to determine whether changes in a dependent variable are caused by an independent variable.

information communications technology (ICT)   information technology blended with communications technology to provide for dissemination of information.

informed consent   consent for treatment that is given based on full disclosure of information.

injury   intentional or unintentional damage to a person resulting from acute exposure to thermal, mechanical, electrical, or chemical energy or from the absence of such essentials as heat and oxygen.

injury risk   a hazardous or potentially hazardous situation that puts people in danger of sustaining injury.

injury surveillance program the ongoing systematic collection, analysis, and interpretation of injury data essential to the planning, implementation, and evaluation of public health practice.

institutional review board (IRB) board of experts, established at all research institutions, that oversees the ethical conduct of research.

intentional tort a civil wrong committed by one person against another based on a willful act. *See also* tort law.

internal validity ability of the research design to accurately answer the research question.

interoperability a feature of the emergency and public safety communications infrastructure that allows personnel from different jurisdictions and systems to communicate with each other effectively.

intervener physician a physician at the scene of an emergency who is not affiliated with EMS or not affiliated with the EMS service that has been dispatched to the scene.

invasion of privacy violation by one person of another person's personal life or personal information.

involuntary consent consent to treatment granted by the authority of a court order.

isometric exercise active exercise performed against stable resistance, where muscles are exercised in a motionless manner.

isotonic exercise active exercise during which muscles are worked through their range of motion.

iterative process process for calculating a desired result by means of a repeated cycle of operations that comes closer and closer to the desired result.

jargon language used by a particular group or profession.

justice the obligation to treat all patients fairly.

legislative law law created by lawmaking bodies such as Congress and state assemblies. Also called statutory law.

liability legal responsibility.

libel the act of injuring a person's character, name, or reputation by false statements made in writing or through the mass media with malicious intent or reckless disregard for the falsity of those statements.

licensure the process by which a governmental agency grants permission to engage in a given trade or profession to an applicant who has attained the degree of competency required to ensure the public's protection.

living will a legal document that allows a person to specify the kinds of medical treatment he wishes to receive should the need arise.

malfeasance a breach of duty by performance of a wrongful or unlawful act.

mean average obtained by adding the objects or items and dividing the sum by the number of objects or items present.

measures of central tendency numerical information regarding the most typical or representative scores in a group.

mechanism of injury (MOI) the force or forces that caused an injury.

median the middle score in a set of scores that have been ordered from lowest to highest.

medical director a physician who is legally responsible for all clinical and patient care aspects of an EMS system.

medical oversight the medical policies, procedures, and practices established by the medical director of an EMS system.

metaanalysis the process or technique of synthesizing research results by using various statistical methods to retrieve, select, and combine results from previous separate but related studies.

minor depending on state law, this is usually a person under the age of 18.

misfeasance a breach of duty by performance of a legal act in a manner that is harmful or injurious.

mission-critical communications information that must get through without fail because a patient's well-being depends on it.

mixed research a research design that contains both quantitative and qualitative properties.

mobile data unit (MDU) vehicle-mounted computer keyboard and display with broadband capacity via radio or wireless connection, capable of sending ambulance status and patient information to the hospital or ambulance quarters.

mode value that occurs most frequently in a data set.

morals social, religious, or personal standards of right and wrong.

morbidity the rate or incidence of a disease.

mortality the number of deaths in a given period.

multiband radio radio or radio system that combines a wide range of radio bands, allowing services that operate on separate bands—such as police, fire, and EMS—to communicate across the separate systems.

multiplex duplex system that can transmit voice and data simultaneously.

National Emergency Medical Services Education Standards: Paramedic Instructional Guidelines Guidelines developed and published in 2009 by the U.S. Department of Transportation for the education of the various levels of EMS practitioner—Emergency Medical Responders, Emergency Medical Technicians, Advanced Emergency Medical Technicians, and Paramedics.

National EMS Information System (NEMSIS) national repository formed to collect and store EMS data from every state in the United States, to create a national EMS database and to create a data dictionary that can be accessed and used by individual EMS systems.

National EMS Research Agenda document describing the history and current status of EMS research and proposing a strategy to guide the research component of EMS into the future; commissioned by the National Highway Traffic Safety Administration and the Maternal and Child Health Bureau of the United States government; published in 2001.

National Highway Traffic Safety Administration (NHTSA) An agency of the United States government established by the Highway Safety Act of 1970 to carry out safety programs to improve motor vehicle and highway safety, particularly to prevent vehicular crashes.

National Incident Management System (NIMS) a system administered by the U.S. Secretary of Homeland Security to provide a consistent approach to disaster management by all local, state, and federal employees who respond to such incidents.

National Transportation Safety Board (NTSB) an independent United States government investigative agency responsible for civil transportation accident investigation, including investigation of aviation accidents and incidents, certain types of highway crashes, ship and marine accidents, pipeline incidents, and railroad accidents.

nature of the illness (NOI) a patient's general medical condition or complaint.

negligence deviation from accepted standards of care recognized by law for the protection of others against the unreasonable risk of harm. In medical practice, negligence is often considered to be synonymous with malpractice. The four elements that must be present to prove negligence in a court of law are duty to act, breach of duty to act, actual damages, and proximate cause. *See also* negligence *per se*.

negligence *per se* negligence committed as a result of violating a statute with resultant injury; automatic negligence. *See also* negligence.

nominal data categorical data in which the order of the categories is arbitrary (e.g., 1 = male, 2 = female).

nonfeasance a breach of duty by failure to perform a required act or duty.

nonmaleficence the obligation not to harm the patient.

nonrandomized controlled trial research protocol in which the subjects are assigned to the study groups by a method other than randomization.

null hypothesis a hypothesis that predicts that an observed difference is due to chance alone and not to a systematic cause.

observational study study in which a phenomenon is described but no attempt is made to analyze the effects of variables on the phenomenon; also called a descriptive study.

odds ratio a measure of association in a case-control study that quantifies the relationship between an exposure and health outcome from a comparative study.

off-line medical oversight medical policies, procedures, and practices established by a system medical director in advance of a call.

on-line medical direction orders directly provided to a prehospital care provider by a qualified physician by either radio or telephone.

Ontario Prehospital Life Support Study (OPALS) a study conducted in the province of Ontario, Canada, of prehospital practices and outcomes.

open access journals scientific publications, typically Internet based, that allow unrestricted access to the contents.

ordinal data a type of data containing limited categories with a ranking from the lowest to the highest (e.g., mild, moderate, severe).

outcomes-based research research designed to understand the end results of particular health care practices and interventions.

P **value** the probability of obtaining by chance a result at least as extreme as that observed, even when the null hypothesis is true and no real difference exists; if it is ≤0.05 the sample results are usually deemed statistically significant and the null hypothesis is rejected.

Paramedic the level of EMS practitioner who provides the highest level of prehospital care, including advanced assessments and care, formation of a field impression, and invasive and drug interventions.

paramedicine the totality of the roles and responsibilities of paramedic practice involving health care, public health, and public safety; the highest level of Emergency Medical Systems practice.

parameter a value that specifies one of the members of a family of probability distributions, such as the mean or the standard deviation.

pathogens microorganisms capable of producing disease, such as bacteria and viruses.

pathophysiology the study of how disease affects normal body processes.

peer review a process of self-evaluation by a profession such as EMS in which qualified individuals within the profession or service assess ongoing practices in order to maintain standards and improve performance.

personal protective equipment (PPE) equipment used by EMS personnel to protect against injury and the spread of infectious disease.

placebo a substance or intervention having no effect but administered or provided as a control in testing, experimentally or clinically, the efficacy of a biologically active preparation.

population group of persons, elements, or both that share common characteristics that are being studied by the investigator.

positional asphyxia lack of oxygen resulting in unconsciousness or death that occurs in a person who is being restrained. Also called *restraint asphyxia*.

post hoc taking place after the fact, as in a review of data after the experiment has concluded.

prearrival instruction instructions from a medically trained dispatcher to a person at the scene of an emergency on how to initiate lifesaving first aid with the dispatcher's help while waiting for the on-scene arrival of emergency personnel.

prehospital care report (PCR) the written record of an EMS response.

primary care basic health care provided at the patient's first contact with the health care system.

primary prevention keeping an injury from ever occurring.

principal investigator (PI) the scientist or scholar with primary responsibility for the design and conduct of a research project.

priority dispatching system that uses medically approved questions and predetermined guidelines to determine the appropriate level of response.

profession a specialized body of knowledge or skills.

professional boundaries   ethical and societal limits to the interactions between members of a profession, such as doctors or paramedics, and the clients or patients they serve.

professionalism   the conduct or qualities that optimally characterize a practitioner in a particular field or occupation.

prospective medical oversight   guidelines established by a medical director in advance of emergency calls, such as those regarding selection of personnel and supplies, training and education, and protocol development.

prospective study   study designed to observe outcomes or events that will occur subsequent to the identification of the group of subjects to be studied.

proximate cause   action or inaction of the paramedic that immediately caused or worsened the damage suffered by the patient.

public health   the science and practice of protecting and improving the health of a community through the use of preventive medicine, health education, control of communicable diseases, application of sanitary measures, and monitoring of environmental hazards.

public safety answering point (PSAP)   any agency that takes emergency calls from citizens in a given region and dispatches the emergency resources necessary to respond to individual calls for help.

PubMed   computerized database operated by the National Libraries of Medicine that allows one to search many of the world's science resources.

qualitative research   research in which the researcher explores relationships using textual, rather than quantitative, data. Case study, observation, and ethnography are forms of qualitative research.

qualitative statistics   the analysis of nonnumeric data.

quality improvement (QI)   an evaluation program that emphasizes service and uses customer satisfaction as the ultimate indicator of system performance.

quality of life   the general well-being of individuals and society.

quantitative research   a study type that quantifies relationships between variables, using numeric terms.

quantitative statistics   statistics that involve analysis of numeric data and are used to make conclusions and future predictions.

quasiexperimental study   study that does not use random assignments to place the subjects into the various study groups.

radio band   a range of radio frequencies.

radio frequency   the number of times per second a radio wave oscillates.

random sampling   sampling in which subjects are chosen by random chance. *See* randomized controlled trial (RCT).

randomized controlled trial (RCT)   study in which subjects are assigned to different treatments, interventions, or conditions according to chance, rather than with reference to some aspect of their condition, history, or prognosis.

reasonable force   the minimal amount of force necessary to ensure that an unruly or violent person does not cause injury to himself or others.

reciprocity   the process by which an agency grants automatic certification or licensure to an individual who has comparable certification or licensure from another agency.

registration   the process of entering one's name and essential information within a particular record, done in EMS to verify the provider's initial certification and to monitor recertification.

repeaters   electronic devices that receive a signal and re-broadcast it at a higher power.

res ipsa loquitur   a legal doctrine invoked by plaintiffs to support a claim of negligence; it is a Latin term that means "the thing speaks for itself."

research   a systematic investigation, including development of the research design, testing, and evaluation, intended to develop or contribute to generalizable knowledge.

response time   time elapsed from when a unit is alerted until it arrives on the scene.

restraint asphyxia   lack of oxygen resulting in unconsciousness or death that occurs in a person who is being restrained. Also called *positional asphyxia.*

retrospective medical oversight   actions of a medical director intended to evaluate ongoing calls or calls that have already taken place, such as auditing a call, directing peer review, conflict resolution, and other quality assurance or improvement processes.

retrospective study   research conducted by reviewing records (e.g., birth and death certificates, medical records, school or employment records) or information about past events elicited through interviews with persons who have, and controls who do not have, the disease or condition, or another characteristic under investigation.

rules of evidence   guidelines that must be followed for permitting a new medication, process, or procedure to be used in EMS.

SafeCom   a communications program of the U.S. Department of Homeland Security that provides research and guidance to emergency response agencies regarding the development of interoperable communications systems.

sampling error   difference between the values obtained from the sample and those that actually exist in the total population.

science   the systematic study of the nature and behavior of the material and physical universe, based on observation, experiment, and measurement, and the formulation of laws to describe these facts in general terms.

scientific method   a method of investigation in which a problem is first identified and observations, experiments, or other relevant data are then used to construct or test hypotheses that purport to solve it.

scope of practice   the range of duties and skills paramedics and other levels of EMS certification are allowed and expected to perform.

secondary prevention   medical care after an injury or illness that helps to prevent further problems from occurring.

semantic   related to the meaning of words.

simplex   communications system that transmits and receives on the same frequency.

single blind study a study in which the investigator, but not the subject, knows the treatment assignment.

situational awareness (SA) perception of all aspects of a scene or situation.

slander act of injuring a person's character, name, or reputation by false or malicious statements spoken with malicious intent or reckless disregard for the falsity of those statements.

smart phone devices that combine the voice capability of a basic cell phone with the ability to perform a variety of data messaging functions such as e-mail and Internet connections as well as taking and sending photos and video.

standard deviation a statistic representing the degree of dispersion of a set of scores around their mean.

standard of care the degree of care, skill, and judgment that would be expected under like or similar circumstances by a similarly trained, reasonable paramedic in the same community.

Standard Precautions a strict form of infection control that is based on the assumption that all blood and other body fluids are infectious.

standing orders treatment procedures preauthorized by a medical director.

statistics mathematical techniques used to summarize research data or to determine whether the data support the researcher's hypothesis.

sterilization use of a chemical or physical method such as pressurized steam to kill all microorganisms on an object.

stress a hardship or strain; a physical or emotional response to a stimulus.

stressor a stimulus that causes stress.

systematic sampling statistical sampling technique in which there is order to the selection of samples for the study. The most common form is where every kth sample is taken (e.g., every 10th name from the phone book).

10-code radio communications system using codes that begin with the word *ten*.

t test a statistical test used to determine if the scores of two groups differ on a single variable.

teachable moment a time shortly after an injury when the patient and observers remain acutely aware of what has happened and may be especially receptive to teaching about how a similar injury or illness could be prevented in the future.

terrestrial-based triangulation a system of location based on the use of three land-based points of observation, such as using the strengths of signals from three cell phone towers to locate a given cell phone signal, or more traditional methods such as the use of sextants in surveying.

tertiary prevention rehabilitation after an injury or illness that helps to prevent further problems from occurring.

tiered response multiple levels of emergency care personnel responding to the same incident.

time sampling statistical sampling technique in which the samples are chosen by a given time interval or time span (e.g., what the subjects were thinking about at intervals of three hours, or what they were doing during the same half-hour each day).

tort law division of the legal system that deals with civil wrongs committed by one individual against another. *See also* intentional tort.

trauma a physical injury or wound caused by external force or violence.

trauma center medical facility that has the capability of caring for the acutely injured patient. A trauma center must meet strict criteria to use this designation.

treatment group the study group in an experimental design that will receive the treatment or intervention being studied.

triage tags tags containing vital information, which are affixed to your patient during a multiple-patient incident.

trunking communications system that pools all frequencies and routes transmissions to the next available frequency.

ultrahigh frequency (UHF) radio frequency band from 300 to 3,000 megahertz.

validity extent to which an investigator's findings are accurate or reflect the underlying purpose of the study.

variance measure of variability indicating the average of the squared deviations from the mean.

very high frequency (VHF) radio frequency band from 30 to 300 megahertz.

voice over Internet protocol (VOIP) technology that provides voice communications through Internet access from a computer or mobile device.

years of productive life a calculation made by subtracting the age at death from 65.

Abandonment, 126
Abbreviations/acronyms, 176–181
Abstract, 90, 91
Accelerometers, 157
Accident scenes, 130
Accreditation, 27
Actual damages, 119
Ad hoc database, 10
Addendum, 184
Administrative law, 115
Advance directive, 127
Advanced automatic crash notification (AACN),
    157, 166–167
Advanced Emergency Medical Technician
    (AEMT), 3
Advanced life support (ALS), 15
Against medical advice (AMA), 188
AIDS (acquired immune deficiency syndrome),
    63, 102
Airway management, 120
Allied health professions, 48
Ambulance operations, 74–75
Ambulances, 29–30
Americans with Disabilities Act (ADA),
    131–132
Analysis of variance (ANOVA), 90
Anchor time, 71
Animal research, 85
Assault, 126
Assessment pearls
        data recording, 174
Assessment/management plan,
        186–187
Automatic crash notification (ACN), 156
Automatic location information (ALI), 156
Automatic number identification (ANI), 156
Autonomy, 139

Back safety, 60–62
Bandwidth, 165
Basic life support (BLS), 15
Battery, 126
Bench research, 85
Beneficence, 139
Bias, 83
Biohazard disposal, 65
Borrowed servant doctrine, 120
Breach of duty, 118
Bubble sheets, 174, 175
Burnout, 71
Bystander, 15

Call incident documentation, 188
Call routing, 156
Case report, 85
Case series, 85
Cells, 163
Cellular telephone system, 163
Certification, 27, 116
Chain of survival, 22
CHART format, 187
Chi square test, 90

Chicken pox (varicella), 63
Children
        prevention needs in, 107
        responses to death, 68
Christian Scientists, 123
Circadian rhythms, 71
Civil law, 115
Civil lawsuit, 115–116
Civil rights, 120
Civil Rights Act of 1964, 132
Cleaning, 65
Clinical protocols, 24
Cognitive radio, 165
Cohort study, 85, 86
Common law, 115
Common operating picture (COP), 160
Communication, 51
        abbreviations/acronyms in,
            176–181
        defined, 152
        in EMS response, 155–159
        format, 153
        future developments, 165–167
        legal issues, 161, 167
        participant's roles in, 151–152
        radio, 153–155, 162–163
        technology, 159–167
        terminology, 154–155
        verbal, 152–154
        written, 154. *See also* Documentation
Communication protocols, 153
Community paramedicine, 165–166
Comparative negligence, 119
Competent, 122
Confidence interval, 88
Confidentiality, 121, 143–144
Consent, 122–123, 126, 144
Constitutional law, 115
Continuous quality improvement (CQI)
        program, 32
Contributory negligence, 119
Control group, 83
Convenience sampling, 93
Corrections medicine, 8
Crime scenes, 130
Criminal law, 115
Critical care transport, 6
Cross-sectional study, 85
Cultural considerations
        elderly and impoverished
            populations, 108
        immunization of at-risk
            populations, 109
        religious beliefs, 123
        responses to death, 67
        responses to illness
            and injury, 137

Data dictionary, 154
Data dredging, 94
Data mining, 94
Dead spots, 159

Death and dying, 67–69
Death in the field, 69, 131
Decontamination, 65–66
Defamation, 121
Defendant, 115
Deontological method, 137
Department of Homeland Security, 20
Dependent variable, 82
Descriptive statistics, 87–88
Digital communications, 163
Diplomacy, 51
Disaster management, 103
Disaster mental health services, 73
Disease surveillance, 103, 104
Disinfection, 66
Do Not Resuscitate (DNR) order, 129–130,
    141–142
Documentation, 46, 131
        abbreviations/acronyms, 176–181
        absence of alterations, 184
        additional resources, 182
        administrative uses, 173
        communications, 176
        completeness/accuracy, 182–184
        formats, 187–188
        improper, consequences of, 191
        legal uses, 174, 191, 193
        legibility, 184
        medical staff uses, 173
        medical terminology, 174
        multiple casualty incidents, 189–190
        narrative sections, 185–187
        oral statements, 182
        patient refusals, 188–189
        pertinent negatives, 176
        prehospital care report, 154,
            172–175, 192
        professionalism, 184
        research uses, 173–174
        services not needed, 189
        timeliness, 184
        times, 176
        uses, 173–174
Double blind study, 84, 85
Duplex, 162
Duty to act, 118
Duty to report, 117, 130

Echo procedure, 154
Elderly patients
        EMS needs in, 108
        prevention needs in, 107
Electronic patient care records, 191–192
Emancipated minor, 123
Emergency departments
        closures, 29
        paramedics in, 9
Emergency medical dispatcher (EMD), 26, 151,
    157–158
Emergency Medical Responder (EMR), 3
Emergency Medical Services: At the Crossroads,
    21–22

Emergency Medical Services for Children
  (EMSC), 20
Emergency Medical Services (EMS) system, 3.
  See also EMS system
Emergency Medical Technician (EMT), 3
Empathy, 50
Employment laws, 131–132
EMS Agenda for the Future, 20
EMS dispatch, 26–27, 157–158
EMS system
  chain of survival, 22
  characteristics, 4
  citizen involvement in, 47
  communications, 25–27, 155–159
  components, 14–15
  evidence-based medicine, 35
  financing, 36
  future directions, 20–22
  as gatekeeper to health care system, 44
  history, 15–20
  legal issues, 31
  licensure/certification, 22–23, 27–28
  local- and state-level agencies, 23
  medical oversight, 23–24
  mutual aid and mass-casualty
    preparation, 31
  patient safety, 33–34
  patient transportation, 28–29
  public health and. *See* Public health
  public information and education,
    24–25
  quality assurance and improvement,
    31–34
  receiving facilities, 30–31
  research, 34–35, 43. *See also* Research
EMT Code of Ethics, 49
Epidemiology, 101–102
Equal Employment Opportunity Act of 1972, 132
Ethical issues in paramedic practice
  allocation of resources, 144
  confidentiality, 143–144
  consent, 144
  EMT code of ethics, 48, 49
  obligation to provide care, 144–145
  in professional relations, 145–146
  in research, 146
  resuscitation attempts, 141–143
  in teaching, 145
Ethical relativism, 137
Ethics
  codes of, 48, 49, 138
  decision making and, 137, 139–141
  defined, 33
  fundamental principles, 138–139
  fundamental questions, 138
  in human research, 87
  impact on individual actions, 138
  in paramedic practice. *See* Ethical
    issues in paramedic practice
  relationship to law and religion, 137
Evidence-based decision making, 96–97
Evidence-based medicine (EBM), 35
Evidence levels, 86–87, 96
Excited delirium syndrome (ExDS), 120
Experiment, 81
Experimental group, 83

Experimental study, 83–85
Exposure, 66
Expressed consent, 122
External validity, 86
Eyewear, protective, 63

Fair Labor Standards Act (FLSA), 132
False imprisonment, 126
Family Medical Leave Act (FMLA), 132
Federal Communications Commission
  (FCC), 168
Federal Emergency Management Agency
  (FEMA), 20
Field diagnosis, 186

Geographic information system (GIS), 160
German measles (rubella), 63
Global positioning system (GPS), 156
Gloves, 63, 174
Good Samaritan laws, 117, 119
Governmental immunity, 119
Gowns, 64

Hand-off (patient transfer), 45–46, 159
Hand washing, 64–65
Health Insurance Portability and Accountability
  Act of 1996 (HIPAA), 121
Health promotion, 103
Helicopter EMS (HEMS), 6–7, 22
HEPA mask/respirator, 63–64
Hepatitis B, 63
Hepatitis C, 63
HIV (human immunodeficiency virus), 63, 102
Hot spot, 163
Hypothesis, 81

Immunity, 117, 119
Immunization. *See* Vaccinations
Impartiality test, 141
Implied consent, 122
In vitro, 85
In vivo, 85
Incubation period, 62, 63
Independent variable, 82
Industrial medicine, 8
Infants, prevention needs in, 107
Infection control, 62–67
Infectious diseases
  incubation periods, 63
  personal protection from, 62–67
  post-exposure procedures, 66–67
  transmission, 63
Inferential statistics, 87–88
Influenza, 63, 65
Information communications technology
  (ICT), 160
Informed consent, 122
Injury, 102
Injury prevention, 103
Injury risk, 102
Injury surveillance program, 102
Institutional review board (IRB), 87
Integrity, 50
Intentional injury, 102
Intentional tort, 117
Internal validity, 86

Interoperability, 26
Interpersonal justifiability test, 141
Interpersonal relations, 73–74
Intervener physician, 24
Invasion of privacy, 122
Involuntary consent, 122
Isometric exercise, 58
Isotonic exercise, 58
Iterative process, 82

Jargon, 185
Jehovah's Witnesses, 123
Justice, 139

KKK-A-1822 Federal Specifications for
  Ambulances, 29–30

Leadership, 50
*Leadership Guide to Quality Improvement for
  Emergency Medical Systems,* 31–32
Legal issues in EMS
  back injuries in EMS
    personnel, 62
  communication systems, 161
  for cross-trained paramedics, 5
  disaster response, 31
  emergency department closures, 29
  EMS as health care system
    gatekeeper, 44
  Health Insurance Portability and
    Accountability Act of 1996, 121
  intervening outside own EMS
    system, 145
  lawsuit risks for EMS
    personnel, 119
  medical research, 87
  patient definition, 46
  privacy of communications, 167
  quality improvement programs, 32
  relationship to ethics, 137
  substance abuse, 61
Legal issues in paramedic practice
  advance directives, 127–129
  confidentiality, 121–122
  consent, 122–123, 126
  crime and accident scenes, 130
  for cross-trained paramedics, 5
  death in the field, 69, 130
  Do Not Resuscitate orders, 129–130
  documentation, 131, 191, 193
  employment laws, 131–132
  legal protection, 117
  licensure and certification, 116–117
  motor vehicle laws, 117
  negligence and liability, 117–120
  organ donation, 130
  patient definition, 46
  patient transportation, 127
  prehospital care report, 174, 192
  problem patients, 124
  professional boundaries, 124
  reasonable force, 126
  refusal of service, 123–124, 125
  reporting requirements, 117, 130
  scope of practice, 116
  withdrawal of consent, 123

Legal system, 115
Legislative law, 115
Liability, 114, 117–120
Libel, 121–122, 185
Licensure, 27, 116
Lifting principles, 61–62
Living will, 128–129

Maleficence, 139
Malfeasance, 118
Malpractice, 117–119
Masks, 63–64
Mean, 88
Measures of central tendency, 88
Mechanism of injury (MOI), 43
Median, 88
Medical direction physician
    communication with, 152, 158–159
    liability concerns, 120, 145–146
Medical director, 23
Medical errors, 33–34
Medical oversight, 23–24
Meningitis, bacterial, 63
Meta-analysis, 84
Minor, 123
Misfeasance, 118
Mission-critical communications, 163
Mixed research, 82
Mobile data unit (MDU), 163
Mode, 88
Morals, 136
Morbidity, 80
Mortality, 80
Motor vehicle collisions
    ambulance involvement in, 75
    prevention, 107
Multiband radio, 165
Multiple-casualty incidents, 189–190
Multiplex, 162

N-95 mask, 63–64
Narrative writing, 185–187
National Emergency Medical Services Education
    Standards: Paramedic Instructional
    Guidelines, 5
National Emergency Medical Services
    Information System (NEMSIS), 154
National EMS Core Content, 23
National EMS Research Agenda, 80
National EMS Scope of Practice, 23
National Highway Traffic Safety Administration
    (NHTSA), 20
National Incident Management System
    (NIMS), 20
National Registry of Emergency Medical
    Technicians (NREMT), 28
National Report Card on the State of Emergency
    Medicine, 22
National Transportation Safety Board
    (NTSB), 22
Nature of the illness (NOI), 43
Negligence, 117–119
Negligence *per se,* 118–119
911 system, 156–157
Nominal data, 90
Nonfeasance, 118

Nonmaleficence, 139
Nonrandomized controlled trials, 84
Null hypothesis, 94
Nutrition, 58–60

Oath of Geneva, 48
Obesity, in EMS personnel, 59
Objective narrative, 185–186
Observational study, 83
Occupational Safety and Health Act
    (OSHA), 132
Odds ratio, 90
Off-line medical oversight, 24
On-line medical direction, 23–24
Ontario Prehospital Advanced Life Support
    Study (OPALS), 24
Open access journals, 91
Ordinal data, 90
Organ donation, 130
Outcomes-based research, 80

p value, 94
Paramedic, 3
    characteristics, 4–5
    cross-trained, 5
    duty to report, 117, 130
    education, 27
    ethical issues. *See* Ethical issues in
      paramedic practice
    expanded scope of practice, 6–9
    as health professional, 5–6
    Internet sites, 28
    legal issues. *See* Legal issues in
      paramedic practice
    legal protection, 117
    licensure/certification, 27, 116–117
    as patient advocate, 4, 52
    professional journals and
      magazines, 28
    professional organizations, 28
    roles and responsibilities. *See* Roles/
      responsibilities of paramedic
    well-being. *See* Well-being of
      paramedic
Paramedicine, 9, 41
Parameters, 88
Patho pearls
    EMS research, 43
    mental disorders, 124
    obesity, 59
Pathogens, 62
Pathophysiology, 41
Patient, 46
Patient advocacy, 4, 52
Patient assessment, 43
Patient management format, 43
Patient safety, 33–34
Patient Self-Determination Act, 127
Patient transfer (hand-off), 45–46, 159
Patient transportation, 28–29, 127
Peer review, 24, 33
Peer-review journal, 82
Personal hygiene, 51
Personal protective equipment (PPE), 62–64
Pertinent negatives, 176
Pertussis (whooping cough), 63

Physical fitness, 57–58
Placebo, 84
Plaintiff, 115
Pneumonia, 63
Population, 88
Positional asphyxia, 120
Post hoc analysis, 95
Prearrival instructions, 26, 158
Prehospital care report (PCR), 154, 172–175, 192.
    See also Documentation
Primary care, 7, 45, 47
Primary prevention, 102
Primum non nocere, 139
Principal investigator (PI), 95
Priority dispatching, 157
Problem patients, 124
Profession, 27, 48
Professional boundaries, 124
Professional journals, 28
Professional organizations, 28
Professional relations, 120, 145–146
Professionalism, 27, 48–52, 185
Prospective medical oversight, 24
Prospective study, 83
Proximate cause, 119
Psychological first aid, 73
Public health
    accomplishments, 100
    EMS organizational commitment,
      103–105
    EMS provider commitment, 105–107
    EMS roles, 102–103
    epidemiology, 101–102
    laws, 100
    prevention needs, 107–108
    prevention strategies, 108–109
    principles, 100–101
Public safety answering points (PSAPs), 156
Public safety communications system, 167–168
PubMed, 81, 91, 92–93

Qualitative research, 83
Qualitative statistics, 90
Quality assurance (QA), 32
Quality improvement (QI), 19, 32
Quality of life, 80
Quantitative research, 82–83
Quantitative statistics, 90
Quasiexperimental study, 83, 84

Radio bands, 161
Radio communication
    procedures, 153–154
    technology, 162–163
    terminology, 155
Radio frequencies, 161
Random sampling, 93
Randomized controlled trial (RCT), 84, 85
Reasonable force, 126
Receiving facilities, 44–45
Reciprocity, 27
Refusal of service, 123–124, 125, 188–189
Registration, 27
Repeaters, 161
Reporting requirements, 117, 130
Res ipsa loquitur, 118

Research, 80
    accessing, 91–93
    application to practice, 94
    documentation use in, 173–174
    EMS system, 34–35, 43
    ethical issues, 87, 146
    format for publication, 90
    participating in, 94–96
    prospective vs. retrospective, 83
    publication process, 91
    quantitative vs. qualitative, 82–83
    reviewing, 91, 93–94
    scientific method in, 80–82
    statistics in, 87–90
    study types, 83–85
    study validity, 86
Respect, 51–52
Response time, 171
Restraint asphyxia, 120
Restraints, 120, 126
Resuscitation
    ethical issues, 141–143
    legal issues, 127–130
Retrospective medical oversight, 24
Retrospective study, 83
Return to service, 46
Roadway safety, 74–75
Roles/responsibilities of paramedic, 4
    administration, 47
    citizen involvement, 47
    community involvement, 47
    continuing education, 52
    documentation, 46. *See also*
      Documentation
    equipment decontamination, 65–66
    health professional, 5–6
    patient advocate, 4
    patient assessment, 43
    patient disposition, 44–45
    patient transfer, 45–46, 159
    personal/professional development,
      47–48
    preparation, 41–42
    primary care support, 45, 47
    professional attitudes, 48–49
    professional attributes, 48–52
    professional ethics, 48, 49. *See also*
      Ethical issues in paramedic practice
    recognition of illness/injury, 43

    response, 42
    return to service, 46
    scene size-up, 42–43
Rules of evidence, 32
Ryan White Comprehensive AIDS Resources
    Emergency (CARE) Act, 117, 132

SafeCom, 153
Sampling error, 88
SARS (severe acute respiratory syndrome), 63
Scene safety, 106–107
Scene size-up, 42–43
Science, 80
Scientific method, 81–82
Scope of practice, 23, 116
Secondary prevention, 102
Self-confidence, 51
Self-motivation, 51
Semantic, 152
Shift work, 71
Simplex, 162
Single blind study, 84
Situational awareness (SA), 160
Slander, 122, 185
Smart phone, 164
Smoking cessation, 60
SOAP format, 187
Sports medicine, 8
Standard deviation (SD or σ), 88, 89
Standard of care, 118
Standard Precautions, 62, 105
Standing orders, 24
Staphylococcal skin infections, 63
Statistics, 87–90
Statute of limitations, 119
Sterilization, 66
Stress, 69
Stress management, 69–73, 105
Stress response, 70–71
Stressor, 69
Subjective narrative, 185
Subpoena, 121
Substance abuse, in EMS personnel, 60, 61
Systematic sampling, 93

T test, 90
Tactical EMS, 7
Target heart rate, 58
Teachable moment, 24, 102

Teaching, 145
Teamwork, 51
Ten-code systems, 153
Terrestrial-based triangulation, 156
Tertiary prevention, 102
Tiered response, 15
Time management, 51
Time sampling, 93
Title VII, 132
To Err Is Human, 33
Tort law, 115
Trauma, 31
Trauma center(s), 19, 31
Trauma center levels, 44–45
Treat and release, 45
Treatment group, 83
Triage tags, 190
Trunking, 162–163
Tuberculosis, 63

Ultrahigh frequency (UHF), 161
Unintentional injury, 102
Universalizability test, 141

Vaccinations, 65, 109
Validity, 86–87
Variance, 89
Very high frequency (VHF), 161
Voice over Internet protocol (VOIP), 157

Well-being of paramedic, 57–75
    back safety, 60–62
    death and dying, 67–69
    habits and addictions, 60, 61
    interpersonal relations, 73–74
    mental health services, 73
    nutrition, 58–60
    personal protection from disease, 62–66
    physical fitness, 57–58
    psychological first aid, 73
    roadway safety, 74–75
    stress/stress management, 69–73
    warning signs of excessive
      stress, 72
    work-related injuries, 57, 62
Whooping cough (pertussis), 63
Work-related injuries, 57, 108

Years of productive life, 102